Health System Strengthening

Published by
ACADEMIC FOUNDATION
in association with

Institute of Public Enterprise

Health System Strengthening

Country Experiences

R.K. Mishra
K.N. Jehangir
Geeta Potaraju
Sobin George

ACADEMIC FOUNDATION
NEW DELHI

www.academicfoundation.com

First published in 2016
by

ACADEMIC FOUNDATION
4772-73 / 23 Bharat Ram Road, (23 Ansari Road),
Darya Ganj, New Delhi - 110 002 (India).
Phones : 23245001 / 02 / 03 / 04.
Fax : +91-11-23245005.
E-mail : books@academicfoundation.com
www.academicfoundation.com

in association with
Institute of Public Enterprise, Hyderabad.

Disclaimer:
The findings/views/opinions expressed in this book are solely those of the authors and do not necessarily reflect the views of the publisher.

Cataloging in Publication Data--DK
Courtesy: D.K. Agencies (P) Ltd. <docinfo@dkagencies.com>

Health system strengthening : country experiences / [editors], R.K. Mishra, K.N. Jehangir, Geeta Potaraju, Sobin George.
pages cm
ISBN 9789332701786

1. Medical care--India. 2. Medical care--South Asia. 3. Medical care--India--Finance. 4. Medical care--South Asia--Finance. 5. Medical policy--India. 6. Medical policy--South Asia. I. Mishra, R. K., 1948- editor. II. Institute of Public Enterprise (Hyderabad, India).

RA529.H43 2016 DDC 362.10954 23

Typeset, printed and bound by The Book Mint, New Delhi.
www.thebookmint.in

CONTENTS

Part II

Health System and Financial Issues

Part III

Health Delivery System: Personnel, Effectiveness and Gender Issues

LIST OF TABLES AND FIGURES

Tables

Figures

About the Editors/Contributors

Editors:

R.K. Mishra, Senior Professor and Dean is the Director of Institute of Public Enterprise (IPE), Hyderabad, is a graduate of International Management Programme, SDA Bocconi, Milan, Italy. He has been a fellow of the British Council and the Commonwealth Secretariat. He has been involved in research and teaching stints at London Business School, Maison Des Sciences De L' Hommes, Paris, University of Bradford, United Kingdom, UN Center on Promotional Enterprises, Ljubljana, as well as University of Ljubljana, Slovenia. He has worked on key assignments with Indian government including Ministry of Finance, Ministry of Power, Ministry of Trade and Commerce, Ministry of Heavy Industry and Public Enterprises, and Ministry of Finance (Department of Disinvestment). He has also worked extensively with international organisations including OECD, United Nations University-World Institute for Economic Development Research, International Civil Service Consortium. His current areas of interest include: corporate finance, corporate governance, international management, management controls, management education, infrastructure development, restructuring, economic reforms, social sector management, good governance and economic environment.

K.N. Jehangir is currently attached to IPE, Hyderabad, as a senior faculty member. Earlier, he was a Director (Research) in Indian Council of Social Science Research (ICSSR), New Delhi, where he was in charge of promoting international collaboration programmes of ICSSR with several countries and international bodies. Dr Jehangir did his PhD from the University of Calcutta on Muslim women. His major area of research interests are: gender, minorities, elections, health systems in India, etc. Some of his publications are: *Muslim Women in West Bengal: Social, Economic and Political Status* (1991), *Minorities in India: Problems and Prospects* (ed.) (2008), *Social Science Research in India and the World* (ed.) (2015).

Geeta Potaraju is currently working as an Assistant Professor at IPE, Hyderabad. She has a PhD in Management with specialisation on public sector enterprises. She has over 15 years of experience in development consulting. Her areas of interests are: participatory governance, health system strengthening, administrative and institutional reforms. Dr Geeta has been involved in a number of key assignments with DFID, UNDP, World Bank, World Bank Institute, Family Health International, Government of India, and state governments. She is an expert on participatory governance tools like Citizens Charters and Right to Information. She has extensively worked on issues of access to information and has developed training manuals for both the supply side as well as the demand side stakeholders.

Sobin George is Assistant Professor at the Centre for Studies of Social Change and Development, Institute for Social and Economic Change, Bangalore. He has an MPhil and PhD in public health from Centre of Social Medicine and Community Health, Jawaharlal Nehru University, New Delhi. His areas of teaching, research and writings cover social gradients of health, marginalities, health behaviour and labour relations

Contributors

Samiha Barkat is Senior Consultant at Cardno Emerging Markets, Australia. As part of her current role, she manages various development programmes worldwide. She has a Masters of Public Health (MPH) from Boston University, and a

Bachelor of Arts in Economics from the University of Virginia. Her areas of interest include: public health, family planning and reproductive health, chronic diseases and health promotion, anti-human trafficking, criminal justice systems, and programme management.

Bula Bhadra was educated at Presidency College, University of Calcutta and McMaster University, Canada. She has been teaching at the Dept. of Sociology, University of Calcutta for last 26 years. Her current areas of specialisation include: sociology of gender, sociology of childhood and sociology of technology. She published both in English and vernacular a large number of articles in these areas.

Biplab Dhak holds PhD degree in Development Studies from University of Mysore through Institute for Social and Economic Change, Bangalore. He also holds MPhil degree in Population Studies from International Institute for Population Sciences, following Masters in Economics from North Bengal University. His area of research has been on health, gender, and migration and poverty issues.

Jonathan Gangbar is Project Manager, mechanisation initiative at NWK Agro services, Zambia.

Pranav Garimella is working as a project associate at the Institute of Public Enterprise, Hyderabad. He works in the areas of public policy, public sector management, law and governance etc.

K. Gayithri is an Associate Professor at the Centre for Economic Studies and Policy (CESP), at the Institute of Social and Economic Change, Bangalore. Her areas of specialisation include: public economics, expenditure planning and management, fiscal policy analysis, programme performance budgeting and measurement of performance.

K.S. James is Professor, Population Research Centre at the Institute of Social and Economic Change, Bangalore. His areas of specialisation are: formal demography including measurement, population and development, mortality and health, and ageing.

Subodh Kandamuthan is currently an Associate Professor and Director of the Centre for Health Care Management at Administrative Staff College of India, Hyderabad. His areas of expertise include: health economics, health financing, health policy, monitoring and evaluation, trade in health services and public private partnerships in social sector.

Barkat-e-Khuda has Bachelor (Honours) and Masters in Economics from University of Dhaka, and PhD in Demography from Australian National University, Canberra. Her major areas of expertise include: Economics, population and development, family planning and reproductive health, health systems, and nutrition.

Swadhin Mondal, a Health Economist, is presently working as a faculty in Economics at the Institute for Studies in Industrial Development (ISID), New Delhi. He completed his PhD in Health Economics from Vidyasagar University, India. His current research area of interests include: health financing, health equity, health system research, economics of ageing, pharmaceutical economics, economic aspect of clinical trials and related fields.

R. Mutharayappa, currently Professor and Head, Centre for Women's and Gender Studies, Institute for Social and Economic Change, Bangalore, was a visiting Fellow at the East-West Center, Program on Population, Honolulu, Hawaii, USA. His research interest and teaching for the last 33 years are on reproductive health, women empowerment, fertility and family planning, population policy, health delivery etc.

M.A.L.R. Perera is a Former Secretary, Ministry of Health, Nutrition & Welfare, Government of Srilanka and Consultant in Health Systems Management & Community Health. He is currently a Senior Fellow Institute for Health Policy, Srilanka.

Swaminathan S. Puwanesh is a Project Management specialist and is currently serving as a IT and web expert at the Institute for Health Policy, Srilanka.

Pavithra Rajan is Research Associate, Injury Division, The Georgia Institute for Global Health, Sydney, Australia and Fellow, Shastri Indo-Canadian Institute, Canada.

P. Satya Sekhar is Professor of Health Management and Bio-Statistics at the Indian Institute of Health and Family Welfare (IIHFW). He is involved in health, demographic and medical research studies. He has a PhD in Agricultural Economics from Andhra University, Visakhapatnam; Master's degree in Statistics from the University of Indore and MBA degree from Sikkim Manipal University (SMU) with Health Care Systems Management as specialisation. Dr Sekhar is associated with many research and consultancy assignments in the areas of quantitative methods, operations research, demography and health management teaching.

U.V. Somayajulu has MSc in Statistics, MA in Sociology, MBA, MPhil and PhD in Population Studies. He has more than 25 years of experience in social and development sector research and has coordinated more than 400 research studies on health, education, gender, rural development, urban development, poverty, sexual health, reproductive health, child health, nutrition, CSR, governance, innovation, HIV/AIDS, water and sanitation, social marketing, climate change, energy, transport etc.

Pawan Kumar Taneja is presently working as Sr. Faculty at Indian Institute of Public Administration (IIPA), New Delhi. His areas of interest include: operations research in public administration, performance measurement and evaluation, public health, health economics, financing health care for marginalised population, corporate social responsibility and performance. He is MCom, MBA, PGDStat and PhD, and has done Certificate courses in Managing Global Health and Health Economics from Johns Hopkins University, USA.

M. Benson Thomas is a Doctoral Scholar at Institute for Social and Economic Change, Bangalore. He has achieved his graduate and post-graduate degrees in Economics from University of Calicut, India through St. Thomas College, Thrissur. His research interests broadly cover the economics of health and populations, demographic dividend, policy issues on health intervention, health care demand and utilisation, epidemiology, bio-demography and population aging.

Introduction

The issues confronting health systems in any country are often complex and challenging especially in the context of its diverse needs and priorities. While delivering effective healthcare to citizens with heterogeneous needs remains a major challenge before any government, the socio-economic factors and the questions of accessibility and affordability to health and related services exert further pressure on the health service delivery systems. Many developing as well as developed countries have set their focus on establishing robust healthcare systems as part of their larger goals of social and economic development, welfare of citizens and in some instances as part of their governance reform agenda. Streamlining health systems also assumes paramount significance in the Millennium Development Goals (MDGs) since several countries are signatories to it. It is important to note that there are slight improvements in child mortality and maternal mortality as well as combating HIV/AIDS, malaria and other diseases, which are part of the goals at a global level. However, such achievements also varied significantly across countries and regions within countries with notable differences among under-developed, developing and developed ones. For instance, the annual number of death among children younger than 5 years of age came down below 10 million in 2006, but its intensity varied as a child born in developing country is 13 times more likely to die within the first five years than one born in a developed country (Holtz, 2013). Similarly, as much as 90 per cent of the maternal deaths occur in the developing and underdeveloped world where Sub-Saharan Africa and South Asia together account for 86 per cent (Holtz, 2013). It points to the huge gaps in health system and health service system of various countries.

Global health issues at present, however, are much deeper and multifaceted than the basic targets of millennium development goals. There are issues of livelihood security, health disparities, exclusion, extreme situation of poverty, nutritional deaths and burden of infectious diseases on one hand, and issues of degenerative diseases, quality healthcare services, equity and new epidemiological transitions on the other. This is not a binary; however coexists within a country across social, religious, ethnic, regional and income groups. The social determinants framework in fact has already flagged the issues such as food and nutrition, inequalities, disparities among and within nations along several markers, aging of population, environment and health, conflicts and violence, which are indicative for countries to design its health and health delivery system. The test therefore for any health system is to address this diverse health landscape where individual to systemic and structural issues play and interplay.

While whether a uniform model of health system is suitable for all countries is in question, World Health Organization's (WHO) definition of health system is an important initial point of reference for several countries. WHO refers to health systems as "all the organizations, institutions, and resources that are devoted to producing health actions." This definition includes the full range of players engaged in the provision and financing of health services including the public, non-profit, and for-profit private sectors, as well as international and bilateral donors, foundations, and voluntary organisations involved in funding or implementing health activities. Health system according to this definition encompasses all levels of service delivery—central, regional, district, community, and household levels. WHO Report (2007) identified four key functions of the health system, which include stewardship, financing, human and physical resources, and organisation and management of service delivery. The health system hence is not just a miscellany of healthcare facilities owned by any particular dominant view or interest. It is also includes issues of access, citizen participation, human resources, role of finances in health sector, coordination among various organisations in health service delivery, skill and capacity within the delivery institutions, etc. The Health

System Strengthening framework of WHO thus revolves around issues of "service delivery, health workforce, information systems, financing issues, and leadership/governance" (WHO, 2007).

This multiplicity of various actors and players, while aiming to explore all possibilities to strengthen the health system, also makes it complex and creates new challenges. Among others, major debates emanating out of these complexities of health system include the public and private dichotomy as well as partnerships, comprehensive and target-oriented approaches, accessibility and affordability, quality and access, and efficiency and coverage. Each country depending on its strengths, weaknesses and multiplicity of needs and priorities responded differently to these questions. We have diverse experience available from various countries the way they deal with such questions. For instance, Sweden, which has one of the best human development index, considers that their healthcare goal is to have equal access to publicly-funded good healthcare, which is provided to all citizens based on the need. Other Scandinavian countries like Norway and Finland also have a streamlined organisational structure, devolution of powers and local level strengthening creating an effective mechanism for health service delivery. When it comes to the United States (US), although Medicare and Medicaid are still important, private sectors play a major role in healthcare financing. This in fact seriously raises the issue of affordable quality healthcare for poor in the US. Similarly, the much-celebrated National Health System (NHS) of the United Kingdom (UK) also saw reduction of primary healthcare trusts and investments from private sector in health infrastructure. Carol Holtz (2013: 103) presents an interesting comparison of healthcare spending of some developed and developing countries, which is worth quoting here:

> The United States leads the world in healthcare spending and spends about seven times as much on total health expenditure per capita as does India....while the government of India spends only $20 per capita annually on healthcare, the US government spends more than 100 times as much. Canada has a universal healthcare system and private spending accounts for only 30% of total spending. In the US, majority is private spending;

in India, three-fourths of all healthcare spending is private. Ukraine, which has a universal coverage, still has a high share of private spending, as the benefits provided are so limited that patients are forced to make sizable out of pocket payments.

Experiences from some developing countries also show the trajectory of skewed public funding and involvement of private sector in a big way. The most striking experience is from China, which had the legacy of rural preventive healthcare programmes and barefoot doctors. The major change in the health system of China is the adoption of market policies for healthcare in rural areas. It reintroduced the system of user charge for clinic visits and hospitalisation, which was completely, borne by the state earlier. Although the rural cooperative medical system in China is dismantled due to the change from community to household production system, the state initiated a social protection scheme to cover health expenditure (Carrin *et al.*, 1999). The New Rural Cooperative Medical Care System (NRCMCS), which was started in 2005, despite being part of the market reform project, also has a thrust on affordable care for the rural poor. Some scholars view that there are serious setbacks within Chinese health sector, especially in rural areas due to the reform project (Messen and Bloom, 2007). The merit, however, of the Chinese health system is their government insurance programmes, huge network of hospitals and healthcare providers, and efficient disease prevention and control systems.

Thailand, another Asian country, introduced universal healthcare for all citizens in 2002. The country has three types of health coverage schemes, which include the civil service welfare system (government employees and families), social security (private employees) and a universal coverage scheme for the rest of the population (Hughes and Leethongdee, 2007). It is estimated that as much as 98 per cent of Thailand's population are covered under such health protection schemes (World Bank, 2012). Thailand has a very strong public health service system with a focus on vibrant primary healthcare, innovative health system development and a progressive health promotion programme. The new national development plan of Thailand also envisages issues of quality healthcare and universal security for all, which shows the trajectory of the country's health system with a focus on universal coverage with quality. South Africa, another developing country, has a large public sector, however, with a rapidly growing private sector in healthcare delivery. In other words, South Africa is embarking on a path of a dual system in healthcare with a parallel public and private system. One of the important aspects of the health system is its decentralised organisation of primary healthcare system. However, studies show that serious regional disparities exist in the system due to differences in the financial capabilities of district and local administration, which adversely affect the population in the rural areas (Harrison, 2004). Quality of affordable healthcare is yet another question that the country faces in the context of the problems of public health delivery and the huge cost at the private sector.

Brazil is often discussed in the health system literature for their apparent success in delivering universal care with the introduction of more decentralised national health system. Literature based on the Brazilian experiments highlight that Brazil improved quality of life of its population significantly with the creation of a national health system (Gragnolati *et al.*, 2013). It further notes that national health system changed the health system remarkably with "decentralisation and new arrangements for sharing of responsibilities across federal, state and municipal levels; and a gradual increase of public spending on health." However, another set of literature shows that there are regional imbalances in the distribution of health infrastructure, which create inequalities in health outcomes of population. For instance, Sousa *et al.* (2012) highlighted that inequalities in Brazil have increased across states and sub-regions in the availability of qualified healthcare professionals due to unequal distribution and the poor regions have the highest deficit.

The South Asian healthcare landscape is more diverse due to the interplays of several factors. It has become increasingly complex with the new public health challenges emanating from issues, such as epidemiological transitions, continuity and re-emergence of infectious diseases, burden of nutrition and degenerative diseases and above all escalating out-of-pocket healthcare expenditure and lower level of social and health protection. This has thrown tremendous challenges on the governments to improve health service delivery systems. Most of the South Asian countries also underwent health sector reforms as part of structural adjustment policies of macroeconomic reforms, which resulted in the strong presence of a private sector in all levels of care. As Islam and Tahir (2001) argue, the health sector reforms, however, in the South Asian countries are not properly informed of the new challenges of continuing communicable diseases, increasing demand for both primary and tertiary levels of healthcare services, population growth in some countries, rapid and unplanned urbanisation, and globalisation and increasing marginalisation of developing countries.

The poor public investment in health and other social sector adds to this situation in several South Asian countries. For instance, the reduction of public expenditure on health and introduction of partnership with private sector were the most notable developments in India. Gupta and Chowdhury (2014), for instance estimates that the total public finances for health in 2010-11 was ₹80,155 crore or $17.6 billion, which was about 1.03 per cent of GDP (gross domestic product). The data on national commission on macroeconomics and health showed that as much as 75 per cent of the per capita healthcare expenditure is met from the household (out-of-pocket) and public spending amounts to only 22 per cent. The ambitious National Rural Health Mission (NRHM) certainly increased the public expenditure on health; however accessibility to quality healthcare services is a continuing question in India due to absence of health protection. One of the reasons is the country's abysmally lower share of workers in the formal sector, where health protection is taken care of by various central government, state government and private insurance schemes. As per the latest estimation from NSSO 68th round data (2011-12), India's 93 per cent labour force is in the informal sector, and as much as 74 per cent are without any social security. If we add non-workers, students, infants and elderly to this group, this would further go up. Although schemes like Rashtriya Swathya Bima Yojana (RSBY) envisage health protection of the poor in the informal sector, it does not answer the entire question of financial burden of healthcare for the poor.

The regional, income and social-religious-ethnic group disparities in health is another important question in India.

Other countries in the region such as Bangladesh, Sri Lanka, Nepal, and Pakistan also have undergone significant changes in their health system and health service system with regard to the general wave of health sector reforms, involvement of international financial institutions and other donour agencies, and the priorities emanating from various interest groups, state and other epidemiological concerns. The health sector reform project in Bangladesh and the Health, Nutrition and Population Sector Programmes (HNPSP) is carried out largely with the involvement of World Bank and bilateral agencies like Department for International Development (DFID), governments of the Netherlands and Sweden, German Agency for Technical Cooperation (GTZ) and Canadian International Development Agency (CIDA). The major thrust of the HNPSP is adoption and integration of essential services with a focus on maternal health, poverty, decentralisation, improved hospital management and NGO (non-governmental organisation) and private sector partnership (WHO, 2004). Like health sector reforms in any other country, there is also an enhanced focus on cost recovery in Bangladesh. The only difference probably is the subsidy given to the vulnerable section in cost recovery. It is debatable in the special context of Bangladesh, whether such market participation in essential healthcare delivery is desirable due to the already inferior health outcomes in the country. Studies have shown that it is essential to regulate the private healthcare sector in the country due to the escalated cost in the sector and also to strengthen redistributive policies of the state (Vaughan *et al.*, 2000).

Nepal also has a strong presence of global and bilateral funding partners in their health system planning, financing and service delivery. The Nepal health sector programme started in 2002 was also in the lines of health sector reforms in general, calling participation from private sector and NGOs, with an emphasis on cost recovery (Government of Nepal, 2011). What happens to the Essential Healthcare Services (EHCS), which is supposed to be free of cost for all, is a crucial question before the Nepal health system. Studies also show that even though EHCS is strengthened in some instances, the question of equity prevails since there is no "mechanism to distribute social determinants of health as equitably as possible which is necessary to ensure the health as human right" (Sapkota, 2012: 39). The structural adjustment and health sector reform programmes in Pakistan also led to a reduction in public expenditure on health and privatisation of healthcare services. These initiatives, as several studies pointed out, lead to widening of disparities across rural and urban areas, across income and socio-religious groups (Ahmed, 1997 as quoted in Baru, 2003).

Sri Lanka, on the other hand, has a strong welfare orientation and hence state involvement in healthcare delivery. This is reflective in the health outcomes of the country, which are better as compared to any other country in the region. The investment in associated sectors like public distribution, drinking water, sanitation, education and housing is also adding to the success story of Sri Lanka. It is also important to note that private sector plays an important role in the healthcare delivery in Sri Lanka. The enhanced role of the state in social sector appears to be levelling the disparities to a certain extent in Sri Lanka. The health sector reforms and entry of private sector, however, are also creating new challenges in the country. Literature from Sri Lanka showed that out-of-pocket expenditure in healthcare increased to 48 per cent in 2005 from 33 per cent in 1953 (Rannan-Eliya and Sikurajapathy, 2009). Another important concern of the Sri Lankan health sector is the differential health outcomes of ethnic groups.

Although we have diverse experience on health system from different countries under different ideological and state regimes, it is important to keep some ethical positions, which refer to humanitarianism, equity, social justice, human rights, citizenship rights, informed choices and freedom of choices in the backdrop. With this backdrop, this volume, at the outset, aims to develop an overall understanding on issues and concerns related to health system of various countries in the very context of the nature of health sector reforms and the new challenges of healthcare delivery system. It attempts to understand how different countries have evolved mechanisms to overcome such challenges and obstacles in health service delivery. It also stresses on understanding what are the ongoing and new experiments in health system and finally to develop a road map to improve the health system. Besides, the volume has a special focus on India by documenting new initiatives and lessons from various Indian states.

Papers in this volume discuss trends, patterns, outcomes, challenges and new experiments that are part of the ongoing health system strengthening projects of various countries. The first part of this volume is on various country experiences with a focus on new initiatives and emerging issues out of healthcare reform processes. Barkat-e-Khuda and Samiha Barkat in their paper discuss the Bangladesh health sector in the special context of MDG 4 and 5. The paper notes that Bangladesh has already achieved the MDG 4 target for under-5 mortality and maternal mortality rate decreased by 40 per cent between 2001 and 2010. However, there are notable inter-group and inter regional differences in such reductions. The reform project as the paper notes has several inefficiencies, which pose challenges to health system strengthening due to lack of coordination among different actors, conflicts among service providers, poor monitoring, weak implementation and above all, resource constraints. The Sri Lankan experience, on the other hand, reveals a successful replicable model. The paper by M.A.L.R. Perera, by the way of showcasing better health indicators of the country, gives an account of the investment in human development, which partly explains this success. The paper discusses initiatives such as universal franchise, free education, free healthcare, primary healthcare, drugs policy/essential drugs, historical evolution of hospitals, devolution/decentralisation, quality assurance programme, and the health master plan, which are components of the strong health and health service system in the country. Another paper by Saminathan Puwanesh showcases the success story of information technology based malaria surveillance system in Sri Lanka. The Bhutan case calls for much deeper and more qualitative indicators of better health. The paper by Tashi Tobgay underscores the need to go beyond the rhetoric of mortality, morbidity and longevity-based articulations in order to have a more nuanced qualitative well-being, often expressed in terms of happiness by individuals. Based on this, the paper provides an account of the status of health happiness in Bhutan under the overarching policy of gross national happiness.

The second part of the volume is on health financing with a special focus on India. Pawan Taneja brings in the discussion of affordable and equitable distribution of healthcare in the context of the higher share of out-of-pocket per capita health expenditure in India. Jonathan Gangbar, Pavithra Rajan and K. Gayithri in their paper bring out the mismatches of priorities and financial outlays of the Integrated Child Development Services (ICDS) programme in the country. The paper argues that regions with a higher prevalence of child malnutrition are not receiving a proportionate level of financial support from both Central and State governments as compared to regions with a lower prevalence. Moreover, the gap between the poorer and richer states seems to have increased over the years. Swadhin Mondal offers an overview of the status of healthcare financing in South Asia and draws corollaries of avoidable health inequalities between groups of people within countries that emanate from social and economic conditions across the region. Veerabhadra Karumunchi discusses the issues and concerns of health sectors with a special focus on financial management from the Indian state of Andhra Pradesh.

The third part of the volume discusses the health delivery system with special reference to human resources, issues of effectiveness, monitoring and evaluation and questions of women's health. Sobin George discusses the challenges of inclusiveness in the health service delivery system due to the persisting caste-based discrimination and the shortage of staff from discriminated groups in the key positions of service delivery. He, highlighting the lowest share of Dalits in the profession of doctors, nurses and associated staff in rural India, argues that the Indian health service system at present is not equipped with addressing the issue of caste-based discrimination in service delivery. P. Geeta and Pranav Garimella draw attention to the monitoring and evaluation of performance of health delivery system in the special context of the recent result framework approach initiated by the Government of India (GoI). Subodh Kandamuthan offers a discussion on the incentive system for retaining health staff, especially at the lower end of the delivery, in the rural India. This, as he notes, is an important concern taking the low enthusiasm of staff for rural health services. This session also has a special focus on women's health. R. Muthurayappa discusses in detail the persisting gender differential in access to health services and outcomes. The paper also puts forth the increased risk behaviour of women to certain diseases like asthma and tuberculosis. Bula Bhadra draws attention to the issue of women's reproductive health in the context of proliferation of the unregulated surrogacy market in India. The paper argues that freedom of choice theory in favour of surrogacy is not valid and it is coming from the disadvantageous position of poor women, which ultimately lead to commodification of their body.

The final part of the volume carries discussions from various Indian states on NRHM, private public partnerships, maternal, neonatal and child care and management information systems in healthcare delivery. The paper by U.V. Somayajulu gives a detailed account of progress of NRHM in the states of Uttar Pradesh, Madhya Pradesh, Bihar, Chhattisgarh, Jharkhand, Rajasthan, Odisha, and Uttarakhand, with a special focus on infrastructure and human resource. P. Satya Sekhar gives an account of the reproductive, maternal, newborn, child and adolescent health initiatives and its performance in the states of Telangana and Andhra Pradesh; whereas M. Benson and K.S. James draw attention to regional disparities in mortality and its causes in Kerala.

We hope that the volume will be useful for all categories of readers, especially those who are policymakers, academicians, medical professionals, as well as common citizens of the developing world.

References

Baru, Rama V. (2003). "Privatisation of Health Services: A South Asian Perspective", *Economic and Political Weekly* 38(42): 4433-37.

Carrin, G., A. Ron, Y. Hui, W. Hong, Z. Tuohong, Z. Licheng, Z. Shuo, Y. Yide, C. Jiaying, J. Qicheng, Z. Zhaoyang, Y. Jun, L. Xuesheng (1999). "The Reform of the Rural Cooperative Medical System in the People's Republic of China: Interim Experience in 14 Pilot Counties", *Social Science and Medicine* 48(7): 961-72.

Government of Nepal (2011). *Nepal Health Sector Program-II.* Kathmandu, Nepal: National Planning Commission, Ministry of Health and Population.

Gragnolati, Michele; Lindelow, Magnus; Couttolenc, Bernard (2013). *Twenty Years of Health System Reform in Brazil: An Assessment of the Sistema Único de Saúde*. Washington, DC:

World Bank.

Gupta, Indrani and Samik Chowdhury (2014). "Public Financing for Healthcare Coverage in India: Who Spends, Who Benefits and at What Cost?, *Economic and Political Weekly* XLIX(35): 59-63

Harrison, S. (2004). "Medical Schemes", in Ijumba and Day (eds.), *South African Health Review:* 291-93. Durban: Health System Trust.

Holtz, Carol (2013). *Global Healthcare: Issues and Policies.* Burlington: Jones & Bartlett Learning.

Hughes, D. and S. Leethongdee (2007). "Universal Coverage in the Land of Smiles: Lessons from Thailand's 30 Baht Health Reforms", *Health Aff (Millwood),* 26(4): 999-1008. July-August.

Islam, Anwar and M.Z. Tahir (2001). "Health Sector Reform in South Asia: New Challenges and Constraints", *Health Policy* 60(2): 151-69.

Meesen, B. and G. Bloom (2007). "Economic Transition, Institutional Changes and the Health System: Some Lessons from Rural China", *The Journal of Economic Policy Reform* 10(03): 209-32.

Rannan-Eliya, R.P. and L. Sikurajapathy (2009). *Sri Lanka "Good Practice in Expanding Healthcare Coverage.* Colombo: Institute for Health Policy. Retrieved from *http://www.ihp.lk/publications/docs/RSS0903.pdf*

Sapkota, V.P. (2012). "Ethical Perspective of Health Sector Reform Process in Nepal", *Health Prospect* No.11. pp.36-39.

Sousa, A., M.R. Dal Poz, C.L. Carvalho (2012). "Monitoring Inequalities in the Health Workforce: The Case Study of Brazil 1991–2005", *PLoS ONE* 7(3), e33399

Vaughan, J.P., E. Karim and K. Buse (2000). "An Overview of the Healthcare System in Bangladesh", *Journal of Public Health Medicine* 22(1): 5-9.

WHO (2004). *Tuberculosis and Health Sector Reforms in Bangladesh: A Concept Paper.* Retrieved from *http://apps.searo.who.int/PDS_DOCS/B0194.pdf.* New Delhi: WHO.

——. (2007). *Everybody's Business: Strengthening Health Systems to Improve Health Outcomes.* Geneva.

World Bank (2012). *Thailand: Sustaining Health Protection for All, World Bank Thailand.* Retrieved from *http://www.worldbank.org/en/news/2012/08/20/thailand-sustaining-health-protection-for-all* on 20 November 2014

Part I

Health System Strengthening: Emerging Issues and Country Experiences

1

BARKAT-E-KHUDA and SAMIHA BARKAT

MDG 4 and 5 and the Health Sector in Bangladesh

Introduction

The 1994 International Conference on Population and Development (ICPD) in Cairo is an important landmark in redefining and addressing the issues of population and reproductive health (RH) within a holistic and human rights-based perspective. The needs of individual human beings, rather than demographic targets, were put at the centre of development agenda.[1]

The 1994 ICPD was an agreement between 179 countries affirming that population dynamics are critical to overall development, and further that women's empowerment and reducing the unmet needs of people in education and health, including RH, are fundamental for both individual and social development, balanced and fair growth, and socio-economic development. Advancing gender equality, eliminating violence against women and ensuring women's ability to control their own fertility are recognised as cornerstones of population and development policies.

The overall objective of the ICPD was to raise the quality of life and well-being of human beings and promote overall development by recognising the inter-relationship between population and development policies and programmes aimed at achieving, by 2015, the eight goals: (i) universal access to RH/FP (family planning) and

---

1. For example, women's health and rights groups used the ICPD as the forum to shift the focus of population programmes from demographic goals and targets to women's lives, including but not limited to, their RH goals (Dixon-Mueller and Germain, 1992; Dixon-Mueller, 1993; Sen *et al.*, 1994; McIntosh and Finkle, 1995).

primary healthcare, (ii) universal access to primary education, (iii) reduce the rate of illiteracy between man and woman, (iv) reduce infant and child mortality, (v) reduce maternal mortality ratio, (vi) halt and reduce HIV/AIDS pandemic, (vii) increase number of births assisted by skilled attendants, and (viii) increase life expectancy (United Nations [UN], 1994).

The international consensus about the mutually reinforcing relationship between population and development was reaffirmed at a number of international conferences, including the Fourth World Conference on Women held in Beijing in September 1995 (UN, 1995).[2] One of the major landmarks influencing policies globally in the 15 years, since the 1994 ICPD, has been introduction of the Millennium Development Goals (MDGs) in 2000 and the subsequent inclusion of MDG target 5.B on universal access to reproductive health. The MDG Declaration was signed by 189 countries in September 2000. Governments and other key actors are working towards implementation of the ICPD Programme of Action (POA) in the context of the MDGs, using a holistic approach. The Doha Declaration, for example, refers to implementation of the ICPD POA in harmony with the MDGs. Commitment to achieving MDG5 is strong, as is the recognition that target 5.A (reducing MMR [maternal mortality rate]) cannot be reached without target 5.B (universal access to reproductive health). Indeed, the MDGs will not be met, if the target of universal access to reproductive health is not met by 2015 (UN, 2010a). Eight MDGs, with 18 targets and 48 indicators, are to be achieved by 2015. The eight MDGs are: (i) eradicate extreme poverty and hunger, (ii) achieve universal primary schooling, (iii) promote gender equality and empower women, (iv) reduce child mortality, (v) improve maternal health, (vi) combat HIV/AIDS, malaria and other diseases; (vii) ensure environmental sustainability, and (viii) develop a global partnership.

---

2. The Beijing Conference identified five strategic objectives related to health. These include: (i) increasing women's access throughout the life cycle to appropriate, affordable and quality healthcare, information and related services; (ii) strengthening preventive programmes which promote women's health; (iii) undertaking gender-sensitive initiatives which address sexually transmitted diseases, HIV/AIDS, and sexual and reproductive health issues; (iv) promoting research and disseminating information on women's health; and (v) increasing resources and monitoring follow-up for women's health (UN, 1995).

Objectives and Data Sources

This paper examines what has been happening in the health sector in Bangladesh, following the ICPD and the MDG. More specifically, it reviews the achievements insofar as MDG 4 and 5 are concerned; identifies the challenges in achieving MDG 4 and 5; and proposes measures to both consolidate the achievements and overcome the challenges.

The paper is based on an extensive review of all relevant documents and data sources. Also, it draws from the meaningful insights gained from discussions with the key stakeholders in the programme, and also draws heavily from the first author's in-depth understanding of the programme and his participation at the ICPD and its Precom and some of the subsequent follow-up meetings as part of the official delegation of the Government of Bangladesh (GoB).

Country Context[3]

With a population of around 160 million people, Bangladesh is now the eighth most populous country in the world and the fifth largest in Asia. With the current annual growth rate of around 1.4 per cent, about two million new faces are being added to the country's population annually. Based on official projections, the population will increase between 170 million and 184 million by 2020 and further to 294 million by 2050 (Khuda and Barkat, 2012a). According to UN estimates, the population of Bangladesh will increase to 185.6 million by 2020 and further to 222.5 million by 2050 (UN, 2010b).

Bangladesh has been rapidly urbanising.[4] In 1974, only 9 per cent of the population lived in urban areas, which is now around 34 per cent. By 2050, it is projected to increase to 56 per cent of the total population (United Nations, 2014). While the annual growth rate of rural population is 0.55 per cent (for 2010-2015),[5] the annual

3. An elaborate discussion on the country context is contained in Khuda *et al.* (2014).
4. The rural-urban migration is largely on account of push factors (Alam and Khuda, 2011).
5. The annual rate of growth of rural population in India and Indonesia during the same period (2010-2015) were 0.79 per cent and -0.61 per cent respectively (UN Population Division, 2012).

rate of growth of urban population is about 2.96 per cent[6] (United Nations Population Division, 2012).

About one-third of the total population is under 15 years of age, 18 per cent are aged 15-24 years,[7] and the elderly population (60 years and above) accounts for around 6 per cent of the total population, indicating a high dependency ratio. Over time, the proportion of the elderly population has been rising with the increase in life expectancy (UN, 2010b). However, the country's health sector is not adequately equipped to meet the challenges of both demographic and epidemiological transitions that the country has been passing through.

The legal female age of marriage in Bangladesh is 18 years; however, a large proportion of marriages take place before the legal age. There has been a slow but steady rise in the age at which Bangladeshi women marry, from a median age at marriage of around 14 years for women who are currently in their late forties to 16.6 years for women in their early twenties.[8] In 2011, about two-third of women aged 20-24 years were married before reaching 18 years, compared to about three-quarter over the past two decades. The female age at marriage is positively associated with female education and their household's wealth status (NIPORT *et al.*, 2013).

---

6. The urbanisation growth rate in Bangladesh is higher than the growth rate of the urban population in India, Pakistan, Sri Lanka in South Asia and Indonesia in South-east Asia (UN Population Division, 2012). See also World Bank (2014a).
7. The youth bulge is often misunderstood to bring in demographic dividend, without clear understanding of the concept. To be able to reap the benefits of demographic dividend, the East Asian experience indicates the need for considerable investments in health and education to be able to produce healthy, skilled workforce. Further, there is need for considerable investment, especially in the industries and services sectors, to be able to create adequate number of high-productive jobs to absorb the healthy, skilled workforce (Khuda and Quibria, 2014).
8. The female age at marriage in Bangladesh is the lowest in South Asia. In 2010, about half of women aged 20-24 years in South Asia reported being married before reaching 18 years (UNFPA, 2012). The prevalence of child marriage varies considerably between and within countries in South Asia. Bangladesh has the highest prevalence of child marriage in the region (66%) followed by Afghanistan and India (46% each) and Nepal (41%) (NIPORT *et al.*, 2013; CSO & UNICEF, 2012, NFHS-2005-06; and NDHS, 2011). It is more prevalent among rural girls, and especially in Bangladesh (70%) and India (56%) (ICRW, 2012). There has been some decline in the prevalence of child marriage among the young adolescents in some South Asian countries. During 1991-2007, Nepal, India and Pakistan recorded significant decline in the marriage of girls under 14 years of age, although there has been no change in the marriage of girls 16-17 years of age for the three counties, except Bangladesh where marriages in this age group actually increased by around one-third (Raj, 2012).

Childbearing also begins early, although it has recorded slight increase in recent years. The median age at birth is about 18 years across all age cohorts, excepting for women aged 20-24 years and 45-49 years. Only 4 per cent of women aged 15-19 years reported having had their first birth in 2010 before reaching 15 years, compared to 11 per cent of women in their forties. Age at childbearing is positively associated with women's education and household wealth status (NIPORT *et al.*, 2013).[9]

The education sector has witnessed considerable improvements. Between 1985 and 2010, primary school enrolment increased from 10 million (6 million boys and 4 million girls) to 17 million (8.4 million boys and 8.6 million girls), and secondary school enrolment increased almost threefold from 2.6 million (1.9 million boys and 0.7 million girls) to 7.5 million (3.5 million boys and 4.0 million girls) (Government of Bangladesh, 2013a).

Since 2006, the Bangladesh economy experienced around 6 per cent average annual growth rate in GDP (gross domestic product). Notable expansion has taken place in the RMG (ready-made garment) sector. Although the sector represents only around 5 per cent of the total labour force (World Bank, 2014b), it accounts for around 80 per cent of total exports and 13 per cent of the GDP (Berg *et al.*, 2011). Bangladesh's garment exports increased from US$ 6.8 billion in 2005 to around US$ 20 billion last year.[10] Export earnings from the garment sector may exceed US$ 30 billion in the next five years.[11] Also, remittances have increased manifold. In 2003, it was US$ 3.18 billion, which quadrupled to US$ 12.87 billion up to November 2012.[12] About 64 per cent of them are coming from migrants working in the Middle Eastern countries (Hussain, 2009). The remittance is the second largest source of income for

9. Studies have identified the factors associated with teenage marital pregnancy among Bangladeshi women, and found that those aged 25-29 years had lower likelihood of experiencing teenage marital pregnancy than those aged 15-19 years. Also, women who desired more than 2 children had significant higher odds and women born in urban areas had significant lower odds for teenage marital pregnancy (Sayem and Nuri, 2011; Haque and Sayem 2009).

10. For a detailed discussion on the growth and contribution of the garment sector in Bangladesh see, Khondhker, Razzaque and Ahmed, 2005; Quddus and Rashid, 2000; Khuda and Barkat, 2014a.

11. Financial Express, 2014.

12. Remittances are 7 times higher than the amount the government receives as foreign aid and 13 times higher than what the government receives as foreign investment.

Bangladesh, next to earnings from the RMG sector.[13] Remittances account for around 11 per cent of the GDP of Bangladesh (Rahim and Alam, 2013).[14]

The per capita GNI (gross national income) is US$ 1,190. The percentage of people living below the poverty line declined over the past decade from about half to less than one-third (Government of Bangladesh, 2011b).[15] At present, it is around 24 per cent. However, the percentage of people living below the poverty line is higher in rural than urban areas, in certain regions of the country, and among the landless and marginal farmers.

The agriculture, industries and services sectors contribute around 17, 30 and 53 per cent respectively to GDP. Both male and female labour force participation rates have increased over time. The increase in employment has largely been in the low-productivity, low-wage informal sector.[16] The current employment generating capacity is unable to provide productive employment to the unemployed and underemployed. Over 2 million new jobs need to be created annually over the next decade to be able to achieve this; indeed, a big challenge for the country, especially given the low overall employment elasticity of the economy with respect to GDP growth (Khuda, 2014).

Health Policies and Plans

Since the independence of the country in 1971, the government has adopted health policies and developed several health programmes

13. See also Ahmed (2010).

14. The position of Bangladesh is 7th in the world remittance income, next to India, China, Philippines, Mexico, Nigeria and Egypt (Rahim and Alam, 2013).

15. Globally, the proportion of people living in extreme poverty (less than $1.25 a day) has been halved. The world reached the poverty reduction target five years ahead of schedule. In developing regions, the proportion of people living on extreme poverty halved from 47 per cent in 1990 to 22 per cent in 2010. About 700 million fewer people lived in conditions of extreme poverty in 2010 than in 1990 (UN, 2013).

The vast majority of people living on extreme poverty reside in Southern Asia and sub-Saharan Africa. In 2010, one-third of the world's 1.2 billion extreme poor lived in India. China ranked second, with around 13 per cent of the global extreme poor, followed by Nigeria (9%), and Bangladesh and the Democratic Republic of the Congo (5% each). About two-third of the extreme poor lived in those five countries in 2010 (UN, 2014).

16. See also World Bank (2006).

and plans to improve health standards of the population, and further reduce the population growth rate.

The Ministry of Health and Family Welfare (MoHFW) is primarily responsible for providing health, population and nutrition services to the people of Bangladesh through its two directorates—Directorate General of Health Services (DGHS) and Directorate General of Family Planning (DGFP), and one project named the National Nutrition Project (NNP).[17] The MoHFW's activities are supplemented by many NGOs (non-governmental organisations) and the private sector, including the Social Marketing Company (SMC). The DGFP provides the following types of services through its field-based network and facility-based service delivery points, the Maternal and Child Welfare Centres (MCWCs): FP (family planning), antenatal care (ANC), postnatal care (PNC), normal vaginal deliveries, C-section deliveries, Expanded Program on Immunization (EPI), behaviour change communication (BCC), adolescent RH services, menstrual regulation (MR), sexually-transmitted infections (STI) screening and treatment, and STI prevention through provision of condoms. The DGHS provides preventive and curative healthcare services, and sexual and reproductive health under separate Operational Plans (OPs), unlike those under which similar RH services are provided by the DGFP. That is, vertical programmes are run under different OPs under the two directorates, with no integration between them.

The Health and Population Sector Programme (HPSP) was formulated as part of the Fifth Five-Year Plan (1998-2003), which called for a single and integrated sector for both health and population (Government of Bangladesh, 1998). The main objective of the HPSP was to ensure universal access to essential healthcare services of acceptable quality and to further slow down the population growth rate. The Essential Services Package (ESP) delivered through different levels of the primary healthcare system included RH services, including FP; child health and immunisation; control on selected communicable diseases; limited curative care; and BCC. The HPSP targets were, however, not achieved (Streatfield *et al.*, 2003).

17. Until made part of the Health, Nutrition and Population Sector Development Program (HNPSDP-2013-2018), the nutrition programme was managed by the National Nutrition Programme (NNP) (Government of Bangladesh, 2011d).

The Health, Nutrition and Population Sector Programme (HNPSP) was launched in 2003 with the goal of achieving sustainable improvement in health, FP and nutrition of the people, particularly of vulnerable groups, through increased availability and utilisation of user-centered, efficient, equitable, affordable and accessible quality of services for a defined ESP along with other related services. Its priority objectives were to reduce: (i) MMR, (ii) TFR (total fertility rate), (iii) malnutrition, (iv) infant and under-five mortality, (v) burden of TB (tuberculosis) and other diseases; and (vi) prevent and control non-communicable diseases, including injuries (Government of Bangladesh, 2004; 2008a; 2011d).

Given that the adolescents in Bangladesh are quite vulnerable to health risks, particularly relating to different aspects of RH because of their lack of access to relevant information and services, the MoHFW identified adolescent health and education both as a priority and a challenge to be addressed under the HNPSP (Government of Bangladesh, 2006).

Under the Health Population Nutrition Sector Development Program (HPNSDP—2011-2016), the government aims to achieve MDGs 4, 5, 6 and part of the MDGs 1 and 8 by developing an efficient and sustainable healthcare service delivery in order to ensure a people-oriented and people-responsive healthcare, particularly emphasising the needs of women, children, adolescents, the elderly, the poor and the marginalised groups. The major objectives are to: (i) expand the access and quality of MNCH (maternal newborn and child health) services; (ii) revitalise the FP programme to attain replacement level fertility, emphasising longer-acting and permanent methods (LAPM) and unmet needs of FP services; (iii) mainstream nutrition within the regular DGHS and DGFP services; (iv) strengthen preventive approaches and control programmes for communicable diseases and non-communicable diseases; (v) strengthen drug management and improve provision of quality drugs; (vi) increase coverage and quality of services by strengthening intra- and inter-sectoral and private sector coordination; and (vii) pursue priority institutional and policy reforms such as decentralisation and local level planning, incentives for service providers in hard-to-reach areas, and PPPs (public-private partnerships) (Government of Bangladesh, 2011d).

Achievements

Family Planning

Knowledge of the family planning method is universal among Bangladeshi couples. Also, there is favourable attitude regarding FP. In terms of use, the Bangladesh FP programme achieved impressive success until the mid-1990s. From about 4 per cent of married couples using FP in 1960s (Sirageldin *et al.*, 1975; Stoeckel and Chowdhury, 1973; Azhar and Hardee, 1977), the contraceptive prevalence rate (CPR) slowly increased during 1970s (Kingdom of Netherlands, 1978; Mia *et al.,* 1978; Bhuiyan, 1980; Khan, Huber and Rahman, 1977; Khuda 1981; 1984). From 8 per cent in 1975, the CPR increased sixfold to 45 per cent in 1994. In 2011, it was 61 per cent (Figure 1.1).[18]

Figure 1.1

Trends in Contraceptive Prevalence Rate Among Currently Married Women Age 10-49 in Bangladesh, 1975-2011

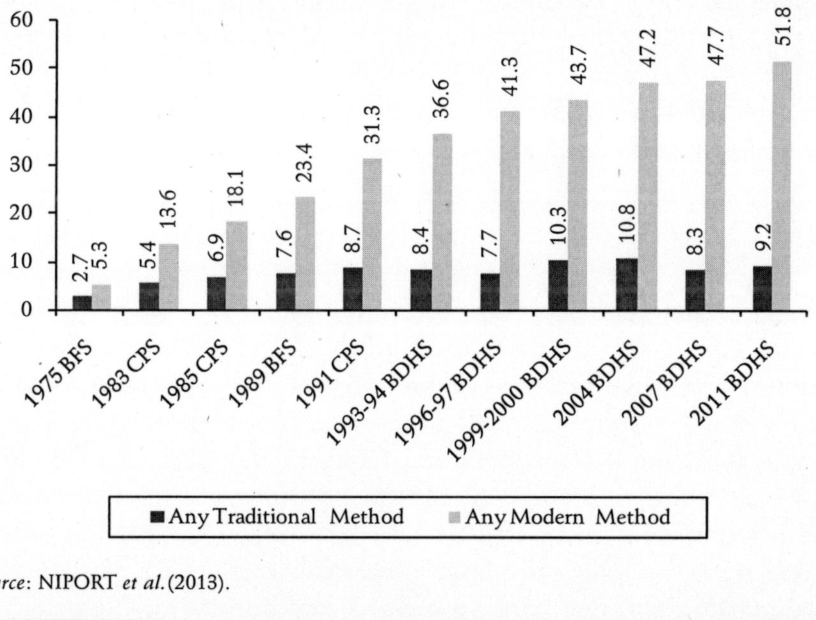

Source: NIPORT *et al.*(2013).

18. The CPR in Bangladesh is higher than in most South Asian countries, except Sri Lanka (64%) and India (64%) (Khuda and Barkat, 2012b). In 2011, 62 per cent of women in developing countries who were married or in union were using some form of contraception, 90 per cent using modern methods. In developing regions, including South Asia, tubectomy and the IUD (intrauterine Device) are the most widely used methods, together accounting for more than half of all contraceptive use (UN, 2013).

The achievements until the mid-1990s can be attributed to strong political will and commitment since the launching of the First Five-Year Plan of Bangladesh in 1973, increase in the demand for FP services, provision of such services by the FP programme, favourable political environment, and socio-economic development (see, Cleland *et al.*, 1994; Caldwell *et al.*, 1999; Caldwell and Khuda, 2000; Khuda *et al.*, 1994b; Khuda *et al.* 2001; Khuda, 2004; Khuda and Barkat, 2012a; 2012b; UNFPA, 2010).

Fertility

During the 1960s, fertility was high, with the TFR of over 7. It declined to 6.3 in 1975, and remained above 6 until 1981. Fertility declined to 5.1 in 1989. Compared to the 1960s and 1970s, fertility declined by 2 children and one child respectively during the 1980s. Between 1989 and 1993-94, fertility declined sharply from 5.1 to 3.4. However, the decline was stalled at around 3.3 during 1994-2000, and then, declined to 2.3 in 2011 (Figure 1.2).[19] Thus, the Bangladesh fertility transition can be divided into four phases: (i) high fertility until the mid-1980s; (ii) rapid decline in fertility between 1989 and 1993-94; (iii) plateuing of fertility decline between 1994 and 2000; and (iv)substantial decline in fertility since the 2000s (Khuda and Barkat, 2014a).

Nutrition

Globally, one in eight people (about 870 million) did not consume enough food on a regular basis to cover their minimum dietary energy requirements during 2010-12, the vast majority (852 million) of whom lived in developing countries. While their numbers continue to be quite high, the proportion of undernourished people in the total population declined from 23 per cent in 1990-1992 to 15 per cent in 2010-2012, indicating that the target of halving the percentage of people suffering from hunger by 2015 is within reach. However, there are large disparities in the rate of reduction in undernourishment among regions and countries. Progress has

19. Fertility is lower in Bangladesh than in most South Asian countries (Khuda and Barkat, 2012b). See also, Haub and Gribble (2011), which had given a TFR of 2.6 for India in 2009; and the Pakistan Demographic and Health Survey 2012-13 gave a TFR of 3.8 for Pakistan.

Figure 1.2

Trends in Total Fertility Rates in Bangladesh, 1975-2011

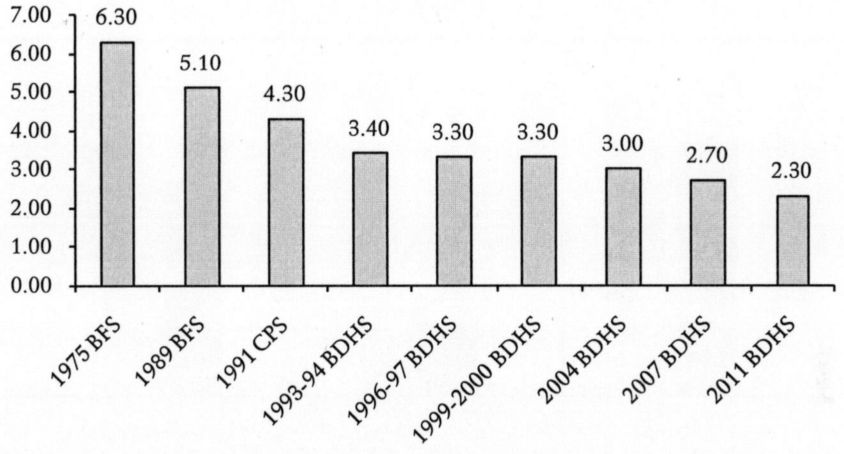

Source: NIPORT, Mitra & Associates and ICF International (2013).

been relatively swift in South East Asia, East Asia, and Central Asia; however, the pace of change in South Asia appears to be too slow to meet the MDG target (UN, 2014).

There has been some improvement in the nutritional status of under-5 Bangladeshi children. Between 2004 and 2011, the level of stunting declined from 51 per cent to 41 per cent, underweight from 43 per cent to 36 per cent,[20] while wasting remained unchanged at around 16 per cent (Figure 1.3). The MDG target for Bangladesh is to reduce underweight among under-5 children to 33 per cent (Government of Bangladesh, 2014).

Malnutrition among ever married women has recorded some decline over time. The mean BMI (body mass index) for ever married women aged 15-49 years is 21.4, which falls in the normal BMI classification. The proportion of women with BMI below 18.5 declined from 34 per cent in 2004 to 24 per cent in 2011. The

20. Around 101 million under-5 children (16% of all under-5 children), worldwide, were underweight in 2011. Between 1990 and 2011, the number of underweight children declined by 36 per cent; however, the prevalence of underweight in 2011 was highest in Southern Asia (57 million or 31%) (UN, 2013).

percentage of women with height less than 145 cm ranged between 13 per cent and 16 per cent (NIPORT *et al.*, 2013: Table 11.10).

Figure 1.3

Trends in Nutritional States of Children Under Five in Bangladesh, 2004-2011

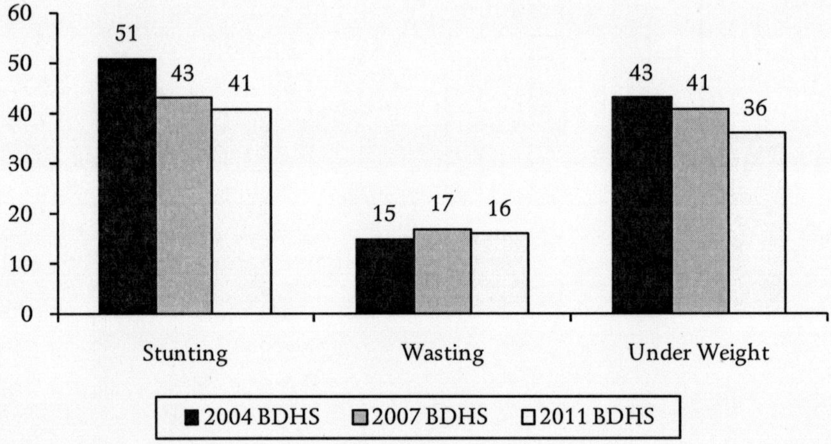

Source: NIPORT *et al.* (2013).

Child and Maternal Health

Child Health

Both the ICPD and the MDG attached high priority to reduction of child mortality. The MDG targeted that child mortality rate should be reduced by two-third by 2015.[21] The targets for Bangladesh are to reduce under-5 mortality and IMR (infant mortality rate) from 133 and 94 respectively in 1990 to 45 and 31.3 respectively by 2015; and to increase the proportion of children immunised against measles from 54 per cent in 1990 to 100 per cent by 2015 (Government of Bangladesh, 2014).

21. Globally, the under-5 mortality rate declined by 41 per cent during the last two decades (from 87 deaths per 1,000 live births in 1990 to 51 in 2011). However, around 6.9 million children (i.e., 19,000 a day) died from mostly preventable diseases in 2011. The overwhelming majority of such deaths occurred in the poorest countries, and in the most disadvantaged areas within countries. Therefore, more rapid progress is needed to meet the 2015 MDG target of a two-third reduction in child mortality, especially in South Asia. Despite steep challenges, however, a number of countries in South Asia (Bangladesh achieving two-third reduction and Bhutan and Nepal 60% each) with very high rates of child mortality in 1990 have defied the odds, showing that progress for all children is within reach (UN, 2013).

Bangladesh achieved considerable success in reducing childhood mortality. Between 1989 and 2011, the IMR declined by half from 87 deaths per 1,000 live births to 43 deaths per 1,000 live births;[22] and the under-5 mortality declined by 60 per cent from 133 to 53[23] (Figure 1.4). Thus, Bangladesh has already achieved the MDG 4 target for under-5 mortality. A matter of concern, however, relates to the slow decline in neonatal mortality (38%); and further that neonatal mortality (32)[24] accounts for three-quarter of infant mortality.

Figure 1.4

Trends in Childhood Mortality in Bangladesh, 1989-2011

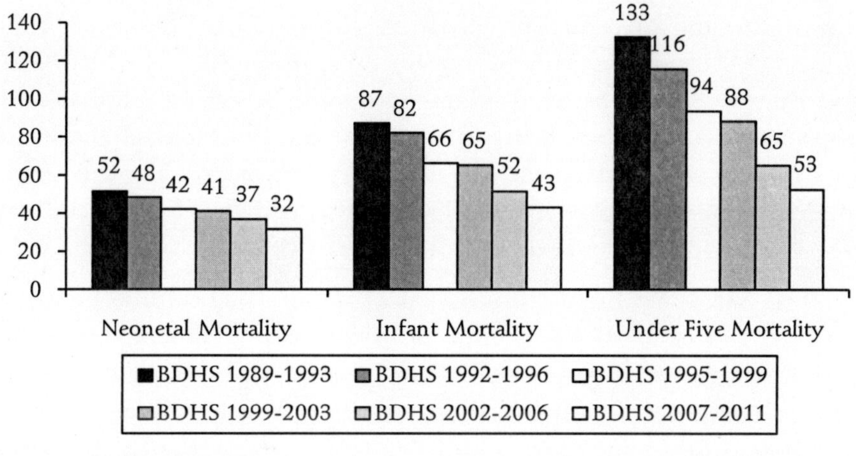

Source: NIPORT et al., 2013.

Vaccination coverage among children under-2 years of age has increased from 59 per cent in 1994 to 86 per cent in 2011. The corresponding increases for BCG, DPT3, Polio3 and measles were from 85 to 98 per cent, 66 to 93 per cent, 67 to 93 per cent, and

22. The IMR in Bangladesh is lower than in all countries of South Asia, except Maldives (14) and Sri Lanka (14) (UNICEF, WHO, The World Bank and UN Population Division, 2011). See also Government of Bangladesh (2013b).

23. The under-5 mortality rate in Bangladesh is lower than in all countries of South Asia, except Maldives (15) and Sri Lanka (17) (UNICEF, WHO, The World Bank and UN Population Division, 2011). See also Government of Bangladesh (2014).

24. The neonatal mortality rate in Bangladesh is lower than in all countries of South Asia, except Maldives (9) and Sri Lanka (10) (UNICEF, WHO, The World Bank and UN Population Division, 2011). See also Government of Bangladesh (2014).

69 to 88 per cent respectively (NIPORT *et al.*, 2013: Figure 10.1). The steady increase in immunisation coverage is largely due to adoption of the Reach Every District (RED) strategy, targeting the low performing districts (Government of Bangladesh 2013b). The HPNSDP has set a target of achieving 90 per cent coverage of measles vaccine by 12 months of age by 2016 (Government of Bangladesh, 2011b).

Maternal Health

Both the ICPD and the MDG attached high priority to reduction of maternal mortality. The HPNDSP has set the target of reducing the MMR to 143 deaths per 100,000 live births by 2015, in line with the MDG goal of reducing MMR by three-quarter between 1990 and 2015. Under the HPNSDP, two OPs, one each, by the DGHS and the DGFP, are being implemented with a strong emphasis on improving access and equity in utilisation of essential maternal and neonatal health services. However, the two OPs are being implemented vertically by the DGHS and the DGFP, without any effective coordination between them.

The MMR declined from 322 deaths per 100,000 live births in 2001 to 194 in 2010,[25] a decline of 40 per cent.[26] During the same period, the pregnancy-related MMR declined by 47 per cent from 382 deaths per 100,000 live births to 201. The MMR declined by half both during pregnancy and delivery and by one-third during post-partum (Figure 1.5; NIPORT *et al.*, 2012).

Antenatal Care (ANC): The percentage of last births that received at least one ANC from a medically trained provider increased from 30 per cent in 1997 to 55 per cent in 2010 (NIPORT

---

25. The MMR in Bangladesh is lower than in all countries of South Asia, except Sri Lanka (74) (WHO 2011a; 2011b). See also Government of Bangladesh 2014.

26. Globally, the maternal mortality ratio declined by 45 per cent between 1990 and 2013, from 380 to 210 deaths per 100,000 live births. Worldwide, almost 300,000 women died in 2013 from causes related to pregnancy and childbirth. In Southern Asia, the decline was 64 per cent. However, meeting the MDG target of reducing the MMR by three-quarter will require accelerated interventions, including improved access to emergency obstetric care, assistance from skilled health personnel at delivery and the provision of antiretroviral therapy to all pregnant women who need it (WHO et al., 2012; UN, 2013; 2014).

Figure 1.5

Pregnancy-related and Maternal Mortality Ratios (per 100,000 Live Births) in Bangladesh, 2001-2010

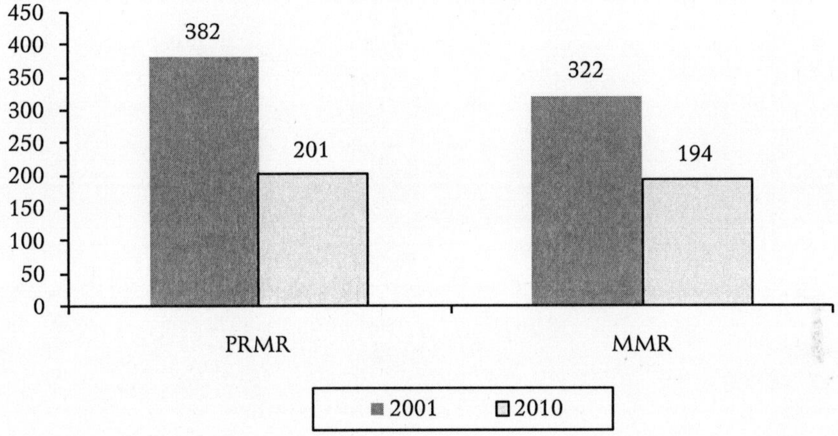

Source: NIPORT et al. (2012).

et al., 2012: Figure 4.1). The major source of ANC in 2010 was doctors (38%), followed by nurses, midwives, and family welfare visitors (15%) (NIPORT et al., 2012: Table 4.1). The proportion of pregnant women receiving the WHO recommended four or more ANC visits increased from 18 per cent in 2005 to over 26 per cent in 2009 (Figure 1.6).[27] The public sector health facilities were the major sources of ANC (42%), followed closely by the private sector (37%) (NIPORT et al., 2012: Table 4.4).

Neonatal tetanus is a leading cause of neonatal deaths in countries like Bangladesh, where a high proportion of births happen at home and by untrained providers. Therefore, tetanus toxoid (TT) injections should be given to women during pregnancy to protect neonatal tetanus. Almost 90 per cent of mothers received TT injections; and 42 per cent received two or more TT injections during their last pregnancy in 2011 (NIPORT et al., 2013: Table 9.4).

27. It is lower than the averages of the developing countries (half) and that of South Asia (36%) (UN, 2013). Over half of the pregnant women in Bangladesh 52 per cent had four or more antenatal care visits during pregnancy in 2012, rising from 37 per cent in 1990 (UN, 2014).

Figure 1.6

Trend in 4+ Antenatal Care Visits in Bangladesh, 2005-2009

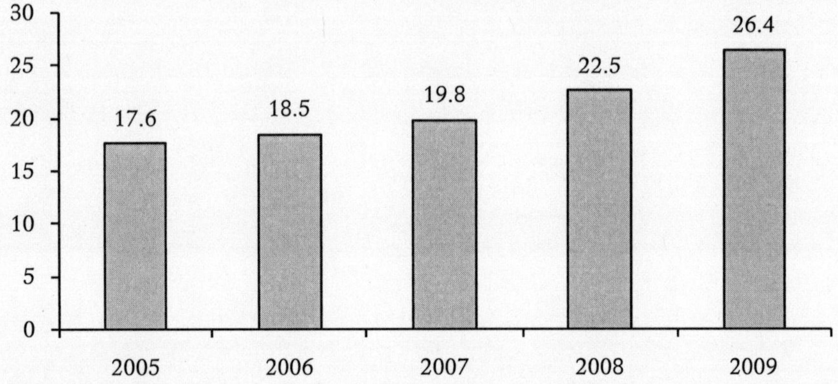

Source: NIPORT et al. (2012).

Delivery Care: Increasing the proportion of births delivered by skilled personnel is one of the important indicators of maternal health in MDG5 (UNFPA, 2010). The percentage of all live births delivered by medically trained provider increased from 12 per cent in 2001 to about 27 per cent in 2010[28] (Figure 1.7), although still low. The rise was primarily due to births attended by doctors. The percentage of births delivered in a facility increased from 9 per cent in 2001 to 23 per cent in 2010 (Figure 1.8), although still low.

Postnatal Coverage (PNC): In 2010, about one-quarter of women with recent deliveries had a postnatal check-up both for themselves and their babies by a medically trained provider (NIPORT *et al.*, 2012: Tables 4.13 and 4.16).

28. In developing regions, the proportion of deliveries attended by skilled personnel increased from 55 per cent in 1990 to 68 per cent in 2012, although only about 50 per cent in Southern Asia, reinforcing the need for rapid expansion of increased access to ANC services; referral to higher levels of care, when required; skilled birth attendance; and emergency obstetric care (UN, 2013; 2014).

Figure 1.7

Percentage of Deliveries by Medically Trained Provider in Bangladesh, 2001-2010

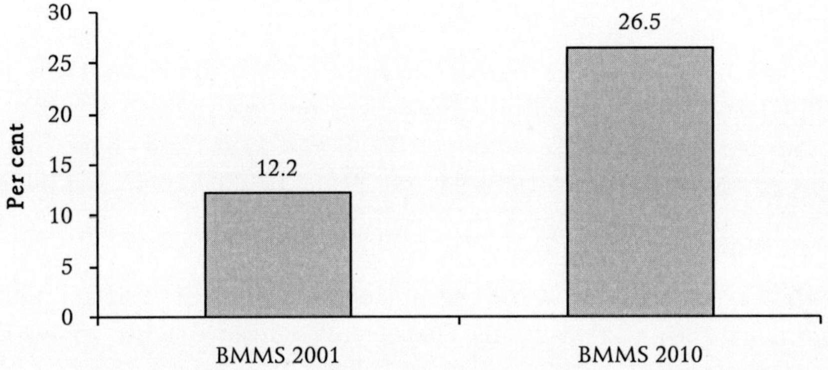

Source: NIPORT, MEASURE Evaluation and ICDDR, B. (2012).

Figure 1.8

Percentage of Births Delivered in a Facility in Bangladesh, 2001-2010

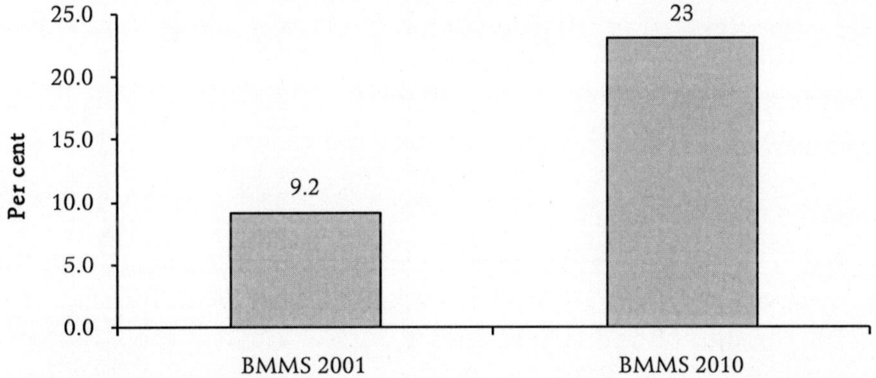

Source: NIPORT *et al*. (2012).

Challenges

Family Planning

The Bangladesh Family Planning Programme (BFPP) is faced with the following major challenges:[29]

Slowing down in the rate of increase in CPR: Between 1975 and 1989, the CPR increased by 1.6 per cent per year, which accelerated to 4.5 per cent annually between 1989 and 1991, and thereafter, it slowed down. Between 1993-94 and 2011, the CPR increased by less than 1 per cent per year. The slowing down in the rate of increase in the CPR is a matter of concern, given that the CPR target is to reach 72 per cent by 2016, i.e., an increase by 2 percentage points annually during 2011-2016. This seems quite difficult, given the trend during 1994-2011.

Regional variations in contraceptive use: Although the CPR has increased nationally, there are pronounced regional variations. In 2011, the CPR was considerably lower in Sylhet (45%) than Rangpur division (69%). Also, the CPR was lower in rural than urban areas. The variations in CPR by region and by place of residence indicate limited access to, and availability of, FP services across the country. Also, this is due to lack of adequate and effective behaviour change communication (BCC) campaigns in the under-served areas of the country.

Low contraceptive use among married adolescents: In 2011, married adolescents accounted for around 13 per cent of currently married women, while less than half of them used contraception. Given the disproportionately high share of such women in the TFR (23%), low CPR among young married adolescents is a major programmatic challenge.

Declining share of longer-acting and permanent methods (LAPM): Over time, the relative share of modern methods has increased, even though the relative use of LAPM has declined.[30] Between 1994

---

29. The challenges are similar to those faced by most South Asian countries (Khuda and Barkat, 2014b).

30. Global experience shows that the most successful FP programmes include considerably high use of LAPM (see, UNFPA, 2010).

and 2011, the relative share of pill increased from 48 per cent to 60 per cent of modern method use, while that of LAPM declined from 32 per cent to only 11 per cent (NIPORT *et al.*, 2013).

The change in the method mix has implications for the FP programme in respect of reliance on fieldworkers, especially among the poor, rural women, for re-stocks of modern temporary methods as well as on the overall programme sustainability. Also, the extremely low fieldworker home visitation, especially in areas with low CPR, and among condom and pill users, adds a new dimension to the problem. In addition, about one-fifth of married women aged 35 years and above and over one-quarter of those with three or more surviving children relies on the pill rather than accepting LAPM, which poses a major problem for efficiency of the programme.

High discontinuation rate: A major problem is the high rate of discontinuation. In 2011, over one-third of the users stopped using a method within 12 months of usage. Discontinuation rate was highest among condom users, followed by pill and injectable users. Most users dropout because of method failure, side effects, health reasons, or because they want to become pregnant. Dropping out on account of side effects and method failure indicates low quality of FP services,[31] thereby contributing to huge system loss for the programme.

Sizeable unmet need for contraception: Although the CPR has increased over time, there is still sizeable unmet need (12% in 2011).[32] Further, if those using traditional FP methods (9% in 2011) are considered, unmet need for effective methods of contraception

31. The high discontinuation is due to poor quality of family planning services. Not surprisingly, therefore, there is high incidence of induced abortions. In 2010, an estimated 647,000 induced abortions and 653,000 MR (menstrual regulation) procedures were performed in Bangladesh (Singh *et al.*, 2012). The 2010 MR rate is similar to the 1995 rate. Combining MR and abortion rates gives an estimated overall pregnancy termination rate of 37 per 1,000 women aged 15-44 years, higher than the equivalent rates for South Central Asia in 2008 (26 per 1,000), although similar to the rate for Southeastern Asia (36 per 1,000) (Sedge *et al.*, 2012).

32. Between 1990 and 2011, unmet need for contraceptives declined from 15 per cent to 12 per cent globally. Current levels of unmet need range from 4 per cent in Eastern Asia to 25 per cent in Oceania and sub-Saharan Africa. This translates into more than 140 million women (married or in union) having unmet need. By 2015, total demand for family planning among married women is projected to grow to more than 900 million, an indication of the unfinished agenda in RH and the scale of efforts needed to keep pace with the demand for contraceptives, especially for more effective modern methods (UN, 2013).

was 21 per cent in 2011, indicating that the target of reducing unmet need to 9 per cent by 2016 seems unachievable.

Fertility

As a country, Bangladesh has achieved near replacement level fertility; however, there are differentials in fertility levels, regionally and by socio-economic characteristics of the women. Chittagong and Sylhet divisions, accounting for around one-fifth of the country's population, have higher fertility (TFR of over 3). Rural women give birth, on an average, to half a child more than urban women (2.5 compared with 2.0 per woman). Women with completed secondary schooling or higher education have already achieved below replacement level fertility (about 2), while those with no education have high fertility (2.9). Women in the highest wealth quintile have already achieved below replacement level fertility (1.9), while those in the lowest wealth quintile have high fertility (3.1) (Khuda and Barkat, 2014a). Also, fertility is higher among non-working women, women belonging to landless households, women without access to mass media, and women belonging to households without electricity connection—an indicator of not only economic condition of the household but also its level of modernisation (Khuda, 2004; Neaz *et al.*, 2004).

A major concern relates to extremely high adolescent fertility in Bangladesh, one of the highest in the world.[33] Thirty per cent of adolescent married women have begun childbearing (24% with live birth and another 6% pregnant). Childbearing among adolescents is higher in rural (32%) than urban (24%) areas; four times higher among those with no education (42%) than those with secondary or higher education; and more than twice as high among those in

33. Adolescent fertility presents a major challenge in developing countries. However, between 1990 and 2010, adolescent fertility declined globally, with the most pronounced decline in Southern Asia. Nevertheless, one in nine (15 million out of 135 million) live births are among adolescent women worldwide, indicating relatively high adolescent fertility, especially in developing countries (UN 2013). Further, in many of the countries with high TFR or high MMR, births to younger women (15-24 years) account for 30-50 per cent of all births. An early transition to motherhood can not only reduce young women's opportunities for their schooling and future employment opportunities, but also, in turn, affect their children's schooling opportunities as well as their children's health and nutrition outcomes (World Bank, 2010a).

the lowest wealth quintile (42%) than those in the higher wealth quintile (Khuda and Barkat, 2014).

Nutrition

Poor nutritional status continues to be a major health problem for many in Bangladesh,[34] especially among young children and women of reproductive ages, who are more vulnerable to nutritional and micronutrient deficiencies than adult males.

Stunting among under-5 children is higher in rural (43%) than urban areas (36%), among those born of very small size (54%) than those born of average or larger size at birth (39%). The stunting is higher in Sylhet (49%) than in Khulna and Rajshahi divisions (34%); and is inversely associated with mother's education and household wealth status. A similar picture is discernible regarding underweight and wasting (NIPORT *et al.*, 2013: Table 20).

Anaemia is a major health problem in Bangladesh, especially among young children and pregnant women. Half of the children aged 6-59 months suffer from some level of anaemia. Boys and those living in rural areas are more likely to be anaemic. It is higher in Barisal (60%) than Dhaka division (48%); and is inversely associated with mother's education and household wealth status (NIPORT *et al.*, 2013: Table 11.7).

Over two-fifth of ever-married women aged 15-49 years are anaemic (36% mild, 7% moderate, and 1% severe). Rural women, those with little or no education and those in the lowest wealth quintile, tend to be shorter. Younger (15-19 years) and older (40-49 years) women are more likely to be thin or undernourished than women in other age groups. Undernourishment is higher among rural than urban women. The proportion of undernourished women is quite high in Sylhet (35%). Malnutrition among women is negatively associated with their education and household wealth (NIPORT *et al.*, 2013: Table 11.11).

34. One of the major problems hindering success in the nutrition sector in Bangladesh is lack of effective coordination among the concerned ministries, especially agriculture, food, and health (Naher *et al.*, 2014).

Child and Maternal Health

Child Health

While the child mortality rates have declined substantially, there are inequalities in terms of access and utilisation of health services among the population subgroups. Neonatal mortality, IMR and under-5 mortality rates are higher in rural than urban areas; and are inversely associated with mother's education and wealth status (NIPORT *et al.*, 2013: Table 8.3).

There are differentials in vaccination coverage among children. Both measles and all basic vaccinations (BCG, measles and 3 dozes each of DPT and polio vaccine, excluding polio vaccine given at birth) are negatively associated with the birth order of children, while they are positively associated with mother's education and wealth status. Both measles and all basic vaccinations are lowest in Sylhet, while they are highest in Khulna division (NIPORT *et al.*, 2013: Table 10.3).

The major challenges in reducing child mortality are: (i) drowning in water, being the leading cause of deaths among under-5 children (42%); (ii) lack of quality services in facility-based child and newborn healthcare; (iii) high neonatal mortality; and (iv) inadequate availability of essential drugs in providing relevant services (Government of Bangladesh, 2013b).

Maternal Health

The major challenges to achieving the MDG5 target are: (i) inadequate coordination between health, family planning and nutrition services preventing the effective use of limited resources and frequently resulting in inefficiencies and missed opportunities; (ii) human resource capacities (acute shortage of manpower of all categories, insufficient skills-mix, and insufficient numbers of health workers especially in rural areas); (iii) low public spending on health; (iv) limited use of public health facilities by the poor due to supply-side barriers; and (v) socio-cultural factors inhibiting use of services by the women (Government of Bangladesh, 2014).

The MMR is not uniform among Bangladeshi women. It rises steeply with age. Compared to an MMR of 130 among women aged 20-24 years, it was about 16 times higher among women aged 45-49 years (1,798) in 2010. The MMR is higher in rural (199) than urban areas (178), in Sylhet (425) than Khulna (64), among women with no education (439) than those with secondary or higher education (90), and almost twice as high among women in the lower wealth quintile (234) than those in the highest wealth quintile (123) (NIPORT *et al.*, 2012: Table 3.3).

The increase in ANC coverage was more rapid between 1997 and 2004 (51%), after which the growth rate slowed down.[35] The proportion of women receiving four or more ANC visits increased between 2005 and 2009 from 18 per cent to 26 per cent, even though still quite low.[36] About one-fifth of the women received ANC at home. Home ANC is more common among women with high birth order; and is inversely associated with mother's education and household wealth status (NIPORT *et al.*, 2012: Table 4.4).

Inequalities in ANC coverage exist by mother's age at birth, place of residence, and household wealth status (Government of Bangladesh, 2013b). The proportions of women receiving any ANC and ANC from a medically trained provider decline with the mother's age at birth; and are lower in rural areas in Sylhet, among women with no education, and those in the lowest wealth quintile (NIPORT *et al.*, 2012: Table 4.1).

The number of pregnant women receiving at least one TT decreases with age and birth order of child. It is lower in rural areas, in Sylhet, among women with no education and those in the lowest wealth quintile. The relationship is in the same direction, even though weaker, when pregnant women receiving two or more TT injections are considered (NIPORT *et al.*, 2013: Table 9.4).

35. Between 1990 and 2011, ANC coverage (at least one visit with a doctor, nurse or midwife during pregnancy) increased from 63 per cent to 81 per cent in the developing regions. Most progress was made in South Asia, North Africa and West Asia over the past decade, while the Caribbean, East Asia, Latin America and South-East Asia already achieved coverage rates of 90 per cent or more (UN, 2013).

36. Although the number of women who receive at least four ANC has increased, these gains will not be sufficient to reach the MDG target set for 2015 (Government of Bangladesh, 2013b).

The proportion of births attended by medically trained providers is not uniformly distributed among all subgroups in Bangladesh, as in various other countries.[37] It was less than half among older women aged 40 years and above (12%) than among women aged 20-29 years. It was almost twice as low in rural (22%) than urban areas, in Sylhet (18%), six times lower among women with no education (11%) than those with secondary complete or higher education, and six times lower among women in the lowest wealth quintile (9%) than those in the highest wealth quintile. Furthermore, two-third of all births were delivered by traditional birth attendants, more common in rural areas, among older women, and among mothers with little or no education and those in the lowest wealth quintile (NIPORT *et al.*, 2012: Table 4.9).

Facility-based delivery varied by characteristics of mothers. It was 2.5 times lower among those aged 40-44 years (10%) than women aged 20-29 years. It was 6 times lower among higher order births (6%) than for first order parity. It was half in rural (19%) than urban areas, and half in Sylhet (15%) compared to Khulna. It was one-sixth among women with no education (10%) than those with secondary and higher education, and one-seventh among women in the lowest wealth quintile (8%) than those in the highest wealth quintile (NIPORT *et al.*, 2012: Table 4.8).

There has been a sharp rise in C-section deliveries, largely driven by financial motives of the providers, more so in the case of the private sector where C-section is the predominant method of delivery. This is a matter of serious concern, given that the private sector is poorly regulated and often charges exorbitant fees (NIPORT *et al.*, 2012: Table 4.9).

Inequity in the use of maternal health services across various groups is, undoubtedly, a major concern in Bangladesh. However, there has been some improvement over the past decade. Women in

37. In 2011, the proportion of deliveries attended by skilled personnel in developing regions increased from 55 per cent in 1990 to 66 per cent. However, in around one-third (46 million of the 135 million) of the live births in 2011, women delivered alone or with inadequate care. There are wide disparities in the level of skilled attendance at birth, from nearly universal in East Asia and Central Asia to only about 50 per cent in South Asia and Sub-Saharan Africa, the regions with the highest levels of maternal mortality (UN, 2013). See also World Bank (2010a).

the highest wealth quintile were 12 times more likely than women in the poorest wealth quintile to deliver in a health facility in 2001, and this declined to by times in 2010 (NIPORT *et al.*, 2012).

The proportions of mothers that undergo postnatal check-up, both for themselves and their babies, are quite low, especially by qualified doctors. Among mothers seeking postnatal check-up for themselves by qualified doctors, it declines sharply with birth order (from 5% at birth order of 6+ to 27% at birth order of one) half in rural (14%) than urban areas, lower in Barisal (8%) than Dhaka (23%), among those with no education (6%) than those with secondary or higher education (48%), and among those in the poorest quintile (5%) than those in the highest wealth quintile (44%) (NIPORT *et al.*, 2012: Table 4.13). A similar picture is discernible regarding seeking postnatal check-up for babies (NIPORT *et al.*, 2012: Table 4.16).

Systemic Problems

Programme Design

Although called 'sector-wide approach program' (SWAP), the HPNSDP and its predecessor programmes, the HNPSP and the HPSP, are not truly SWAPs. Such programmes consisted of a number of Operational Plans (OPs)—HPSP (25), HNPSP (38), and HPNSD (32), with each OP being designed as a separate unit, independent of each other. The problem is further complicated by the bifurcation of services between the DGHS and the DGFP. Thus, the OPs are implemented vertically without any meaningful integration. For example, the DGHS and DGFP each have several OPs dealing with RH, without any meaningful integration between and among the OPs. All these result in duplication of efforts and wastage of resources. Also, to be truly SWAP, the programmes should also have included projects/activities implemented by the NGOs and the private sector.[38]

38. For more elaborate discussion, see Government of Bangladesh (2011c).

Stewardship Role of MoHFW

The MoHFW is not only the public service provider, but also the regulator for all service providers: public, private, and NGOs. With the fast growth of the private sector, the stewardship role of MoHFW has become even more important, especially in ensuring that the private sector adheres to acceptable standards and provides quality services at affordable rates, so that there is no exploitation, particularly among the poor. The MoHFW exercises its regulatory role through enactment of laws and through institutions specifically created to administer those laws for example, the Bangladesh Medical and Dental Council (BMDC) and the Bangladesh Nursing Council (BNC) for registration of doctors and nurses respectively. However, the fast-expanding private sector is making demands on the limited capacity and resources of the regulators. Accreditation and standard-setting are crucial for ensuring quality for both the private and the public sector. However, the MoHFW failed to take major steps during the HNPSP period to convince that its stewardship role was up to the desired level.[39]

Monitoring and Supervision

Like planning, monitoring of implementation is concentrated at Dhaka, with limited delegation of authority to the lower tiers of the MoHFW structure. As a result, quality of service suffers; and the process of good governance and accountability remains weak.

Gaps in Commodity Security

Before 1998, most RH commodities and contraceptives were supplied by donors. However, under the HPSP and the subsequent plans, procurement is to be carried out in line with International Development Association (IDA) and World Bank procurement guidelines. The procurement and supply of goods under IDA guidelines, World Bank procedures and the GoB (Government of Bangladesh) Public Procurement Regulations is a complex and time-consuming process. Despite the government taking measures to simplify and modernise the public procurement policy and

39. For more elaborate discussion, see Government of Bangladesh (2011c).

procedures, delays continue to hamper the procurement process largely due to: (i) limited technical capacity of the concerned officials and the Tender Evaluation Committee members; (ii) high turnover of concerned and trained staff; and (iii) considerable time involved for MoHFW and World Bank review process as well as for actual decision-making (Khuda and Barkat, 2012a).

Lack of Adequate Support for BCC

The Information, Education and Motivation (IEM) Unit of the DGFP and the Health Education Bureau (HEB) of the DGHS prepare various types of communication materials; however, most such materials are not updated on a regular basis and are often not adequately tailored to meet the specific needs of different clientele groups. Also, there is no separate cadre of BCC officials at the district level.

According to the concerned officials, the major constraints to effective BCC include: (i) lack of adequate support from the higher level decision-makers, (ii) inadequate funding, and (iii) absence of adequate number of trained staff. As a result, both the users and the service providers do not get access to relevant information from a coherent national BCC strategy.[40] Consequently, provider knowledge is relatively low, resulting in poor quality of service.

Gaps in Programme Efficiency

The programme is inefficient due to a number of factors: lack of integration between DGHS and DGFP, infighting between medical and non-medical staff within DGFP, staff vacancies,[41] absence of career planning, low staff morale, inadequate training, poor monitoring and supervision, lack of leadership and management, limited funding, weak implementation capacity, and non-involvement of other concerned ministries. All these result in considerable system loss.

---

40. See also Government of Bangladesh (2008b).
41. Currently, there are only 0.300 physicians, 0.280 nurses or midwives and 0.020 dentists per 1,000 people in Bangladesh.

Limited Funding

Between 1997 and 2007, the THE (total health expenditure) increased threefold to Tk. 159.91 billion (US$2.32 billion), rising from 2.7 per cent of the GDP during 1997-2000 to only 3.4 per cent in 2007.[42] Per capita spending on health almost doubled from Tk. 391 (US$9) in 1997 to Tk. 1,111 ($16), although still one of the lowest in the world.[43] The main source of finance for the THE is out-of-pocket spending by households (64%),[44] followed by government spending (26%)[45] and external resources (8%).[46] Households' relative

---

42. In 2008, THE as percentage of GDP was lower in Bangladesh (3.4%) than in Sri Lanka (4.1%), India (4.2%), Nepal (6%) and Maldives (13.7%), though higher than in Pakistan (2.6%) (WHO 2011b; Government of Bangladesh, 2010a).

43. The WHO Report of the Commission on Macroeconomics and Health (2001) strongly recommended increasing investment in health to promote economic development and poverty reduction. According to the report, the least developed countries need a minimum of US$34 per capita (i.e., half of what is being spent in Bangladesh) to introduce the essential health interventions. According to a more recent estimate, US$54 per capita is needed to attain a fully functioning health system and to cover a basic package of services, including interventions targeting non-communicable diseases by 2015 (WHO, 2010). The results of the MDG Needs Assessment and Costing study (2009-2015) show that US$19 per capita is required to achieve only the health-related MDGs during 2009-2015 in Bangladesh (Government of Bangladesh, 2010b).

44. In Bangladesh, the well-off pay more out-of-pocket for healthcare; spend proportionally more of their household resources on healthcare; and receive more or better care. The poor pay less because they cannot afford to pay, and hence, cannot often seek treatment, thereby obtaining less healthcare (O'Donnell *et al.*, 2008). As a consequence, they experience loss of health, with its adverse effects on productive capacity. Furthermore, although the government has targeted 60-65 per cent of total resources towards *upazila* and lower administrative levels providing primary healthcare, the proportion of development expenditure going to *upazilla* and lower levels to total development expenditure has actually declined from 65 per cent in 2001/02 to 52 per cent in 2007 (Government of Bangladesh, 2010b). In most cases subsidies to hospital care is pro-rich, while non-hospital care is pro-poor (O'Donnell *et al.*, 2007). Also, the utilisation of out-patient services by the poor is likely to be affected because of their reliance on unqualified providers (O'Donnell *et al.*, 2008).

45. Increased and sustained investment in sexual and reproductive health services in developing countries can bring about considerable benefits to women, families and societies. In addition to improved health, investment in sexual and reproductive health services contributes to economic growth, societal and gender equity, and democratic governance (Singh *et al.*, 2003). Also, investment in family planning yields considerable benefits. For each US$ invested in family planning in Bangladesh, there is US$6.5 savings—about half in education, followed by about one-third in maternal health, and about one-fifth in water and sanitation (Smith *et al.*, 2009). Hence, policymakers should find enough justification to increase spending in sexual and reproductive health and family planning services.

46. In 2012, net official development assistance (ODA) from developed countries was $125.6 billion (i.e., 0.29% of donors' combined gross national income), a 4 per cent drop in real terms from 2011. The decline is attributed to the economic and financial crisis and eurozone turmoil. Despite current fiscal pressures, some countries belonging to the Development Assistance Committee (DAC) of the Organisation for Economic Co-operation and Development (OECD) have maintained or increased their aid budgets in pursuit of the set targets. Net ODA increased in real terms in 9 of the 24 DAC countries, with the largest increases by Australia, Austria, Iceland, Luxembourg and the Republic of Korea (UN, 2013).

share of the health expenditure increased, while that of the GoB decreased (Table 1.1).

Table 1.1

Data on Health Expenditure in Bangladesh, 1997-2007

	1997	*2007*
Total Health Expenditure (THE)	Tk. 48.47 billion (US$1.1 billion)	Tk. 159.91 billion (US$2.32 billion)
THE as % of GDP	2.7	3.4
Per capita spending on health	Tk. 391(US$9)	Tk. 1,111(US$16)
Households' share of health spending as % of THE	57	65
GOB's share of health expenditure as % of THE	36	26

Source: Government of Bangladesh (2010a).

Other sources of financing include NGOs, CBHI (community-based health insurances) or MHI (micro health insurances) (Bangladesh Health Watch, 2012); and fees charged for services, private firms[47] (spending only 0.8% of THE), and private health insurance (only 0.2% in 2007).

The trend during 1997-2007 showed: (i) continuing low levels of public spending[48] (including donors) compared to other South Asian and Asian countries; (ii) flat public, including donor, spending (below 1% of GDP) throughout the period; and (iii) high out-of-pocket spending, especially relating to purchase of medicines. The implication of low public spending is that it forces households to spend more on healthcare. In Bangladesh where social protection is inadequate, the low public spending leads to further impoverishment of households.

Actual expenditure from the Revenue Budget is generally over 90 per cent in most years; however, expenditure from the Development Budget ranges between 62 per cent to 89 per cent (Khuda and

47. Commercial banks, mostly private, spent BDT 689 million on health in 2010 as part of its Corporate Social Responsibility (CSR), which is 10 times higher the amount spent in 2007, thus showing increasing contribution from this source (Bangladesh Bank, 2011).

48. Only 4.4 per cent and 5.3 per cent per cent respectively of the total and the development budget have been allocated to the health sector in the Bangladesh 2014-15 budget (Government of Bangladesh, 2013c).

Barkat, 2012a). Thus, not only is allocation to the maternal, child and RH and FP programme inadequate, the programme is also unable to spend the funds allocated to it, thereby not being able to achieve its desired objectives. Inefficiencies in public spending remain the health sector's most immediate challenge. Widespread system inefficiencies, weak planning capacity and overly centralised approval process lead to under-spending of available funds. Further, weak accountability and weak governance inevitably lead to underperformance in the delivery of public services, resulting in inefficient use of existing resources (World Bank, 2010b).

Conclusions and Recommendations

Since Independence, the country's population has more than doubled. Also, the country is faced with both a demographic and an epidemiological transition, which the health sector is not adequately equipped to deal with. The government has adopted health policies and developed several health programmes with the overall objective of improving health standards of the population and further containing the rate of population growth, giving special consideration to the needs of the disadvantaged and marginalised groups.

The Bangladesh FP programme achieved impressive success until mid-1990s. The CPR increased almost sixfold from 8 per cent in 1975 to 45 per cent in 1994. In 2011, it was 61 per cent. However, since the mid-1990s, the Bangladesh FP Programme has been faced with a number of critical challenges: (i) slowing down in the rate of increase in CPR, (ii) regional variations in contraceptive use, (iii) low contraceptive use among married adolescents, (iv) declining share of LAPM, (v) high discontinuation rate, and (vi) sizeable unmet need for contraception.

Fertility declined by about half from 6.5 in 1975 to 3.4 in 1994. In 2011, Bangladesh achieved near replacement level fertility. However, fertility decline is not uniform. There are differentials, by regions and by socio-economic status of the women.

Vaccination coverage and that of measles among children under-2 increased to 86 per cent and 88 per cent respectively in

2011. However, there are differentials in vaccination coverage among children. Both measles and all basic vaccinations are lowest in Sylhet, and are negatively associated with the birth order of children.

Child and maternal malnutrition continue to be major problems, especially in rural areas and Sylhet division; and are inversely associated with education and wealth status.

Both the ICPD and the MDG attached high priority to reduction of child and maternal mortality. Bangladesh has already achieved the MDG 4 target for under-5 mortality. Between 2001 and 2010, the MMR and pregnancy-related MMR declined by 40 per cent and 47 per cent respectively to 194 and 201. However, decline in childhood mortality has not been uniform. Neonatal mortality, IMR and under-5 mortality rates are higher in rural areas; and are inversely associated with mother's education and wealth status. The MMR is not uniform among all women, being considerably higher among older women, in rural areas, in Sylhet division; and is inversely associated with women's education and wealth status.

The percentage of last births that received at least one ANC from a qualified provider increased from 30 per cent in 1997 to 55 per cent in 2010. Almost 90 per cent of mothers received TT injections; and over two-fifth received two or more TT injections during their last pregnancy in 2011. One-quarter of women with recent deliveries reported to have undergone postnatal check-ups, both for themselves and for their babies. The percentage of live births delivered by qualified provider and at a facility increased to 27 per cent and 23 per cent respectively in 2010, although still low. However, the increase in ANC coverage was more rapid between 1997 and 2004, after which the rate of increase slowed down. Although the proportion of women receiving four or more ANC visits increased, it is still quite low. About one-fifth of the women received ANC at home. The proportion of women receiving ANC from a qualified provider declines with the mother's age at birth; and it is lower in rural areas and Sylhet division, and among mothers with little or no education and those belonging to lower wealth quintiles.

The proportion of births attended by qualified providers is lower among older women, in rural areas, in Sylhet division, and among mothers with no education and those in the lowest wealth quintile. Furthermore, two-third of all births were delivered by traditional birth attendants, more common in rural areas, among older women, among mothers with little or no education and those in the lowest wealth quintile. The proportions of mothers having postnatal check-up, both for themselves and their babies, by qualified doctors are unacceptably low.

The HPNSDP and its predecessor programmes are not truly SWAPs. They consist of a number of OPs, each designed as a separate unit and implemented vertically by DGHS and DGFP, resulting in duplication and wastage of resources.

The fast-expanding private sector is making demands on limited capacity and resources of the regulatory institutions. However, the stewardship role of the MoHFW is not up to the desired level.

Like planning, monitoring of implementation is concentrated at the headquarters Dhaka, thereby failing to achieve desired improvement in service delivery.

Despite efforts by the government to simplify and modernise the public procurement policy and procedures, delays continue to hamper the procurement process.

Communication materials are not updated on a regular basis, and are not tailored to meet the specific needs of different clientele groups, resulting in poor quality of service.

The programme is inefficient due to a number of factors: (i) lack of integration between DGHS and DGFP, (ii) infighting between medical and non-medical personnel within DGFP, (iii) human resources (HR) issues (such as staff vacancies, absence of career planning, low staff morale and inadequate training), (iv) poor monitoring and supervision, (v) lack of leadership and management, (vi) limited funding, and (vii) weak implementation capacity. All these result in considerable system loss.

Per capita spending on health is still one of the lowest in the world. The main source of financing is out-of-pocket spending by households. In Bangladesh where social protection is inadequate, the low public spending leads to further impoverishment of households.

There is not only inadequate allocation, but also the programme is unable to spend the allocated funds, thereby not being able to achieve its desired objectives. The health sector financing is faced with four challenges: (i) heavy reliance on out-of-pocket spending, (ii) inadequate financing, (iii) inequity in health financing and utilisation, and (iv) inefficient use of existing resources.

While progress has been made, nonetheless, there is need for accelerated action to both further consolidate the achievements and also overcome the challenges.

The government's political will and commitment to strengthening the health sector must be clearly reflected in its policy documents, enhanced budgetary allocations, and needed reforms (for good governance, improved transparency and accountability), thereby enhancing implementation capacity to achieve the desired results in the sector.

Repositioning FP as an essential element of RH is a priority task. Greater priority must be given to improved coverage and quality of services, with major emphasis given to policies and programmes to reduce inequities in access to services and health outcomes.

With early ages at marriage and childbearing, there is need to attach high priority to adolescents and youth with better sexuality/family life education and youth-friendly information and services. The MoHFW should, therefore, establish meaningful links with the youth, education and other concerned ministries, because reducing adolescent pregnancy will contribute to the overall socio-economic development and prevent intergenerational transmission of poverty.

There is need to integrate service delivery, especially insofar as RH is concerned, by ensuring that OPs dealing with RH services under DGHS and DGFP are brought under a unified command in order to not only enable more people to get services but also considerably reduce overlap and wastage of resources. The RH care should be provided through the PHC (primary healthcare) system, and the government should work to increase the accessibility, availability, acceptability and affordability of healthcare services and the facilities to provide access to basic healthcare for all. Therefore, there is need to ensure that health systems support integration of RH in PHC and improved coordination in support of the full continuum of care, and to further ensure that services are expanded to reach poor and vulnerable population groups. Also, greater emphasis should be given to health systems strengthening and health sector reform. Decentralisation and privatisation should be encouraged. In addition, health systems should be made gender- and culturally-sensitive and community-oriented, and transparency and accountability should be ensured.

The most critical challenge for the health sector in Bangladesh is the absence of a dynamic and proactive stewardship role of the MoHFW to be able to design and enforce policies so as to further strengthen and enhance the overall health system in the country. Such strong leadership should be able to bring about meaningful, effective, and efficient health system reforms to work for improvement of the health of the people, and which should be built upon the values of equity and accountability. Also, such reforms should ensure that the NGOs and the private sector maintain standards in the provision of quality services and control over excessive charges, without, however, curtailing the freedom of NGOs and the private sector.

More specifically, the MoHFW should: (i) improve access to quality services, especially among the priority groups and in under-served areas, including urban slums; (ii) strengthen overall supervision, monitoring and evaluation; (iii) address human resource issues: filling in vacant posts, ensuring required training and re-training, developing career path to boost staff morale; (iv) ensure commodity security and logistics; (v) implement a coherent BCC strategy; (vi) increase budgetary allocation; (vii) enhance programme efficiency; and (viii) enhance implementation capacity.

Reference

Ahmed, M.S. (2010). "Migrant Workers Remittance and Economic Growth: Evidence from Bangladesh", *ASA University Review* 4(1). Dhaka.

Alam, N., and B. Khuda (2011). "Out-Migration from Matlab—A Rural Area of Bangladesh: Directions, Levels and Differentials", *Asian Population Studies* 7(1). March.

Azhar, M. and M.S. Hardee (1977). *Changes and Differentials in Men's Knowledge of Attitude towards and Practice of Family Planning in Pakistan during the Sixties*. Karachi: Pakistan Institute of Development Economics.

Bangladesh Bank (2011). *Review of CSR Initiatives in Banks (2010)*. Dhaka.

Bangladesh Health Watch (2012). *Bangladesh Health Watch Report 2011: Moving Towards Universal Health Coverage*. Dhaka: James P Grant School of Public Health, BRAC University.

Berg, A., H. Saskia, K. Sebastian and T. Thomas (2011). *Bangladesh's Ready-made Garments Landscape: The Challenge of Growth*. New York: McKinsey & Company.

Bhuiyan, K.C. (1980). "Some Aspects of the Family Planning Programme in Rural Bangladesh", *The Journal of Family Welfare*. September.

Caldwell, B. and B. Khuda (2000). "The First Generation to Control Family Size: A Micro-study of the Causes of Fertility Decline in a Rural Area of Bangladesh", *Studies in Family Planning*. 31(3): 239-51.

Caldwell, J.C., B. Khuda, B. Caldwell, I. Pieris and P. Caldwell (1999). "The Bangladesh Fertility Decline: An Interpretation", *Population and Development Review* 25(1).

Cleland, J., J.F. Phillips, S. Amin and G.M. Kamal (1994). *The Determinants of Reproductive Change in Bangladesh: Success in a Challenging Environment*. Washington, DC.: The World Bank.

Central Statistics Organisation (CSO) and UNICEF (2012). *Afghanistan Multiple Indicator Cluster Survey 2010-2011: Final Report*. Kabul.

Dixon-Mueller, R. (1993). *Population Policy and Women's Rights: Transforming Reproductive Choice*. New York: Praeger.

Dixon-Mueller, R. and A. Germain (1992). "Stalking the Elusive 'Unmet Need' for Family Planning", *Studies in Family Planning* 23(5).

Financial Express (2014). "Export Earnings from RMG May Exceed US$ 30 Billion in the Next 5 Years", *Financial Express*. Dhaka. 1 March.

Government of Bangladesh (2014). *The Millennium Development Goals Bangladesh Progress Report 2013*. Dhaka: Planning Commission, General Economic Division.

———. (2013a). *Statistical Yearbook of Bangladesh-2012*. Dhaka: Bangladesh Bureau of Statistics.

———. (2013b). *The Millennium Development Goals Bangladesh Progress Report 2012*. Dhaka: Planning Commission, General Economic Division.

———. (2013c). *Bangladesh Budget 2013-14*. Dhaka: Ministry of Finance.

———. (2011a). *Report on Household Income & Expenditure Survey-2010*. Dhaka: Bangladesh Bureau of Statistics.

———. (2011b). *Health, Population and Nutrition Sector Development Plan (HPNSDP) (2011-2016), Programme Implementation Plan (PIP)*. Vol. 1. Dhaka: Ministry of Health and Family Welfare, Planning Wing.

———. (2011c). *Final Report on End-Line Evaluation of Health, Nutrition and Population Sector Programme (HNPSP)*. Dhaka: Ministry of Planning, Implementation Monitoring and Evaluation Division.

———. (2011c). *Final Report on End-Line Evaluation of Health, Nutrition and Population Sector Programme (HNPSP).* Dhaka: Ministry of Planning, Implementation Monitoring and Evaluation Division.

———. (2011d). *Health, Population and Nutrition Sector Development Plan (HPNSDP)* (2011-2016), *Programme Implementation Plan (PIP).* Vol.1. Dhaka: Ministry of Health and Family Welfare, Planning Wing.

———. (2010a). *Bangladesh National Health Accounts: 1997-2007.* Report prepared for MoHFW by Data International Ltd. Dhaka.

———. (2010b). *Millennium Development Goals Needs Assessment & Costing 2009-2015 Bangladesh.* Dhaka: GED, Planning Commission.

———. (2008a).*Health, Nutrition and Population Sector Programme (HNPSP), 2nd Revised Programme Implementation Plan: July 2003-June 2011.* Dhaka: Ministry of Health and Family Welfare, Planning Wing.

———. (2008b). *The National Communication Strategy for Family Planning and Reproductive Health.* Dhaka: DGFP, Ministry of Health and Family Welfare.

———. (2006). *Adolescent Reproductive Health Strategy.* Dhaka: MoHFW.

———. (2004). *Health, Nutrition and Population (HNP) Strategic Investment Plan: July 2003-June 2010.* Dhaka: MoHFW.

———. (2003). *Population Census 2001: National Report*. Dhaka: Bangladesh Bureau of Statistics.

———. (1998). *Health and Population Sector Programme 1998-2003: Programme Implementation Plan.* Dhaka: MoHFW.

Haque, M.A.and A.M. Sayem (2009). "Socioeconomic Determinants of Age at First Birth in Rural Areas of Bangladesh", *Asia-Pacific Journal of Public Health* 21: 104-11.

Haub, C. and J. Gribble (2011). "The World at 7 Billion", *Population Bulletin* 66(2). Washington DC: Population Reference Bureau.

Hussain, Z. (2009). *Remittances in Bangladesh: Determinants and 2010 Outlook. End Poverty in South Asia.* Washington, DC: The World Bank.

International Center for Research on Women (ICRW) (2012). *Child Marriage in Southern Asia: Context, Evidence and Policy Options for Action.*

International Institute for Population Sciences (IIPS) and Macro International (2007). *National Family Health Survey (NFHS-3), 2005-06: India: Volume I.* Mumbai.

Khondhker, B., A. Razzaque and N. Ahmed (2005). *Exports, Employment and Working Conditions: Emerging Issues in the Post-MFA RMG Industry.* Paper prepared for the International Labour Office.

Kingdom of the Netherlands (1978). *Bangladesh: Rural Development in Four Thanas in Kushtia District, A Study on the Problems of the Rural Poor Appraisal of an Experimental Programme.* Ministry of Foreign Affairs, International Technical Assistance Department.

Khan, A.R., D.H. Huber and M. Rahman (1977). "Household Distribution of Contraceptives in Bangladesh-Rural Experiences", *Rural Demography* IV(1 & 2). Dhaka.

Khuda, B. (2014). "Labor Force and Employment in Bangladesh", *Asian Profile* 43(2). Canada.

———. (2004). "Fertility Decline in Bangladesh: Role of Family Planning Programme and Socio-Economic Changes", in G.W. Jones and M. Karim (eds.), *Fertility Decline in Muslim Countries*. London: Hurst and Company.

———. (1984). "Population Control in Bangladesh: The Prospects", in G.W. Jones (ed.), *Demographic Transition in Asia*. Singapore: Maruzen Asia Pvt. Ltd.

———. (1981). "Family Planning in Rural Bangladesh", *DERAP Working Paper* No. 229. Norway: Chr. Michelson Institute.

Khuda, B. and M.G. Quibria (2014). "Reaping Benefits of Demographic Dividend", *The Daily Star*, 3 April. Dhaka.

Khuda, B., S. Barkat and D. Roy (2014). "Population and Development Challenges in Bangladesh", in Mishra, Jayasree and Jehangir (eds.), *Social Science Research in India and Selected Geographies*. Routledge.

Khuda, B. and S. Barkat (2014a). *Fertility Decline in Bangladesh*.

———. (2014b). "Repositioning Family Planning Programmes in South Asia", *Asian Profile*, Canada : Richmond, BC.

———. (2012a). "The Bangladesh Family Planning Programme: Achievements, Gaps and the Way Forward", in W. Zaman, H. Masnin and J. Loftus (eds.), *Family Planning in Asia and The Pacific: Addressing The Challenges*, ICOMP/UNFPA, Malaysia.

———. (2012b). "Unmet Contraceptive Need and Family Planning Programmatic Challenges in South Asia", in W. Zaman and H. Masnin (eds.), *Report on the Regional Workshop on Operationalizing the Call for the Elimination of Unmet Need for Family Planning*. Kaula Lumpur, Malaysia: International Council on Management of Population Programmes (ICOMP) and UNFPA.

Khuda, B., J.C. Caldwell, B.K. Caldwell, I. Pieris, P. Caldwell and S. Ahmed (2001). "Determinants of the Fertility Transition in Bangladesh", in Z. Satthar and J. Phillips (eds.), *Fertility Transition in South Asia*. New York: Oxford University Press Inc.

Khuda, B., A. Barkat, J. Helali, P. Miller and J. Haaga (1994a). *Population Policy in Bangladesh: A Review of Ten Priority Areas.URC (Bangladesh) and Population Council*. Dhaka.

Khuda, B., A. Barkat, B. Robey, M.A. Mannan, J. Helali, A. Sultana and S.A. Salam (1994b). *Bangladesh Journalists Reporting on Population and Family Planning: Study Results*. Baltimore: Center for Communication Programs, Johns Hopkins School of Public Health.

McIntosh, C.A. and J.L. Finkle (1995). "The Cairo Conference on Population and Development: A new paradigm?" *Population and Development Review* 21(2).

Mia, M., A.L.M.S. Zoha, M. Haq, M.R. Khan, M.M. Rahman and M.Z. Hossain (1978). "Basic Information of Family Formation and Family Planning in Rural Bangladesh", *Rural Demography* 5(1 and 2). Dhaka.

Ministry of Health and Population, New ERA and ICF International Inc. (2012). *Nepal Demographic and Health Survey 2011*.

National Institute of Population Studies, MEASURE DHS and ICF International (2013). *Pakistan Demographic and Health Survey-2012-13, Final Report*. Islamabad.

NIPORT, MEASURE and ICDDR, B. (2012). *Bangladesh Maternal Mortality and Healthcare Survey 2010-Final Report*. Dhaka.

NIPORT, Mitra and Associates and ICF International Inc. (2013). *Bangladesh Demographic and Health Survey-2011*. Dhaka.

Naher, F., B. Khuda, S.S. Ahmed and M. Hossain (2014). "How Nutrition-friendly are Agriculture and Health Policies in Bangladesh?" *Food and Nutrition Bulletin* 35(1). The Nevin Scrimshaw International Nutrition Foundation.

Neaz, A., Ahmed Al-Sabir and M.A. Khan (2004). *Review and Identification of Gaps in the Current Knowledge and Understanding on the Leveling of Total Fertility Rate in Bangladesh* (unpub.). Dhaka: Centre for Integrated Development Studies.

O'Donnell O, van Doorslaer E, Rannan-Eliya RP *et al.* (2008). "Who Pays for Healthcare in Asia?" *Journal of Health Economics* 27.

———. (2007). "The Incidence of Public Spending on Healthcare: Comparative Evidence from Asia" *The World Bank Economic Review* 21(1): 93-123.

Quddus, M. and S. Rashid (2000). *Entrepreneurs and Economic Development: The Remarkable Story of Garment Exports from Bangladesh*. Dhaka: The University Press Limited.

Rahim, S.A., and M.A. Alam (2013). "Foreign Remittance Income in Bangladesh: Opportunities and Challenges", *Asian Business Review* 2(2). Dhaka.

Raj, A. (2012). "Changes in Prevalence of Girl Child Marriage in South Asia", *The Journal of the American Medical Association*.

Sayem, A.M. and A.T. Nuri (2011). "Factors Associated with Teenage Marital Pregnancy among Bangladeshi Women", *Reproductive Health* 8: 16.

Sedge G., S. Singh, I.M. Shah, E. Ahman, S. Henshaw and A. Bankole (2012). "Induced Abortion: Incidence and Trends Worldwide from 1995 to 2008", *Lancet* 379 (9816): 625-32.

Sen, G., A. Germain and L.C. Chen (eds.) (1994). *Population Policies Reconsidered: Health, Empowerment, and Rights*. Cambridge, MA: Harvard University Press.

Singh, S., J.E. Darroch, M. Vlassoff, J. Nadeau (2003). *The Benefits of Investing in Sexual and Reproductive Healthcare.* New York and Washington: The Alan Guttmacher Institute and UNFPA.

Singh, S., A. Hossain, I. Maddow-Zimet, H.U. Bhuiyan, M. Vlassoff and R. Hussain (2012). "The Incidence of Menstrual Regulation Procedures and Abortion in Bangladesh, 2010", *International Perspectives on Sexual and Reproductive Health* 38 (3): 122-32.

Sirageldin, I., M. Hossain, M.T. and Cain. 1975. "Family Planning in Bangladesh: An Empirical Investigation", *Bangladesh Development Studies*, Dhaka.

Smith, R., L. Ashford, J. Gribble and D. Clifton (2009). "Family Planning Saves Lives", 4th Edition. Washington DC: Population Reference Bureau.

Stoeckel, J. and M.A. Chowdhury (1973). *Infant Mortality and Family Planning in Rural Bangladesh*. Dhaka: Oxford University Press Limited.

Streatfield, K., A. Mercer, A.B. Siddique, Z.U.A Khan and A. Ashraf (2003). *Health and Population Sector Programme 1998-2003, Bangladesh: Status of Performance Indicators 2002*. Dhaka: ICDDR.

UNICEF, WHO, and The World Bank and UN Population Division (2011). *Levels and Trends in Child Mortality: The UN Inter-agency Group for Child Mortality Estimation*.

United Nations (2014). *The Millennium Development Goals Report 2014*, New York.

———. (2014). *World Urbanization Prospects: The 2014 Revision*. New York: Department of Economic and Social Affairs.

———. (2013). *The Millennium Development Goals Report 2013*, New York.

———. (2012). *World Urbanization Prospects: The 2011 Revision*. New York: Department of Economic and Social Affairs.

———. (2010a) The Millennium Development Goals Report 2010, New York.

———. (2010b). *World Urbanization Prospects: The 2008 Revision*. New York

———. (1995). Report of the Fourth World Conference on Women, New York.

———. (1994). *Programme of Action of the International Conference on Population and Development*. New York.

UNFPA (2012). *Marrying too Young, End Child Marriage*, New York

———. (2010). *Revitalizing the National Family Planning Programme in Bangladesh: Towards Replacement Level Fertility and the Achievement of MDGs 4 and 5 by 2015*. Dhaka.

United Nations Population Division (2012). *World Urbanization Prospects: The 2011 Revision*. New York.

World Bank (2014a). *World Development Indicators*. Washington, DC: The World Bank.

———. (2014b). *Bangladesh Development Update*. April.

———.(2010a). *Better Health for Women and Families: The World Bank's Reproductive Health Action Plan 2010-2015*. Washington.

———.(2010b). *Bangladesh Country Assistance Strategy, 2011-2014*. Dhaka.

———. (2006). *Establishing Social Protection for Women Garment Workers in Bangladesh*, Social Protection Policy Briefs, Manila.

WHO, UNICEF, UNFPA and The World Bank (2012). *Trends in Maternal Mortality: 1990 to 2010*, Geneva.

World Health Organization (2011a). *Global Health Observatory Data Repository*.

———. (2011b). *World Health Statistics 2011*.

———. (2010). *Responding to the Challenge of Resource Mobilisation-mechanisms for Raising Additional Domestic Resources for Health.* World Health Report, Background Paper 13.

2

M.A.L.R. PERERA

Blazing a Trail for the World Health Development in Sri Lanka

Introduction

Sri Lanka is recognised as a country with good healthcare and outstanding health indicators comparable to those of developed countries. The country has met the Millennium Development Goals (MDG) target of halving extreme poverty and is on track to meet most of the other MDGs, outperforming other South Asian countries (World Bank). A number of major innovations in healthcare management has blazed a trail at times followed by the world. The achievements in healthcare provision have been on a platform of overall socio-economic development policy with the emphasis on human development (long before the concept of HDI (human development index), based on fundamental values as found in Oriental and Buddhist philosophy. Some of the innovations have subsequently been enshrined in the international arena with popular captions (ex-PHC [primary healthcare]). The achievements are reflected in the current health status in Table 2.1.

Table 2.1

Health Status

•	CBR 17.9 (2013)*	•	CDR 5.2 (2013)*
•	IMR 8.8 (2013)**	•	NMR 6.5(2013)**
•	MMR 22.3 /100,000 LBs (2009) *	•	Life expectancy (2001) 68.8 (M) 77.2 (F)*

Sources: * Dept. of Census & Statistics; ** Family Health Bureau/Ministry of Health.

Broad Health Policy

Western, Ayurveda, Unani, Siddha and Homoeopathy systems are legally recognised. PPP (private-public partnership) in healthcare is based on the premise that those who can afford, should access the private sector. Public sector services are free at the point of delivery with universal access to public Western system, geographically and socially. Guiding principles of health policy are respect of the dignity of individuals, recognition of the right of individual involvement in management of care, quality, equity and accessibility, optimal utilisation and acknowledgement of the inter-relationship with other sectoral development (sector wide approach: SWAP). Policy is reflected in the vision and mission of the Health Ministry.

Vision of the Ministry of Health

"A healthier nation that contributes to economic, social, mental and spiritual development." Spiritual aspect of health has been emphasised in Ayurveda. It is interesting to note that in recent times, this aspect has relatively been incorporated into the World Health Organization (WHO) definition of health.

Mission

To achieve the highest attainable health status by responding to people's needs and working in partnership to ensure access to comprehensive, cost-effective and sustainable health services (Health Master Plan, 2007-2016).

Reasons for Satisfactory Health Status

Sri Lanka's notable achievements in the sphere of social development can be considered exceptional in the context of her relatively low level of income, and a relatively weak economic performance. In sharp contrast to the economic performance, there has been steady and exceptional improvement in Sri Lanka's health and health-related social indicators. These significant improvements in the health indicators have been the outcome not only of the performances within the health sector itself but also of major socio-economic developments in the non-health sectors such as universal franchise (1931), free education (1938) and free food supplements.

Socio-cultural factors have also played an important leverage role in the evolution of the modern health system and its adaptation. Thus, emphasis had been on human development, a concept introduced by Amartya Sen in 1990. The culture of the country has been predominantly shaped by its adherence to the Buddhist way of life which accords a high place to human well-being and health. High priority was given to health service and healthcare in a value system in which the alleviation of pain and suffering and compassion towards all living creatures occupied a central place and in which religion, education, and health also received high priority. These social and economic changes in Sri Lanka have taken place within a vigorous political process which in stages produced a representative form of government and political institutions over a considerable period of time. Universal adult franchise and the competitive political process have enabled the vast rural majority to make their demands on the system and secure their due share of the various social welfare benefits extended by the state. It also promoted the active involvement of women in the political process and gave them the political weight which enabled them to make the political elites respond to their concerns.

Primary Healthcare

The first health unit was established in Kalutara in 1926 and provided all elements of PHC, but the term was coined at the Alma Ata conference in 1978. The Public Health Midwife/Family Health Workers play a pivotal role in MCH (maternal and child health) care. In the aftermath of the Alma Ata declaration, the national charter for Health Development was signed on 7 February 1980 and the concept of national health development network was established. These two are land marks for the region.

Drugs Policy

Prof Senaka Bibile, a respected pharmacologist is the father of the essential drugs concept (Wickremasinghe and Bibile, 1971), subsequently enshrined by WHO in 1977. The origin dates back to the National Formulary Committee that was established in 1958. The principle of the EDL (essential drugs list) emerged when the committee recommended that public hospitals confine the drugs used to 500 by generic name. In keeping with recommendations in the Wickremasinghe-Bibile Report, the State Pharmaceutical Corporation (SPC) was set up in 1971, and functioned as the sole importer of drugs to the public and private sectors at that time (economy of scale). With the country embracing open economic policy in 1977, the supply of pharmaceuticals by the SPC was confined to the public sector mainly. The State Pharmaceuticals Manufacturing Corporation (SPMC) was set up in the year 1987 with grant aid received from the Japanese government through the Japan International Cooperation Agency (JICA), with the stated objective to manufacture quality, effective and safe medicinal drugs. This far-sighted decision was proposed in the Bibile-Wickremasinghe report. The first formal national EDL was published in 1985 and has been revised regularly.

Place in Historical Evolution of Hospitals

Ancient cultures linked religion, social care and medicine, early hospitals being set up by non-state actors such as religious/ social care organisations. Earliest ones documented were in ancient Egyptian temples. In ancient Greece, temples dedicated to the healer-God Asclepius performed the role. *Vaisya* (merchant) families in India established houses for dispensing charity and medicine. In 325 A.D., the Christian church constructed a hospital in every cathedral town. London Dispensary established in 1696, was the first Government clinic in the British Empire to dispense medicines to poor sick people. The realisation that it is the duty of governments to provide health services dawned much later. The French Government secularised healthcare institutions in 1900.

The global perspective in the evolution is depicted in Table 2.2.

In complete contrast, in Sri Lanka, the *Mahawamsa* (historical chronicle) provides the earliest documentary evidence of institutions specifically dedicated to the care of the sick anywhere in the world set up by state actors. King Pandukabhaya of Sri Lanka (437 BC to 367 BC) built lying-in-homes and hospitals (*Sivikasotthi-Sala*) in various parts of the country. Mihintale Hospital is considered the oldest one in the world.

Devolution/Decentralisation of Health services

Health services were decentralised to Superintendents of Health Services in 1954 (later designated as Regional Directors). With the setting up of provinces (13th Amendment to the Constitution), healthcare was devolved to the nine provinces and placed under Provincial Directors in 1987.

Table 2.2

Global Perspective in the Evolution of Hospitals

Time	*Role of hospital*	*Characteristics*
7th century	Healthcare	Byzantine empire, Greek and Arab theories of diseases
10th to 17th century	Nursing, spiritual care	Hospitals attached to religious foundations
11th century	Isolation of infectious diseases	Nursing of infectious diseases such as leprosy
17th century	Healthcare for poor people	Philanthropic and state institutions
Late 19th century	Medical care	Medical care and surgery, high mortality
Early 20th century	Surgical centres	Technological transformation of hospitals, entry of middle-class patients, expansion of outpatient departments
1950s	Hospital-centred health systems	Large hospitals, temples of technology
1970s	District general hospitals	Rise of district general hospital, local, secondary and tertiary hospitals
1990s	Acute care hospital Ambulatory surgical centres	Active short-stay care, expansion of day admissions, expansion of minimally invasive surgery

Source: Healy and McKee (2001).

National Commission on Macroeconomics & Health (NCMH)

Sri Lanka was one of the first countries in the world to set up a NCMH (2002) in the wake of the publication of the WHO report on Macroeconomics and Health in December 2001. The Terms of Reference of the report were:

1. Advice Government and the Minister of Health on all broad policy issues, policy options and directions in relation

to investments in health, both in the public and private sectors so that health could make an optimal contribution to development of the country.

2. Recommend new approaches and strategies for scaling up health interventions, particularly those aimed at the poor, and increasing the investments in health for human development.
3. Commission appropriate studies in different aspects of macroeconomics and health, which will support the work of the Commission.
4. Recommend modalities for mobilising increased external resources for health development and for advicing on broad policies and strategies for their optimal utilisation.
5. Advice the Minister on all aspects related to economics and health for overall health and human development in Sri Lanka.

The structure is depicted in Figure 2.1.

Figure 2.1

Structure of National Commission on Macroeconomics and Health

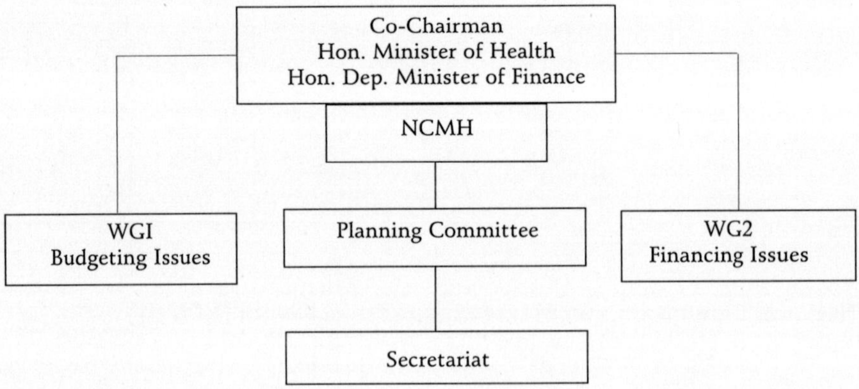

A major responsibility thrust upon the Commission was the development of a health finance policy for equity, efficiency and sustainability with emphasis on:

- Improvement of the equilibrium among equity, efficiency and sustainability of health finance.

- Development of a health finance policy for national, provincial and district levels.
- Development of a plan to reorient procedures and formats towards performance-based planning and budgeting.
- Cost effectiveness studies.
- More autonomy.
- Community involvement.

Social Marketing

Sri Lanka carried out a successful social marketing programme in leprosy control (with resources from the Novartis Foundation) to generate and satisfy the demand for leprosy diagnosis and treatment. The programme was in response to some systemic issues such as, free and effective treatment available but not widely known, one-third of newly diagnosed patients could not come to terms with diagnosis, limited access to leprosy services, fear and high stigma. Underlying strategy was to use commercial marketing techniques to change behaviour. Expected outcomes were that patients would self-examine for insensitive patches and seek professional care; healthcare providers to 'think leprosy' when examining skin patches and refer for treatment; and the community to encourage patients to seek prompt treatment. The communication challenge was to create interest in a disease which most people were indifferent to/disgusted with. The main messages were, leprosy is curable sans deformities; free treatment is available in the healthcare system; and seek care immediately. The approach was positive and attractive with powerful language projecting simple messages. The thrust was consistent use of layout, colours, fonts, design, logos that enabled people to easily perceive all materials as dealing with leprosy, and provision of synergistic effect aimed at easy recall. The communication mix (TV and radio) gave high visibility *via* soaps, spots, dramas, talk shows; use of print campaign (newspapers advertisements, brochures, posters); billboards at bus shelters as point of 'sales' of messages; and interpersonal communication to reinforce messages and trigger action. Anecdotal evidence pointed to changed perception of leprosy, in the public as well as stakeholders, triggering of action as shown by people coming forward for diagnosis (every second new patient reported voluntarily) and establishment of a link between an insensitive patch and leprosy. In addition, the campaign seemed to have brought leprosy to the public health agenda and created a sense of pride for all involved. It is also credited for expanding the network of leprosy care, detecting hidden cases and eliminating leprosy as a public health problem. The ripple effects claimed are adoption of concepts by the WHO, and adoption of approach by Brazil, India, Nepal and Madagascar. The approach was also adopted, adapted, and scaled up by BBC World Service Trust (Williams *et al.,* 1998).

The National Quality Assurance Programme (NQAP)

The formal initiative in quality assurance started in 1988 was based on "Quality Assessment and Assurance in Primary Healthcare" (M.I. Roemer and C. Montoya Aguilar, WHO Geneva, 1988). Two pilot projects were undertaken in the same year and a decision was taken by Ministry of Health (MoH) to initiate a QAP (quality assurance programme) for the health sector. A national consultative meeting was held in December same year and a National Programme with 32 sets of indicators and standards formulated (Ministry of Health, 1995). This programme mostly concentrated on availability of services and improving quality in the areas of basic patient needs, cleanliness (responsiveness), health education and maternity care. The programme was extended in a phased manner to selected Teaching and Provincial hospitals. A review of the programme, held in 1994, felt that the programme needed more focus. Accordingly, five critical areas of care were selected, fresh indicators and standards developed (Ministry of Health, 1995). The next important landmark is the launch of the programme at the Castle Street Hospital for Women (CSHW), using the Japanese concept of 'five-S' as the entry point to the QAP, presently followed by all institutions. For the first time in the history of health services, the CSHW won a national award for quality of care and productivity in 2001. The Ministry was quick to use the opportunity to fill a long felt void and named the CSHW the focal point for the national QAP by General circular no: 02–109–2003 of 8 October 2003 (Perera, 2004).

The Directorate of Healthcare Quality and Safety was commissioned on 18 September 2012. National guidelines have been published for improvement of quality and safety of healthcare institutions (for line ministry and provincial hospitals), improvement of quality and safety of healthcare institutions (for primary medical care units), improvement of quality and safety of healthcare institutions (for offices of medical officer of health, improvement of quality and safety of healthcare institutions (for specialised public health units and campaigns), improvement of quality and safety of healthcare institutions (for health management units) and improvement of quality and safety of healthcare institutions (for training institutions) (Ministry of Health, 2012).

Four institutions have so far won Sri Lanka Standards Institution awards for Quality and 146 for productivity. The Directorate is an international centre for training and so far, 21 such programmes have been conducted and many more are in the pipeline (Director, Healthcare Quality and Safety, 2014).

Health Master Plan (HMP) 2007–2016

HMP is based on dialogue and discussions involving all stakeholders; officials of national and provincial ministries of health, the private health sector, professional associations, trade unions, NGOs, consumer groups etc. A SWAP was thus followed. In addition, evidence from community and facility-based studies as well as reports of expert committees, enriched the plan. It aims to build on successes and experiences of the past, and address the challenges facing a health sector in transition (demographic, epidemiological transition, resource constraints, increased demand and expectations of the public, the need for equity and development of a management ethos for good governance and ensured quality of services). The HMP supports overall economic and social goals. The aim of improving health status and reducing inequalities is to be achieved by five strategies, namely:

1. To ensure the delivery of comprehensive health services, which reduce the disease, burden and promote health.
2. To empower communities (including households) towards more active participation in maintaining their health.

3. To improve the management of human resources for health.
4. To improve health financing, resource allocation and utilisation; and
5. To strengthen stewardship and management functions of the health system.

The master plan profiles strategic programmes to achieve each strategic objective. HMP profiles a number of strategic programmes to achieve immediate objectives and packages of projects to be implemented for the corresponding programmes. A participatory approach is maintained to continuously review strategy and work out detailed activity profiles for priority projects, the required inputs, and indicators with means of verification and budgets (Ministry of Health, 2007).

Conclusion

On the way towards achieving outstanding health indicators, which even developed countries can be proud of, Sri Lanka has blazed trails in health development—some of which have subsequently set the tone for regional/global initiatives.

References

Healy, J. and M. McKee (2001). "The Evolution of Hospital Systems", in M. McKee and J. Healy, *Hospitals in a Changing Europe*. Oxford: Open University Press.

Ministry of Health (1995). *Quality Assurance of Patient Care Services*. Colombo.

———. (2012). *Quality & Safety of Healthcare Institutions*. Retrieved on 18 September 2012, from: *http://www.health.gov.lk/QSHI.htm*

———. (2007). *Health Master Plan Sri Lanka: Healthy & Shining Island in the 21st Century—Summary*. Retrieved on 14 September 2012, from: *http://203.94.76.60/HMP-Guidlines/HMP-07- 16/1%20Original%20Documents/HMP%20Summary.pdf*

Perera, M.A.L.R. (2004). *Current Status and Outcomes of the National Quality Assurance Programme*.

Wickremasinghe, S.A. and S. Bibile (1971). "Pharmaceuticals Management in Ceylon", *Br Med J*. 3(5777): 757-58. 25 September.

Williams, P.G., D. Dewapura, P. Gunawardene and S. Settinayake (1998). "Social Marketing to Eliminate Leprosy in Sri Lanka", *Soc. Mar.* Q. 4(4): 27-31 (Summer).

World Bank *http://www.worldbank.org/en/country/srilanka/overview,* Accessed 12 October 2014.

Others:

Director, Healthcare Quality, Ministry of Health, Personal communication dated 16 October 2014.

Health Master Plan 2007-2016. http://www.health.gov.lk/en/index.php?option=com_content&view=article&id=327&Itemid=102, Accessed on 12 October 2014.

http://www.who.int/social_determinants/thecommission/finalreport/en/ accessed 18 October 2014.

3

SAMINATHAN S. PUWANESH

Enhancing Surveillance for Malaria through Improving Public-Private Participation

Introduction

This paper describes an innovative PPP (public private partnership) to address a major constraint in Sri Lanka's quest to eradicate malaria. Malaria was a major public health problem in Sri Lanka. Anti Malaria Campaign (AMC) was set up in 1911 to eliminate indigenous transmission of plasmodium falciparum malaria. Present objective is to eliminate indigenous transmission of malaria by the year 2014, maintain zero mortality from malaria and prevent reintroduction of malaria from other countries.

Sri Lanka is on the verge of eliminating malaria and strengthening malaria surveillance system is an essential component of the proposed malaria elimination programme strategy. For this purpose, it is necessary to strengthen malaria case surveillance in both government and private sector healthcare facilities. Strengthening surveillance will contribute to detecting and investigating all malaria cases and suspected malaria infections. The strengthened surveillance should be complemented by increasing diagnostic capacity, better case management, and preliminary investigation and follow up activities.

The strengthening of case notification has been planned through the use of several interventions aimed at actively seeking parasite carrying individuals in the community. Establishment of a real time notification and reporting system is also a priority. It is observed that although the surveillance system in the government sector is functioning satisfactorily the private health sector reporting is inadequate. Therefore, developing a complementary notification system for the private health sector will facilitate and enable early reporting of cases. Thereby, real time surveillance of cases that is at present not notified and missed out, will take place. Hence, this mechanism will make it possible to carry out effective containment strategies through the establishment and deployment of rapid response teams at district level for control activities.

Since the present routine surveillance system has not been able to successfully deal with this problem, special efforts to enhance the system of reporting by the private sector was thought to be necessary. The Institute for Health Policy (IHP) developed and established a complementary reporting system for this sector and piloted it in Monaragala and Anuradhapura districts. This system has now been implemented for the whole country to be used as a national complementary reporting system for malaria by the private health sector providers. The project is described next.

Project Activities

The activities were carried out in two phases:

Phase 1

Phase 1 involved setting up of the database and obtaining the services of a telecommunication service provider and piloting of the system in two districts.

Phase 2

Phase 2 saw implementation of the system in other districts and maintenance and supervision of the implementation of the system at national and district levels. The activities involved are detailed chronologically as follows:

Establishment of a database of all private health sector establishments dealing with patients and laboratory investigations

In phase one, four categories of private healthcare sector providers were identified to be included in the database, namely, full time private GPs (general practitioners) who are graduate medical officers; private laboratories; private hospitals; full time

RMPs (registered medical practitioners) who are a category of non-graduate medical staff trained by the Department of Health.

Establishment of a call centre at AMC, for enhancement of private health sector surveillance for malaria

Space in the computer room at AMC was allocated to set up the call centre. A medical officer was assigned to function as head of the Information Centre of the unit and to monitor the notifications via the dedicated telephone number. Information Technology manager at AMC was identified to be the call centre manager and was given the responsibility to handle and maintain software and hardware items of the call centre.

Selection of a service provider

IHP project team evaluated all the available telecommunication services providers in Sri Lanka to select the best with the capacity to provide this project with an appropriate solution. Requests for proposals for required services were submitted to all the leading service providers. "Dialog" a leading provider, responded with a solution and it was noted that this was the only institute which had the capacity to develop a solution and help in implementing the same. Dialog allocated a dedicated platinum number (0117 626 626) for the project.

As per request made by IHP, Telephone Regulatory Commission Sri Lanka (TRCSL) authorised Dialog in May 2011 to carry out this activity as a CSR (corporate social responsibility) project with the following benefits to AMC, namely, waiving off initial payment and the monthly rental for provision of services or providing it at a reduced rate

Purchasing hardware and software items for the call centre

Vence Technology, a private company, was selected for provision of hardware and software as recommended by Dialog. Voice prompts which were needed to be played once the number is dialed were recorded in three languages i.e. Sinhala, Tamil, and English. Scripts were edited by medical officers at AMC for final recording and editing.

Setting up of the dedicated communication system

Vence Technology provided the hardware and software support to manage and maintain the information by using a PBX (private branch exchange) database system. PBX is an IP (internet protocol) system enabling users to send and receive calls from their IP phones and providing advanced features such as call hold, call transfer, voicemail and auto-attendant.

Data structure

This IP-HUB (HUB is a common connection point for devices in a network) communication solution has facilities for provision of extension information, call information, favourites information (extension, queue, attendant), as well as for operator methods, call parking methods, and storage methods.

Voice data is stored into the PBX database in terms of the following variables.

1. Status: shows whether the voice was recorded, not recorded, queued or altogether failed.
2. From: shows the information of the originator of the call.
3. To: information of destination of the call (AMC head quarters).
4. Date and Time: originator's date and time (peak and off peak hours).
5. Duration: voice recorded time (minutes/seconds).

The important feature of the PBX database is, it can export all the data to other applications such as excel, access etc for the analytical work. IHP designed and installed two databases; one is MS-Access and the other, My-SQL for the above purpose at AMC.

These two databases now have 3257 data files in terms of GPs, RMPs, private hospitals, and medical laboratories and are geared to update every month. To enhance the tracking of information about malaria cases, IHP also introduced a WebLog Expert method in corporation with Lanka Communication Services (Pvt.) Ltd. This is a fast and powerful access log analyser giving information about AMC website's visitors' activity statistics, accessed files, paths through the site, information about referring pages, search engines, browsers, operating systems etc, this also produces easy-to-read reports that include both text information (tables) and charts.

Development of Standard Operational Procedures (SOP)

Initial manuscript of the SOP for the new surveillance system was piloted at the two pilot training programmes held in Monaragala and Anuradhapura which ran for 6 weeks, and finalised.

The solution was then institutionalised and monitored as discussed in the next section.

Orientation training of general practitioners and advocacy meetings to introduce the enhanced surveillance system for malaria

These orientation training and advocacy meetings were organised by the Independent Medical Practitioners Association.

Finalising the enhanced surveillance system for the private health sector and handing over the responsibilities to AMC for maintaining the system.

After the maintenance phase was over on 31st of December 2011, responsibility of taking forward the system established at the AMC was handed over to the AMC management with the assurance of assisting them with any technical assistance if needed from IHP.

Monitoring and Evaluation

Regular monitoring of the functioning of the call centre and the project was carried out to:

1. Ensure the proper functioning of the hardware and software items in the system.
2. Identify shortcomings and areas to be improved.
3. Assess whether the IT manager at AMC has attended to the incoming calls, retrieved the recordings, and contacted the relevant RMOs (regional malaria officers) to inform about notifications. RMOs are the technical officers responsible for all AMC activities at the District which is the second sub national level in the administrative structure of the country.

4. Generate reports from information received after establishment of the call centre at AMC.

PBX Database Login

The database has three login areas in terms of the languages Sinhala, Tamil, and English. The Database Administrator or authorised person has the authority to control the system. Every transaction of the voice data is saved in the system and converted into the text format. This is the most prominent platform in the PBX system, for information for decision-making.

Table 3.1 shows an example of the saved data in the database according to the variables. The data can be exported to other applications such as MS-Excel, MS-Access, MS-SQL, and My-SQL for further analysis.

Examples of Case Notifications

Following cases have been notified in the districts Mullaitevu and Negombo in 2011.

1. The Mulliaitevu call has been recorded in the system on 19th November 2011 at 11.03 a.m. and the call duration is 1 min. and 10 sec.

2. The Negombo call was recorded in the system at 7.58 a.m. on 03rd October 2011 and the same day the call re-originated at 9.33 a.m. and instructions on treatment given over the phone by the Medical Officer at the AMC.

Database Summary

1–30 November 2011		*1–27 December 2011*	
Classification of Data	*Number of calls*	*Classification of Data*	*Number of calls*
Recorded to HDD	16 (20.5%)	Recorded to HDD	4 (11.1%)
Call Failed	3 (3.8%)	Call Failed	2 (5.5%)
Not Recorded	59 (75.6%)	No Recorded	30 (89.3%)
Total	78	Total	36
Call back from AMC	3	Call back from AMC	1
Queue	6	Queue	3

Table 3.1

Data Received

Status	*Notes*	*From*	*From Name*	*To*	*To Name*	*Date and Time*	*Connection*	*Duration, min:sec*
• * No Record		0718246270	(...)	Auto Attendant	MAIN VR	10/24/11 11:33 AM	DBN	0:05
• * Recorded to HDD		0772647423	XXXXXX	5001	VM-SINHALA	10/22/11 6:15 PM	DBN	0:27
• * Call failed		5010	OPERATOR	03122	OPERATOR	10/17/11 3:45 PM	DBN	0:00

Notes: 1. * indicates new data is recorded in the database. 2. The variable Status "Not Recorded" means that the Malaria officer has physically answered the call through the toll free number. 3. "Recorded to HDD" means that the voice has been recorded in the Hard Disk for subsequent processing. 4. "Call failed" means that the call had failed due to some error by the originator, but the number can be traced by the call centre officer and followed up.

Table 3.2

Data Reviewed

Status	*Notes*	*From*	*From Name*	*To*	*To Name*	*Date and Time*	*Connection*	*Duration, min:sec*
£ No Record		0718246270	(...)	Auto Attendant	MAIN VR	10/24/11 11:33 AM	DBN	0:05
£ Recorded to HDD		0772647423	XXXXXX	5001	VM-SINHALA	10/22/11 6:15 PM	DBN	0:27
£ Call failed		5010	OPERATOR	03122	OPERATOR	10/17/11 3:45 PM	DBN	0:00

Note: £ reflects that the Data Manager reviewed the data.

Handing Over of Completed Project to the AMC for Institutionalisation

During the initial implementation of the project, database showed 3257 records from GPs in 2011. The records were analysed by institutional and patient levels for further study. At the end of 2011, all data were transferred to My-SQL (Web database) for online archiving and officially handed over to the AMC.

References

Dalpatadu, K.C.S., S.S. Puwanesh, S.R. Kumara and S. Gamage (2012). "Innovative Approach for Notification of Malaria Cases from the Private Health Sector", *Nineteenth Annual Scientific Sessions*, The College of Medical Administration of Sri Lanka, p.14.

http://www.ihp.lk/research/project.html?project_id=CD-002

Part II

Health System and Financial Issues

4

PAWAN K. TANEJA

Financing Healthcare to Achieve Equitable Universal Health Coverage

Issues and Challenges in India

Introduction

OOP (out-of-pocket) expenses/user fees for utilisation of healthcare services exist in majority of the developing countries. Worldwide every year, 150 million people face catastrophic healthcare costs because of direct payments, while 100 million are pushed into poverty—the equivalent of three people every second (Xu *et al.,* 2007). For ensuring universal coverage of health in a country, the policymakers needs to ensure that everyone in the population has access to appropriate promotive, preventive, curative and rehabilitative healthcare when in need and at an affordable cost. Inequities in health systematically put groups of people who are already socially disadvantaged (for example, by virtue of being poor, female, and/or members of a disenfranchised racial, ethnic, or religious group) at further disadvantage with respect to their health; health is essential to well-being and to overcoming other effects of social disadvantage. Equity in health financing means people contribute for health on the basis of ability to pay rather than according to whether or not they fall ill. Therefore, once a person falls ill and accesses services, a major source of health funding needs to come from prepaid and pooled contributions rather than from fees or charges levied.

Affordable and equitable distribution of healthcare is a key issue in most countries. Governments throughout the world are increasingly realising the value of developing health systems that provide healthcare, while financially protecting the people in the fairest way possible. In high-income countries, increasing costs, financial constraints of public budgets and economic considerations regarding international competitiveness have all made social health protection reform a political priority. On the other hand, middle-and low-income countries, providing equitable and affordable healthcare is high on the development agenda, given the large numbers of people lacking sufficient financial means to access health services; worldwide, millions of people are pushed into poverty every year by the need to pay for healthcare.

Approaches to Healthcare Financing

Broadly, there are two broad approaches to finance healthcare, i.e., market-based and government-financed system. Both of these approaches offer different advantages and disadvantages and neither of them is perfect in all aspects. Most of the nations innovate and choose a mix of both of these approaches in order to provide basic and advanced healthcare as per prevailing needs of its citizens.

In market-based healthcare systems, medical care is generally delivered through private organisations and individuals. All healthcare providers are part of a system in which they compete with each other to provide services to patients at competitive price and quality. In this system, there are many different payers, healthcare service providers and suppliers, and people with insurance can choose which ones serve their needs best. Healthcare service providers are provided with overall best-practice guidelines that indicate when, for whom and which treatments should be used. However, they (service providers) are free to make care decisions on a case-by-case basis, considering the needs of each patient. The main advantage of market-based systems approach is it offers financial incentives to healthcare service providers to spend on research and development in the field of medicine and medical technology so as to obtain/maintain competitive edge over competitors. As a result, new advances are available to patients sooner.

On the other hand, government-financed systems tend to provide everyone living in the country with coverage that offers access to some basic level of care. In this system, people pay for health services through taxes and other charges. In government-financed healthcare, sometimes the government delivers the care itself and sometimes it contracts with other providers to do so. These systems typically have more power to place limitations on the care offered to patients and doctors in order to keep costs down due to their wider coverage. But at the same time, it tends to take longer for new advances to be accepted in these systems, which is why the level of diagnostics, quality of care and treatments offered under these systems are not be the same as those available in a market-based healthcare system.

In recent past, SHI (social health insurance) and community-based health insurance schemes have emerged as another mechanism for financing and managing healthcare to achieve universal healthcare coverage through pooling of health risks of its members on one hand, and the financial contributions of enterprises, households, and the government, on the other. Evidence across globe clearly highlights that universal health coverage cannot be achieved in low- and middle-income countries just through voluntary or contributory-based health insurance schemes like in developed nations. Governments, policymakers and funders have to adopt context-specific health financing mechanisms that address the needs of the poor as well as the rich in their countries.

In recent past, many developing countries have initiated the process of building domestic need based financing systems to advance universal healthcare coverage. These countries are not just blindly deploying healthcare financing models used in high-income countries, rather these low- and middle-income countries like Thailand, Mexico, Sri Lanka, and Kyrgyzstan are focusing on building own universal health coverage success stories (Oxfam, 2013). Although modus operandi to achieve universal healthcare coverage differ in these countries, they follow the basic principle of universal healthcare services, i.e., healthcare is provided on the basis of citizenship and/or residency and not on the basis of employment status or financial contributions to public exchequer.

Healthcare Financing Scenario In India

The provisions of healthcare services are divided under State list and Concurrent list in India. As per Constitution of India, issues related to public health and hospitals fall under the State list and issues such as population control and family welfare, medical education, and quality control of drugs are included in the Concurrent list. The Union Ministry of Health and Family Welfare (UMoHFW) is the central authority responsible for implementation of various programmes and schemes in areas of family welfare, prevention, and control of major diseases.

Historically, the Indian state has always been an insignificant player in the financing of healthcare. Private providers, both current and traditional, as well as informal providers, have been the dominant players in the healthcare market. Role of the government in financing of healthcare in India was limited to two forms. First, to cover urban populations and those working in the organised sector under some form of social security, such as the Employee State Insurance Scheme (ESIS) or Central Government Health Scheme (CGHS) and have unlimited access to medical services. Secondly, the rural population and those working in the unorganised sector have been provided with the free or subsidised tax-based financed public healthcare facilities. Inability to access, informal payment and non-availability of above two forms of financing forced a major chunk of population to depend upon out-of-pocket expenditure for utilising services of private providers depending on their ability to pay. This system of healthcare financing has raised serious concerns of inequity of health services across population. Further, tax-based public facilities were also not able to provide a similar quality of care as provided under the SHI Scheme (like ESIS/CGHS) due to low funding that heightens inequality. In, the year 1999, public health expenditure in India has declined from 1.3 per cent of GDP (gross domestic product) in 1990 to 0.9 per cent of GDP. The Union Budgetary allocation for health was 1.3 per cent while the State's budgetary allocation was 5.5 per cent (National Institute of Rural Development and Panchyati Raj, 2005). The district-level household survey and facility survey (DLHS 2003) reported that only 76 per cent of first referral units and 63 per cent of CHCs (community health centres) had adequate infrastructure, 61 per cent of the first referral units and 46 per cent of CHCs had adequate equipment, 32 per cent of first referral units and 24 per cent CHCs had adequate supply, and 37 per cent of first referral units and 14 per cent of

CHCs had adequate staff. During the three months preceding the survey only, 58 per cent of the PHCs (primary health centres) conducted deliveries, 6 per cent conducted medical termination of pregnancy, 22 per cent provided neo-natal care and 65 per cent performed intrauterine device insertion and 41 per cent conducted sterilisations. If the percentage of PHCs having adequate staff was more than 90 per cent in Tamil Nadu, Maharashtra, and Kerala, it was less than 20 per cent in Odisha, West Bengal, and Bihar.

Figure 4.1

Healthcare Financing India Year 2010

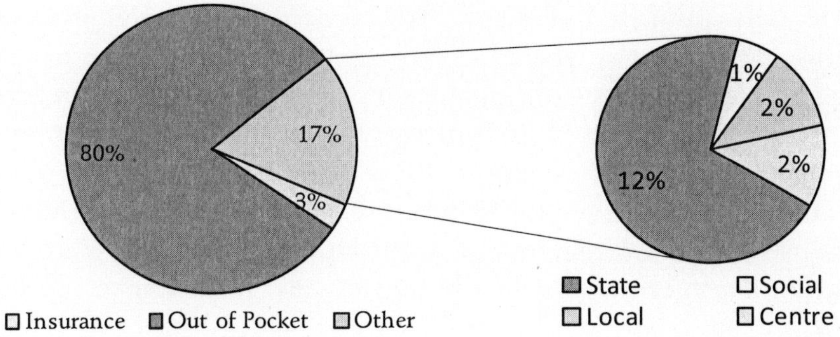

Source: *World Health Statistics 2010.* Geneva.

In year 2005, on recognising the importance of health in the process of economic and social development and in improving the quality of life of our citizens, the GoI launched the National Rural Health Mission (NRHM). The main objective of the Mission is to carry out necessary architectural correction in the basic healthcare delivery system. The Mission adopted a synergistic approach by relating health to determinants of good health *viz.,* segments of nutrition, sanitation, hygiene and safe drinking water. It also aimed to mainstream the Indian systems of medicine to facilitate healthcare. The main focus of NRHM was to provide accessible, affordable and quality healthcare to the rural population, especially the most vulnerable.

On 1 May 2013, the NRHM, along with the recently launched National Urban Health Mission (NUHM), has been subsumed under the National Health Mission (NHM). With recent change in the government at Centre under the leadership of Narendra Modi, it is being considered to roll out a National Health Assurance Mission (NHAM) to reduce the OOP spending on healthcare by the common man (Press Information Bureau, 2014). Despite making significant progress especially since the launch of NRHM, challenges to related availability, accessibility and quality of healthcare services are found to persist. The major areas of concern in achieving equitable universal health coverage in India are listed below.

Heavy Out-of-Pocket Expenditure

Due to the lack of extensive and adequately funded public health services, a large proportion of the population incurs heavy OOP expenditure on services purchased from the private sector. Figure 4.2 shows that the OOP expenditure as a proportion of total health expenditure is very high at 60 per cent in India as compared to the global average of 20.5 per cent. This picture has improved significantly after introduction of Rashtriya Swasthya Bima Yojana (RSBY) and few other state-initiated health insurance schemes, because prior to implementation of this scheme, OOP rate was nearly 80 per cent and contribution of health insurance schemes was just 3 per cent (See Figure 4.2).

Figure 4.2

Out-of-Pocket Expenditure as % of Total Expenditure on Health

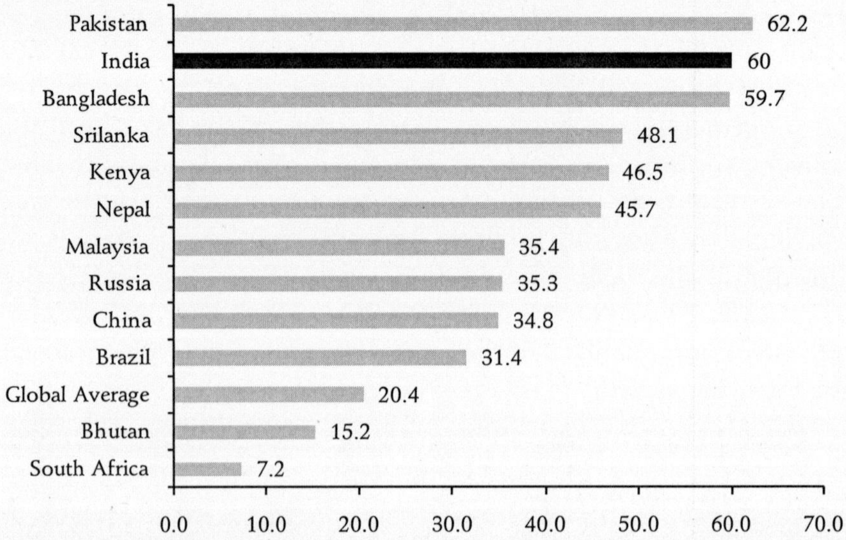

Source: World Health Statistics 2013, Geneva.

Limited Public Health Spending

The total expenditure on healthcare in India, including public and private expenditure is broadly comparable to other 4developing countries at similar levels of per capita income. The total expenditure on healthcare (both public and private together) is 3.7 per cent of the GDP. However, according to the *World Health Statistics 2013*, public expenditure on health is very low constituting 28.2 per cent of total health expenditure. According to the GoI's 12th Five Year Plan, public health expenditure in the country was only 1.04 per cent of GDP in 2011-12 as compared to the global average of 5.4 per cent (See Figure 4.3)

Figure 4.3

Government Expenditure on Health as % of GDP

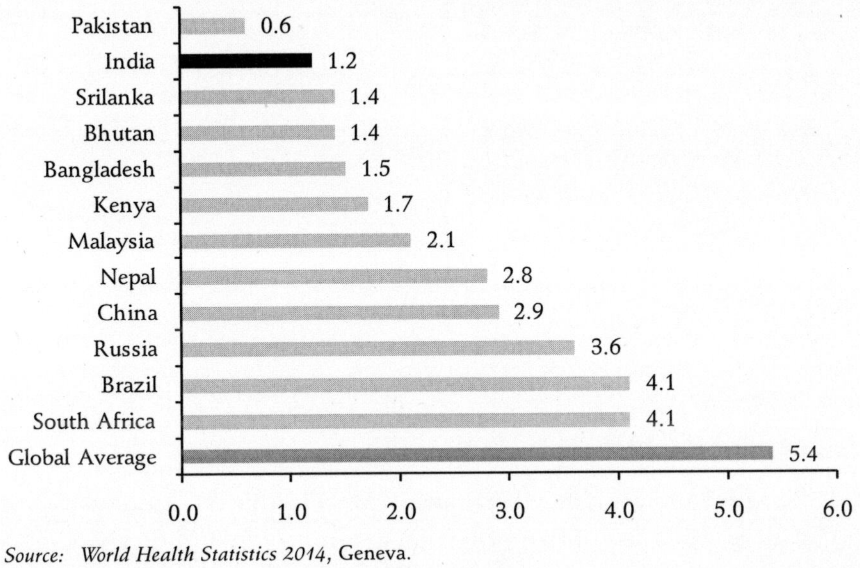

Source: World Health Statistics 2014, Geneva.

Limited Role of Health Insurance Schemes

According to an estimation by High Level Expert Group Report on Universal Health Coverage for India, the Union Government funded insurance schemes cover just an estimated population of 181 million through the ESIS (60 million); CGHS (3 million); and RSBY (118 million), etc. While ESIS and CGHS provide for comprehensive healthcare, RSBY provides for only hospitalisation cover with a benefit limit of ₹30,000 (US$500 approximately) per enrolled household per year (See Figure 4.3). Further, an estimated population of 20 million is covered under Indian Railway and Defence services health network. In addition, 110 million people in the South Indian states including 70 million in Andhra Pradesh, 35 million in Tamil Nadu, and 5 million in Karnataka receive coverage under state government funded health insurance schemes. However, most of these schemes cover only inpatient care, mainly at the tertiary level.

Figure 4.4

Population Coverage Under Various Health Schemes in India

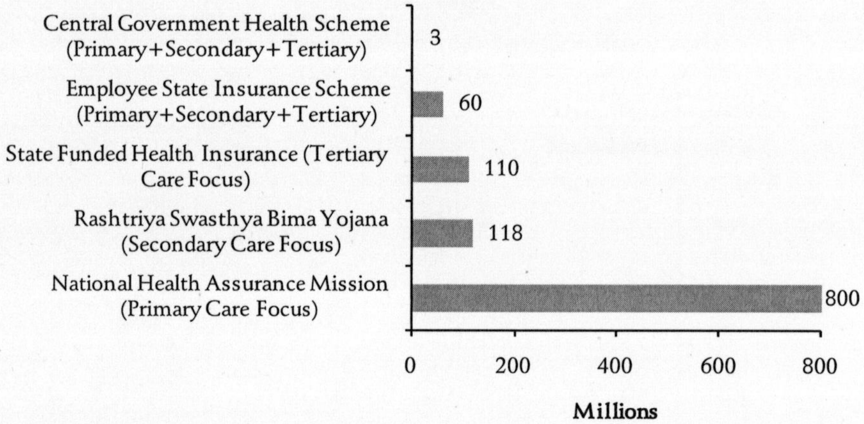

Source: United Nations, *Universal Health Coverage,* India. *http://www.in.one.un.org/img/uploads/figure3.jpg*

Variation in Health Insurance Coverage

According to another estimation by Planning Commission, in India, as of 2010, any form of health insurance, including the CHGS, ESIS, government sponsored schemes and private health insurance, together covered approximately 302 million individuals or 25 per cent of the total population (See Figure 4.5). The state of Andhra Pradesh with highest level of coverage has 85 per cent of its population covered by the state sponsored Rajiv Aarogyasri health insurance scheme (out of the total population of 84 million). Any form of health insurance covers 62 per cent of population in Tamil Nadu (out of which Kalaignar covers 84%). These are two states where state-sponsored health insurance schemes are strongest in their outreach.

But on the other hand, states like Rajasthan, Assam and Madhya Pradesh has only 3 per cent health insurance coverage.

Lack of Confidence on Community Based Health Insurance (CBHI) Schemes

Literature from developing world recognised CBHI as one of the potential ways to extend healthcare equity to the poor and near poor and the workers in unorganised sector (Purohit, 2014). As under these schemes, community members prepay for health services by pooling their resources to share the financial risks of healthcare, own the scheme and control its management, including the collection of premiums, the payment of healthcare providers, and the negotiation of benefits package, etc. However, most of these studies evaluating impact of these schemes highlighted the inability of these schemes to include the poorest of the poor or improve access to inpatient care in Indian circumstances (Ranson, 2003). Recently, a study by Devadasan *et al.* (2011) on patient satisfaction related to quality care on two leading CBHI schemes, Action for Community Organisation, Rehabilitation and Development (ACCORD) and Kadamalai Kalanjiam Vattara Sangam (KKVS), found no significant difference in the levels of satisfaction between the insured and uninsured patients (Devadasan *et al.,* 2011).

Issues and Challenges in the Way to Achieve Equitable Universal Health Coverage in India

The High Level Expert Group (2011) on UHC suggested that the GoI should rely primarily on general tax revenues, rather than trying to collect explicit insurance contributions from the informal sector. Healthcare financing scenario in India highlighted in above section suggests that funding tertiary care through health insurance schemes like RSBY and funding primary care through systems like NHM/NHAM are two predominant pathways available to ensure equitable universal health coverage in India. In this section, we have tried to uncover the current issues and challenges with the way of RSBY and NHM.

Figure 4.5

National and State-wise Health Insurance Coverage in 2010

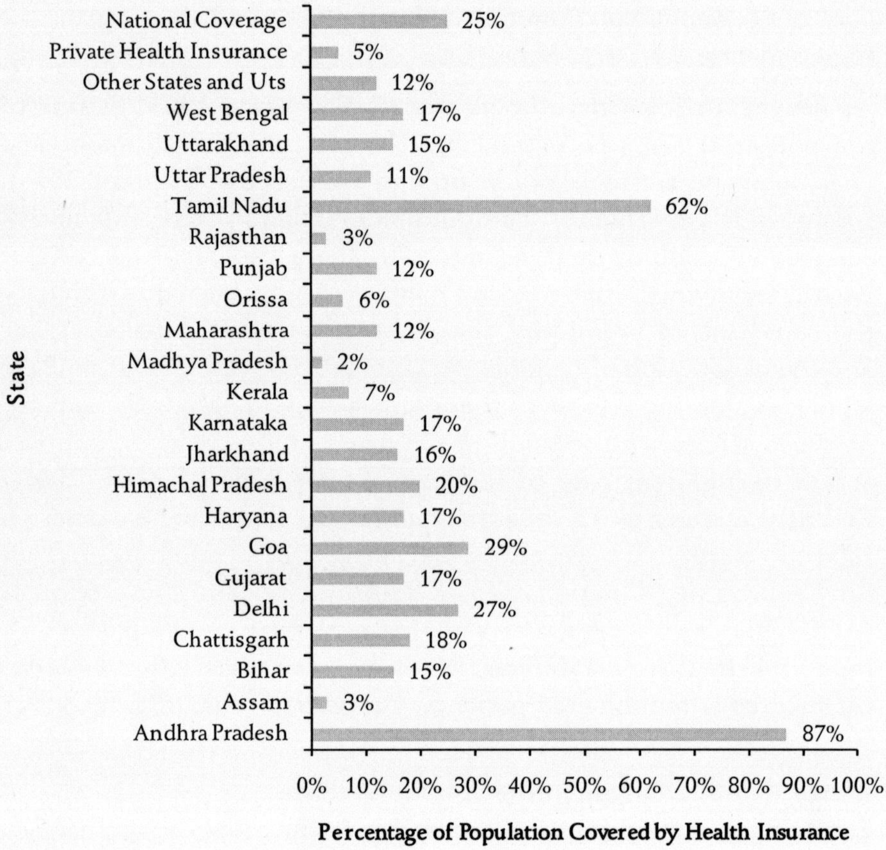

Source: Planning Commission (2011).

Issues and Challenges for RSBY Scheme

- *Depth and Breadth of the Social Protection*: Initially, only the BPL (below poverty line) families were covered under RSBY scheme. Further, using decade-old lists based on the Census of 2001 as criteria for selecting the beneficiaries, the government ended up spending money on undeserving people. To address this challenge Ministry of Labour extended the scope of the scheme from BPL families to Mahatma Gandhi National Rural Employment Guarantee

Act (MGNREGA) workers, domestic workers, *beedi*[1] workers and street vendors. Further, on 23 July 2011, the GoI expanded the RSBY coverage to seven more unorganised segments including ragpickers, rickshaw pullers, taxi and auto-rickshaw drivers, miners, sanitation workers and toddy workers. These steps notwithstanding, nearly 50 per cent or more of the identified eligible beneficiaries are yet to be enrolled for the scheme in almost every state (Figure 4.6). However, some of the state governments, such as Kerala and Andhra Pradesh extended the cover of the health insurance schemes to the non-poor as part of its strategy to ensure universal health insurance coverage.

- *Benefit on outpatient care (OPD): The Global Burden of Diseases* Report of WHO[2] highlighted the issue of shifting, burden of disease to non-communicable diseases in India, which require mainly OPD treatment. It was estimated that out of the estimated 10.3 million deaths that occurred in India in 2004, nearly 50 per cent of deaths were due to chronic diseases[3] and nearly 11 per cent were due to injuries. According to another study estimate in 2004, the people of India spent US$9.1 billion OOP on tests, treatments and medical devices to manage these chronic diseases (Taylor, 2010). Another study estimated that of the total OOP medical expenses of an average individual just 25 per cent were on inpatient care (IPD) and remaining 75 per cent of were on OPD and medicines (Kapila, 2011). But, the RSBY scheme was designed to benefit people living below poverty line for inpatient care only, which required minimum 24-hours hospitalisation. Consequently, both beneficiary as well as healthcare service provider had motivation to convert a regular OPD case into an IPD case, resulting in fake utilisation of services. The major challenge

1. A *beedi* is a thin, Indian cigarette filled with tobacco flake and wrapped in a tenduor possibly even Bauhinia racemosa leaf tied with a string at one end.
2. WHO (2004). The Global Burden of Disease: 2004 Update. Accessed on 20 June 2012, available at *<http://www.who.int/healthinfo/global_burden_disease/GBD_report_2004update_full.pdf>*
3. Includes cardiovascular diseases, mental health disorders, diabetes and cancer.

in providing insurance coverage on OPD care was the difficulty in administration resulting from high volume and diversity of transactions. Further, the RSBY coverage of a maximum of ₹30,000 for a family was far less than other SHI schemes (see Table 4.1). This became a major issue in the case of acute diseases.

Table 4.1

Package Rates for Similar Procedures, 2009-10

(in ₹)

Procedures	*Rajiv Aarogyasri Scheme (AP)*	*Kalaignar (TN)*	*Yeshasvini (KN)*	*Vajapayee Arogyasri Scheme (KN)*	*RSBY*
Coronary bypass surgery	95,000	90,000	60,000	95,000	Up to 30,000
Coronary Angioplasty	60,000	60,000	25,000	60,000	
Transurethral Resection on prostate	30,000	25,000	12,000	20,000	14,250
Nephrolithotomy	10,000	25,000	14,000	10,000	10,000
Nepherectomy	40,000	40,000	14,000	10,000	10,000
Appendectomy	18,000	NA	9,000	NA	6,000
Cholecystectomy	20,000	25,000	9,000	NA	10,000
Hysterectomy	20,000	25,000	6,000	NA	10,000
Tympanoplasty	15,000	NA	3,500	NA	7,000
Normal Delivery	NA	NA	NA	NA	2,500

Note: NA: Not Applicable, Service Not Covered; AP: Andhra Pradesh; TN: Tamil Nadu; KN: Karnataka.

Source: Scheme documents and websites of various schemes.

To address this issue, the Ministry of Labour, in collaboration with the International Labour Organization (ILO) and ICICI Foundation,[4] launched an RSBY pilot project in the district of Puri, Odisha, covering both outpatient and inpatient cares for beneficiaries from July 2011 (Sen, 2011). Punjab Health Systems

4. ICICI Foundation for Inclusive Growth (ICICI Foundation) was founded by the ICICI Group in early 2008 to carry forward and build upon its legacy of promoting inclusive growth. ICICI Foundation works within public systems and specialised grass-roots organisations to support developmental work in four focus areas i.e., primary healthcare, elementary education, skill development and sustainable livelihoods, and financial inclusion.

Corporation (PHSC)[5] also submitted a detailed plan report to the GoI for launching the scheme in three districts of Punjab—Ferozepur, Bhatinda and Ropar—as a pilot project to cover both OPD and IPD services (Hindustan Times, 2012).

- Utilisation of services and financial unsustainability: Under RSBY, reporting and incentives were based on number of cards distributed/number of families enrolled. The limit of enrolling five people per card was an incentive structure to issue more number of cards leading to issuance of multiple cards per household[6] and falsification of enrolment rate.[7] An independent evaluation in three districts of the eastern part of Uttar Pradesh found that less than 50 per cent beneficiaries who were insured under RSBY were aware of the scheme benefits and entitlements. Only 37 per cent females in these households were found to be aware of the scheme. A study initiated by State Nodal Agency RSBY, Chhattisgarh (Council for Tribal and Rural Development, 2012) in 2011-12 showed that none of the non-RSBY household was aware of the RSBY scheme.

The hospitalisation rate at the all-India level was about 20 per thousand beneficiaries in year 2012. But this was marked by extreme variation from about 38 per thousand in Kerala to as low as 1 per thousand in Assam, in comparison with the national average of 31 per thousand (Public Health Foundation of India, 2011). The claim ratio also varied across districts from 2 per cent to 157 per cent[8] and 0.01 per cent to 89 per cent across states (Taneja and Share, 2012). Low level of awareness among beneficiaries and masses appeared to

5. The nodal agency implementing the RSBY in Punjab state.
6. A household may include more than one family.
7. During an independent evaluation in 3 districts of the eastern part of Uttar Pradesh, it had been found that average family size of the insured families comes to 2.3 members as against 5 permissible under RSBY.
8. Lower claims ratio is certainly a welcome situation from an insurer's perspective but, if looked at from the Government's viewpoint, denote sub-optimal utilisation of benefits. Similarly, the higher the claims ratio is better for customer/society. But claims ratios above 100 per cent are too high as they signal that the product is not financially sustainable. The high level of variance between the highest and lowest is certainly an eyebrow raiser, should be considered for medical surveillance as it senses presence of malpractices.

Figure 4.6

State-wise RSBY Card Issued (in '000) to BPL Families

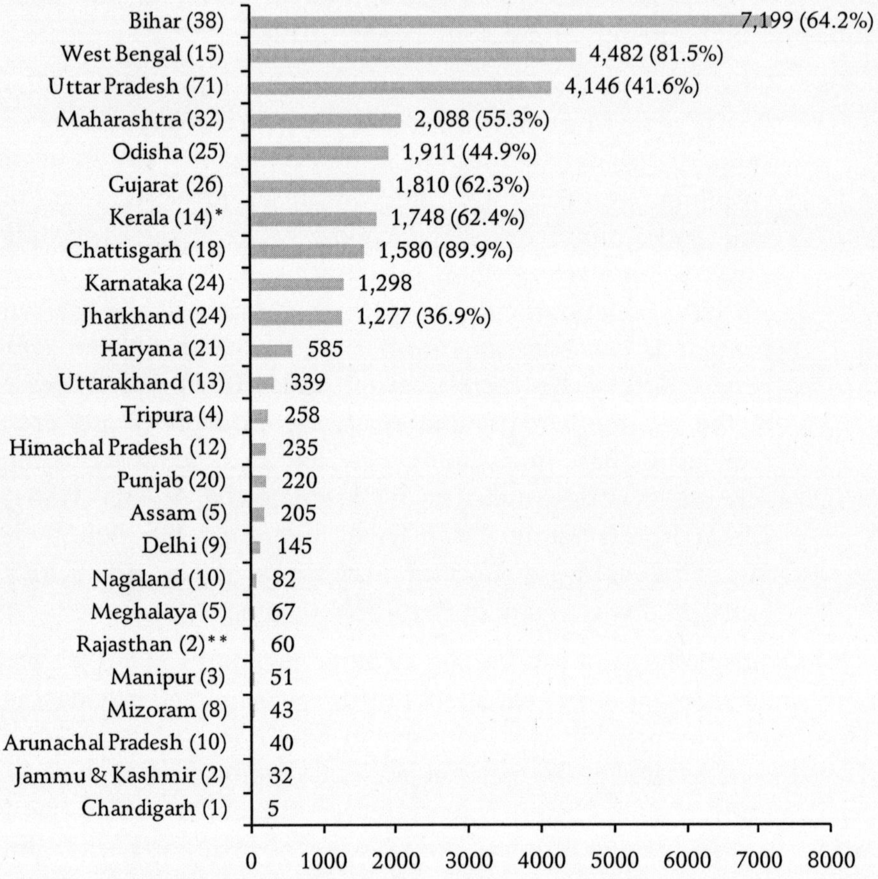

Note: Data are provisional. Length of bars in the chart is not-to-scale. Percentages denote the conversion rates in enrolment. Numbers in the bracket with name of the states denote number of active district(s).

* Data for Kerala includes state BPL families.

** Data for Rajasthan pertain to Families under MGNREGA.

Source: *http://www.rsby.gov.in/overview.aspx* cited on 19 June 2012.

be the root cause for the uneven healthcare services utilisation rate, uneven claim ratios, and frauds (Vasisht and Pandit, 2012).

To address these concerns, GoI instructed insurance companies to take the help of local NGOs (non-governmental organisations) to create awareness about RSBY during the enrolment process. Further,

GoI, with the help of state governments, took several measures such as tracking daily online claims submitted by healthcare facilities, physical verification of records by conducting various audits such as communication audit, process audit, hospital documentation audit, transaction audit, random concurrent audit, random survey of users' experiences, and hospital empanelment process audit of healthcare service deliveries, etc. As of March 2012, 273 hospitals had been de-empanelled from RSBY on grounds of poor performance in terms of service delivery or cases of fraud detection.

Issues and Challenges for NHM

- *Poor absorption capacity*: The GoI had increased allocations for health through the NRHM since 2005, by bringing Reproductive and Child Health and Universal Immunisation programmes under the NRHM umbrella. But the total budget allocations for NRHM under the 11th Plan period for the five-year period (from 2007-08 to 2011-12) was just 73.9 per cent of originally recommended ₹89,478 crore for the Mission by Planning Commission of India (Planning Commission, 2013).

  Further, financial allocations under the NRHM were based on Programme Implementation Plans (PIPs), which were prepared by state governments and subject to approval by the Union Government. Although the first two instalments were released unconditionally, subsequent ones were released subject to expenditure of at least 50-60 per cent (UNICEF and Center for Budget Governance and Accountability, 2011). States that had failed to spend their previous instalments did not receive subsequent tranches. The unspent balance of the previous year was incorporated into the next year's allocation. Most states that were not able to spend their funds efficiently, therefore, did not get more funds in subsequent rounds, even though financial allocations under the NRHM were based on needs (See Figure 5.7). Figure 5.7 shows that overall, NRHM expenditures were reasonably high with about 89 per cent of the funds released for the programme from 2005-06 to

Figure 4.7

Spending of NRHM Funds During 11th Five Year Plan Across States

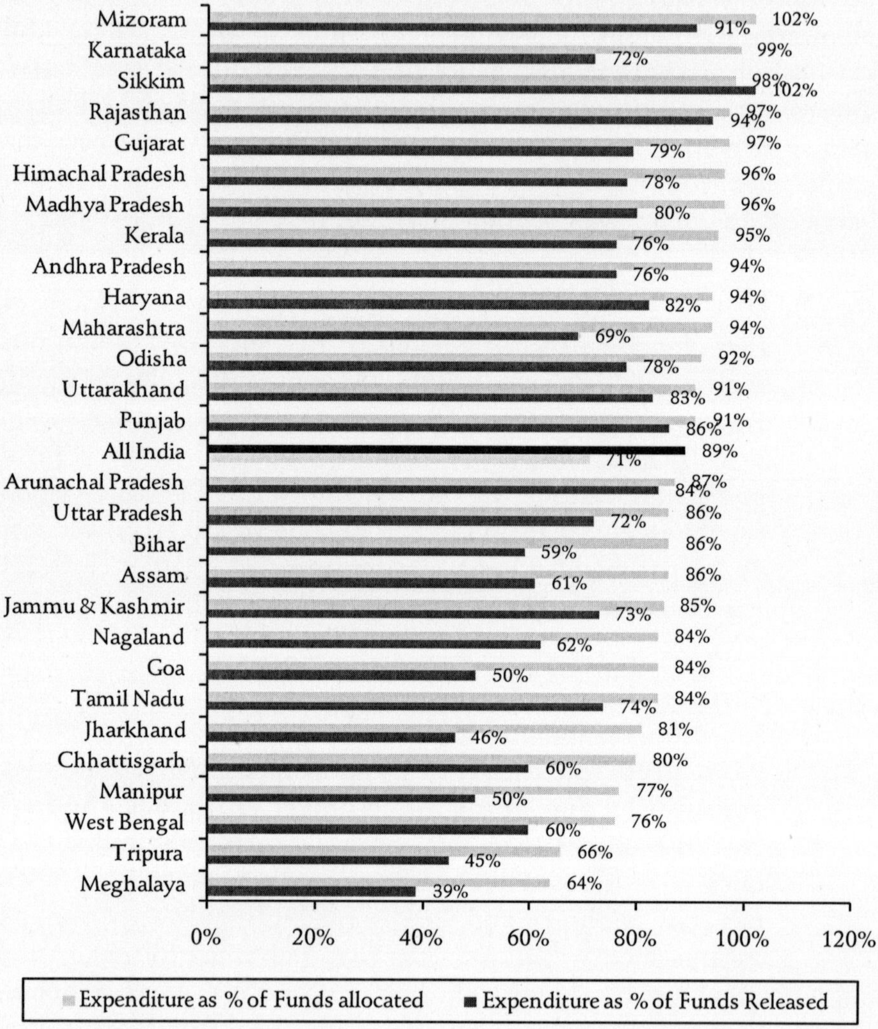

Notes:* Total expenditure includes additional funds provided by the state government (if any).

\# Total expenditure figures presented here are not strictly comparable with the funds released by the Union Government because expenditure includes additional funds provided by the state government (if any).

Source: Compiled by CBGA from data available on *http://mohfw.niuc.in/NRHM.htm*

2009-10 being utilised at an all-India level. But there is room for improvement for states like West Bengal, Tripura and Meghalaya, given that states like Rajasthan, Gujarat and Karnataka were able to achieve near full utilisation. Further, the figure highlights that states like Jharkhand were able to utilise less than half of the allocated funds against the original budgetary allocation approved. The main cause of this 'absorption' problem is the rigid public sector financial management system, with strict line item controls, which constrain the authority of line managers to reallocate resources to other heads/scheme where more money is needed (Duran *et al.,* 2013).

- Poor Quality of Fund Utilisation: An in-depth study of Health Management Information System (MIS) data of NRHM, by UNICEF and Center for Budget Governance and Accountability highlighted that utilisation of funds at the state and district is not uniform across components of i.e. Reproductive and Child Health (Family Planning and Janani Suraksha Yojana (JSY)), flexible pool funds i.e., additional funds for institutional strengthening and immunisation activities. Some of the states and districts had spend money mainly on Family Planning, Intensive Pulse Polio Immunisation activities and other had spend funds for mainly for Janani Suraksha Yojana (JSY) and funds for other areas remained idle. The report also observed that most of the NRHM funds spending were concentrated in the last two financial quarters of the year.
- Lack of Human Resources and Service Quality at Primary Care: Another related issue to money with NRHM is that of providing quality services with sufficient workforce who has right knowledge, skills and attitudes. The qualified doctors are predominantly concentrated in urban areas. Therefore, a realistic human resources plan catering to the need for both clinicians (doctors, nurses, paramedics, etc.) and health system workers (managers, economists, lawyers, etc.), such as continuing education, and incentives to work in remote and underserved areas, should be made.

The Way Forward

The poor population was always exposed to catastrophic spending and distress financing during illness. The availability, acceptability, financial and geographical accessibility are four major determinants to remove inaccessibility to healthcare for poor people (Jacobs *et al.*, 2012).

On tertiary care front, RSBY, a poor-friendly health insurance scheme has shown a pathway for promoting poor people's access to healthcare by its innovative mechanism. Independent evaluations have shown that poor people are facing several problems in enrolment and hospitalisation processes.[9] There is an urgent need to initiate appropriate corrective measures in form of consorted effort to reach poor people, healthy involvement of civil society organisations for effective IED (information, education and communication) and BCC (behaviour change communication) activities to ensure extensive enrolment coverage, empanelment of more clinics and hospitals in rural areas, careful monitoring, and proper distribution of drugs and others supplies to the health facilities to add to the robust strength to the scheme. Further, in order to ensure UHC, the scope of the scheme should be extended to the non-poor i.e., APL (above poverty line) population as well. This will improve financial sustainability of the scheme by widening the pool of financial resources. The scope of the scheme can also be extended by offering scheme benefits to vulnerable group of school children who are already covered under mid-day meal scheme. The administration of the scheme may be transferred to Ministry of Health and Family from Ministry of Labour and Employment in order to improve the convergence of funds for NHAM and RSBY.

With increasing burden of disease from non-communicable diseases, on primary and secondary care front, department of

---

9. Such as no coverage for expensive special diagnostic test like CT scan, MRI etc., and treatments like blood transfusion, no coverage for expenses on buying prescribed drugs which are not available at facility Complicated Procedural Formalities, patient admitted at night are deprived off due medical attendance and care, and delay in distribution of smart cards has sabotaged the process of healthy implementation of the scheme and multiplied out-of-pocket expenses of poor on healthcare, moral hazards, discrimination in treatment by doctors; list of empanelled hospitals is not given along with smart cards, inadequate capacity building intervention for grass-roots facilitators, and inadequate enrolment of beneficiaries in several areas.

AYUSH Care should be further strengthened under NHAM funding for improving promotive and preventive healthcare. To strengthen the public health surveillance system, CHIS (citizen health information system) should be designed by merging information with Adhaar and RSBY disease database. In order to resolve the issue of human resources for health, learning from Assam government for rural health practitioners' course should be implemented in other states as well where there is shortage of human resources. However, before implementing this course, career advancement pathway for these rural health practitioners to mainstream should be devised so that they feel integrated with the system.

References

CBGA and UNICEF India (2011). *National Rural Health Mission (NRHM): Budgeting for Change Series.* New Delhi.

Council for Tribal and Rural Development (CTRD) (2012). *Final Report on Evaluation of RashtriyaSwasthyaBimaYojana Scheme in Chhattisgarh*. May. Available at: *www.rsbychhattisgarh.in/WebSite/UploadDoc/70.pdf*> Cited on 10 September.

Devadasan, N., B. Criel, W. Van Damme, P. Lefevre, S. Manoharan and P. Van der Stuyft (2011). "Community Health Insurance Schemes and Patient Satisfaction-evidence from India", *The Indian Journal of Medical Research* 133(1): 40.

Duran A. *et al. (2013). Universal Coverage Challenges Require Health System Approaches: The Case of India. Health Policy, http://dx.doi.org/10.1016/j.healthpol.2013.11.009*

Hindustan Times (2012). "Punjab Moots Plan to Add OPD Patients under RSBY", *Hindustan Times,* 20 May.

Jacobs, B., P. Ir, M. Bigdeli, P.L. Annear and W. Van Damme (2012). "Addressing Access Barriers to Health Services: An Analytical Framework for Selecting Appropriate Interventions in Low-income Asian Countries", *Health Policy and Planning* 27(4): 288-300.

Kapila, S. (2011). "RSBY-An Upgrade Required", *Prayas: Towards Improved Social Protection in India, Special Issue Health for All,* April 2011 accessed on June 20, 2012, available at *www.swasthindia.in/RSBY-UpgradeRequired.pdf*

National Institute of Rural Development and Panchyati Raj (2005). "*National Rural Health Mission 2005-12: Mission.* Document" available at: *http://www.nird.org.in/brgf/doc/Rural%20HealthMission_Document.pdf*

Oxfam (2013). "Universal Health Coverage: Why Health Insurance Schemes are Leaving the Poor Behind", in *Oxfam briefing paper* 176. Available at: *http://www.oxfam.org/sites/www.oxfam.org/files/bp176-universal-health-coverage-091013-en_.pdf*

Planning Commission (2013). Twelfth Five Year Plan (2012–2017) Social Sectors Vol. III Sage Publication pp. 5 available at *http://planningcommission.gov.in/plans/planrel/12thplan/pdf/12fyp_vol3.pdf*

Press Information Bureau (2014). "Rolling out of National Health Assurance Mission", Ministry of Health and Family Welfare, Government of India, 15-July-2014.

Public Health Foundation of India (PHFI) (2011). *A Critical Assessment of the Existing Health Insurance Models in India.* 31 January. Available at: *www.planningcommission.nic.in/reports/sereport/ser/ser_heal1305.pdf*

Purohit, B. (2014). Community Based Health Insurance in India: Prospects and Challenges. Health, 6, 1237-1245. *http://dx.doi.org/10.4236/health.2014.611152*

Ranson, M.K. (2003). "Community-based Health Insurance Schemes in India: A Review". *National Medical Journal of India* 16(2): 79-89.

Sen, A. (2011). "Soon, Your Visit to Doctor too could be covered by Insurance", *The Economic Times*, Daily Newspaper, Jul 18, 2011.

Taneja, P.K. and H. Sihare (2012). "Pros & Cons of Micro Health Insurance to Eradicate Health Problems in the Below Poverty Line (BPL) Population: Empirical Evidence from India", *Italian Journal of Public Health* 8(4).

Taylor, D.W. (2010). "The Burden of Non-Communicable Diseases in India", *Hamilton ON: The Cameron Institute*.

UNICEF and Center for Budget Governance and Accountability (2011). National Rural Health Mission: Budgeting for Change Series 2011. Delhi. 7-9 December. *http://www.cbgaindia.org/files/working papers/NRHM.pdf*

Vasisht, S. and N. Pandit (2012), "Experiences of RSBY Beneficiaries in a District of Western India: A Qualitative Study", *International Journal of Exclusive Management Research* 2(2): 1-8.

Xu, K., D. Evans, G. Carrin, A.M. Aguilar-Rivera, P. Musgrove, T. Evans (2007). "Protecting Households from Catastrophic Health Spending", *Health Affairs* 26(4): 972-983.

5

JONATHAN GANGBAR, PAVITHRA RAJAN and K. GAYITHRI[1]

Integrated Child Development Services in India

A Sub-National Review

Introduction

India's Integrated Child Development Services (ICDS) is one of the world's largest child development programmes. It is a centrally sponsored scheme that has been the Government of India's (GoI) flagship programme since 1975 for addressing the holistic needs of the child. The ICDS programme offers a comprehensive range of services that aim to improve the nutritional and health status of children within 0-6 years, as well as pregnant and lactating women. More recently, the programme was extended to cover adolescent girls. Also, ICDS lays the framework for overall physical and mental development of children within 0-6 years through non-formal pre-school education (for those within 3-6 years) and through the provision of nutritional and health education to their mothers.

Since inception, ICDS and its efficacy have been greatly hindered by an apparent policy-implementation gap, which continues to remain a challenge today, and has affected overall performance of the programme at the all-India level. Factors that perpetuate this policy-implementation gap and the effective performance of ICDS, as highlighted in the current research on

1. The authors would like to express their deep gratitude to the Canadian International Development Agency and the Shastri-Indo Canadian Institute for their funding support and the Institute for Social and Economic Change, India for providing the necessary support for completion of this study. An earlier version of this paper was published as an ISEC Working paper.

ICDS, are attributable to: (i) poor resource allocation, (ii) poor governance, and (iii) programmatic deficiencies (refer to Appendix A-5.1 for further information regarding ICDS's programmatic deficiencies). Compounding the aforementioned challenges is the fact that in 2001, the Supreme Court of India issued an interim order stating that the ICDS programme was to be universalised and that implementation of this order was to come into effect by 2004 (Mohmand, 2012). The universalisation of ICDS has created a new challenge for implementing bodies of the programme as there is a need to not only expand the programme, but to ensure expansion with quality. As highlighted in the fairly recent research on ICDS, its universalisation and the effectiveness of its implementation hinges on the quality with which the programme is universalised (Drèze, 2006). A fair amount of research has been produced that highlight programmatic deficiencies of the ICDS programme (i.e., overemphasis on Supplementary Nutrition Programme, neglect of children within 0-3 years, regressive programme coverage and overburdened/undertrained human capital at the field level) that are overtly affecting its quality implementation; however there are opportunities for further research that investigate ways to remedy these deficiencies and improve service quality throughout the universalisation process.

The ICDS programme has been widely investigated and studied; however there are several gaps that exist amongst the available research. First, it is important to recognise that the research produced or commissioned by affiliates of the ICDS programme, such as National Institute of Public Cooperation and Child Development (NIPCCD) or The World Bank, are not independent in nature. These organisations represent their own and/or another organisation's interests, and hence are likely to produce research that often adheres to an external agenda. This can influence what is studied regarding ICDS and how it is reported. Second, most of the ICDS research undertaken in recent years has taken place at the micro-level and is either project-specific and/or focused on a particular geographic region in the country (state, district, block and/or village). Third, although some research has been produced in recent years that focuses on the efficacy of ICDS from a national and sub-national perspective, there has been extensive focus on issues as they relate to poor governance and programmatic deficiencies. There is a need to explore issues affecting ICDS as they relate to resources: adequacy, allocation and utilisation.

First, this paper presents an overview of the relevant sections of the ICDS policy, followed by a snapshot of ICDS's performance at the national level with emphasis on its performance since the programme has been universalised. From there, this paper analyses the funding patterns of the ICDS programme over time and compares resource adequacy, allocation and utilisation at the sub-national level.

ICDS: Policy Overview

As mentioned earlier, the ICDS scheme, a centrally sponsored initiative, has been designed to address the holistic developmental needs of the child. The comprehensive set of services delivered *via* ICDS, targets children (0-6 years), pregnant and lactating women and adolescent girls. Outlined below are important elements of the ICDS policy that are discussed in greater detail in further sections.

Infrastructure

ICDS delivers services specifically focused on health, nutrition, and education, which are delivered by Anganwadi Workers (AWWs) at Anganwadi Centres (AWCs) at the village level. AWCs are established based on the number of beneficiaries in the area. The norms surrounding AWCs dictate that one AWC is meant to cover between 400-800 beneficiaries. However, in remote areas in the country such as the northeast, the norms change to one AWC for 300-800 beneficiaries.

Funding Patterns

The funding patterns under the ICDS scheme follows a top-down model that bifurcates the programme into two components: ICDS General (G), which is meant to cover the operational costs of the programme and ICDS Supplementary Nutrition (SN), which is provided for the supplementary nutrition component of ICDS.

The norms that dictate how funding is provided for these two components differ, and have also evolved over time. Since 2009, 90 per cent of funding for ICDS (G) has come from the Central government and the remaining 10 per cent covered by each respective state government. Prior to 2009, the Central government was responsible for providing 100 per cent of the funding for ICDS (G). For ICDS (SN), the norms have evolved from no central assistance (prior to 2005-06) to a 50:50 central-state contribution (from 2005-06–2008-09). This norm is still applicable across all states with the exception of the north-eastern states, where the norm from 2009-10 was changed to 90:10 central-state contribution for SN.

Nutritional Component

The ICDS (SN) component is the largest element of the ICDS programme. Supplementary feeding is provided to all eligible beneficiaries for 300 days per year. The purpose of this component is to bridge the protein-energy gap and average dietary intake of children and pregnant and lactating women. The norms for ICDS (SN) expenditure per beneficiary per day fall under 3 categories: (i) children aged 6-72 months (ii) severely malnourished children 6-72 months and (iii) pregnant and lactating women. The year 2008 onwards, these norms have been revised. The daily expenditure for category 1 has increased from ₹2 to ₹4; category 2 from ₹2.7 to ₹6; and category 3 from ₹2.3 to ₹5. For children within 0-6 months, exclusive breastfeeding is emphasised; whereas for those between 6 months and 3 years, a THR (take home ration) in the form of wheat or rice is given. Lastly, for children within 3-6 years, hot cooked meals are provided at the AWCs.

Policy Goals and Measurement

The primary goal of the ICDS policy is to improve health and nutrition of children aged 0-6 years, pregnant and lactating mothers and adolescent girls. Key output indicators of the scheme relate to anthropometric measurements and infant mortality rate.

The aforementioned elements of the ICDS policy outline the normative framework for implementing this programme. It is necessary to examine how these norms are translating into practice.

ICDS at the All-India Level: Post-Universalisation

ICDS and its efficacy have long been hindered by a policy-implementation gap, which is evident from the state of the key indicators pertaining to child and maternal health and nutrition in India. Although it cannot be said that there is a direct link between these indicators and ICDS *per se*, it is fair to infer that a programme, with the resources, coverage and extensive history of ICDS should have been in a position to help improve such indicators. However, it is projected that India will miss its targets in relation to child health and nutrition, as per the MDG India Country Report published in 2011. This is substantiated by the Ministry of Women and Child Development, which highlights that between 2006 and 2010, in India, the percentage of children that were underweight and severely underweight was reported at 43 per cent and 16 per cent respectively. The same can be said for the child health indicators, such as IMR (infant mortality rate) and CMR (child mortality rate), which were reported at 48 per 1000 and 63 per 1000 respectively, *versus* their targets of 30 per 1000 (IMR) and 31 per 1000 (CMR).

The Supreme Court of India's mandate to universalise the ICDS programme and its further order in 2002 to monitor the progress of its implementation and impose penalties on those states that were failing to universalise the programme, placed a significant amount of pressure on the GoI to begin establishing the required 1.4 million AWCs that were necessary to achieve universalisation (Mohmand, 2012). In order to deal with the massive resource requirements that universalisation would entail, while also dealing with the consistent issue of persistent underfunding for ICDS, it was recommended that the Government of India (GoI), as well as the international community, substantially increase their financial support of ICDS (Gragnoloti *et al.,* 2006). In fact, between the fiscal years 2007-08 and 2013-14, the GoI has increased their support by approximately 66.39 per cent (Kapur, 2013). As well, in 2012, The World Bank approved its ICDS System Strengthening and Nutrition Program[2] in India, which would contribute USD $106 million to be used towards the improvement of nutrition in India under the ICDS programme (The World Bank Group, 2012).

However, increasing the expenditure on ICDS will not translate into an increase in the programme's effectiveness. Firstly, it is likely that expenditure on ICDS would need to increase as the programme expanded, as a result of the universalisation process. What needs to be examined is whether the increase in the resources provided is adequate, considering the new needs of the programme and the norms laid in the ICDS policy. More importantly, effective implementation of the ICDS programme depends upon how efficiently available funds and resources are utilised (Nayak *et al.*, 2006). The efficient utilisation of resources once again highlights the importance of universalisation with quality; however given that expansion the ICDS programme, based upon a design, is largely considered inefficient, it seems that universalisation with quality is likely to be neglected at the expense of simply achieving the mandated targets for universalising the programme. This is evidenced in the budget brief released for FY (financial year) 2013-14, whereby it was noted that the number of AWCs fell short of the sanctioned targets for the previous fiscal year. Furthermore, most of the existing AWCs across India lack basic infrastructure like clean drinking water facilities, hygienic toilet facilities and separate kitchen (Kapur, 2013).

Based on the aforementioned statement, it can be inferred that with regard to the actual delivery of ICDS services, there is greater emphasis (at present) on ensuring physical establishment of the mandated AWCs *versus* understanding how the resources that are

2. This programme falls under The World Bank's broader strategy—Scaling Up Nutrition: A Framework For Action, which outlines priorities for addressing the persistent issues related to under-nutrition and to facilitate Millennium Development Goals (MDGs) achievement. The ICDS System Strengthening and Nutrition Improvement Program will seek to improve nutritional outcomes of children in India and will do so by focusing on four key areas: (1) institutional and systems strengthening, (2) community mobilisation and behaviour change, (3) convergent nutrition action, and (4) project management and monitoring and evaluation. On 6 September 2012, a USD $106 million credit was issued to support the GoI for improving nutritional outcomes for children under 6 years (The World Bank Group, 2012).

required to run the programmes that take place in the AWCs can be most efficiently used to achieve intended outputs and outcomes. Granted, it is necessary for the GoI to meet its mandated targets and ensure that AWCs are available for beneficiaries across the country, but by simply focusing on expansion targets, the inefficiencies that add to the financial burden and ineffectiveness of the ICDS programme, such as the disporportionate amount of funding for the Supplementary Nutrition Programme (SNP), and poorly trained and overburdened human capital, can only worsen in the long run. There is a substantial need to start allocating funds towards initiatives that address the issue of malnutrition as opposed to continuing to over-budget for interventions related to food provision and infrastructure development (Mohmand, 2012). In effect, universalisation *versus* quality universalisation can potentially detract from the effectiveness of the ICDS programme and its objectives.[3] Given the diversity of the country and the regional disparities that exist, it is more effective to look at ICDS from a sub-national perspective. This is because the performance of poor performing regions tend to bring down the national performance of the ICDS programme. There are region-specific factors that are responsible for why certain regions are performing better or worse, and hence it is necessary to undertake an evaluation of ICDS at the sub-national level and review the financial patterns that have developed over time. As well, there are also opportunities to conduct research that appraises the technical efficiency[4] of ICDS, although it may be better to examine this at the individual state level.

---

3. Objectives of the ICDS programme: (i) improve nutritional and health status of children of 0-6 years (ii) lay the foundation for proper psychological, physical and social development of the child (iii) reduce the incidence of mortality, morbidity, malnutrition and school dropout (iv) achieve effective co-ordination of policy and implementation amongst the various departments to promote child development (5) enhance capability of the mother to look after normal health and nutritional needs of the child through proper nutrition and health education (Ministry of Women and Child Development, Government of India: *http://wcd.nic.in/icds/icds.aspx*).
4. "Technical efficiency refers to the physical relation between resources (capital and labour) and [a particular] outcome. A technically efficient position is achieved when the maximum possible improvement in outcome is obtained from a set of resource inputs. An intervention is technically inefficient if the same (or greater) outcome could be produced with less of one type of input" (Palmer and Torgerson, 1999: 1136).

Regional Breakdown

The classification of Indian states was done region-wise, taking into consideration the socio-economic differences that exist between states. The regions consist of the south, the northeast, the poor north, the rich north and the other north (Das Gupta *et al.*, 2005).

The South	Andhra Pradesh, Karnataka, Kerala and Tamil Nadu
The Northeast	Arunachal Pradesh, Assam, Manipur, Meghalaya, Mizoram, Nagaland and Tripura
The North: "Poor"	Bihar, *Jharkhand, Uttar Pradesh, *Uttarakhand, Orissa, Madhya Pradesh and Rajasthan
The North: "Rich"	Punjab, Haryana, Gujarat and Maharashtra
The North: "Other"	Himachal Pradesh, Jammu and Kashmir and West Bengal

Note: * Jharkhand and Uttarakhand—in the study by Das Gupta *et al.,* 2005, Jharkhand and Uttarakhand were not included in the analysis; however they are included in this study and are considered a part of the 'poor north' because of their relation to Bihar and Uttar Pradesh respectively, which both belong to the 'poor north' category.

Resource Allocation and Funding[5]

ICDS programme comprises two major components: ICDS-General (G) and ICDS-Special Nutrition (SN). ICDS (G) is meant to cover operational costs and ICDS (SN) is for funding the Supplementary Nutrition component of ICDS. There has been a significant increase in the allocation of resources to the ICDS programme during the period under reference. While ICDS (G) has increased by 78 per cent, that of ICDS (SN) has risen by a much larger margin of 227 per cent. In terms of per cent composition too, there is a clear incline towards ICDS (SN) as revealed by the per cent distribution of ICDS (G) and ICDS (SN); the former has declined from 63.92 per cent in 2006-07 to 49.11 per cent in 2010-11 and the latter has increased from 54.23 per cent to 65.68 per cent during the reference period (Table 5.1) Increase in the number of operational projects and AWCs, coupled with revision of the financial norms, has resulted in such a large increase (Government of India, 2013).

---

5. Data from the Comptroller Auditor General's (CAG) Report (2013) on *Performance Audit of ICDS Scheme was* used in order to conduct the secondary data analysis for this report.

Table 5.1

Release and Expenditure on ICDS

(₹ *in crores)*

Years	ICDS (General)		ICDS (SN)		Total	
	Release	Expenditure	Release	Expenditure	Release	Expenditure
2006-07	2691.94 (63.92)	2618.34 (45.76)	1519.22 (36.08)	3102.51 (54.23)	4211.16	5720.85
2007-08	3108.82 (60.12)	2992.94 (40.29)	2062.29 (39.88)	4433.83 (59.71)	5171.11	7426.77
2008-09	4045.78 (63.94)	3967.37 (44.6)	2281.32 (36.06)	4928.34 (55.4)	6327.1	8895.71
2009-10	4390.80 (54.07)	4839.66 (36.99)	3730.13 (45.93)	8242.96 (63.01)	8120.93	13082.62
2010-11	4794.41 (49.11)	5306.91 (34.32)	4968.72 (50.89)	10153.69 (65.68)	9763.13	15460.6
Total	19031.75 (56.65)	19725.22 (38.99)	14561.68 (43.35)	30861.33 (61.01)	33593.43	50586.55

Note: Figures in brackets represent percentage to the respective totals.

Source: Computed using CAG Report (2013) on *Performance Audit of ICDS Scheme*.

Between the time periods 2006-07 and 2010-11, the norms regarding how financial assistance is provided by the Central government to the states has changed for both of the categories respectively.

ICDS (G)

With respect to ICDS (G), between 2006-07 and 2010-11, the Central government has gone from providing 100 per cent financial assistance to providing 90 per cent and requiring the states to supplement the additional 10 per cent of costs.

It is quite noticeable that there has been a substantial incremental increase in per capita funds released and per capita expenditure over time with a growth rate of 25.58 per cent and 36.99 per cent respectively (Table 5.2). The region that stands out is the north poor. In per capita terms, the north poor region is receiving the least amount of funds in both 2006-07 and 2010-11. As well, the north poor appears to have had a lesser rise in per

Table 5.2

Per Capita Funds Released and Expenditure (₹ in crore): ICDS (G) and ICDS (SN)

Region	2006-07						2010-11						Growth Rate (%)					
	ICDS (G)			ICDS (SN)			ICDS (G)			ICDS (SN)			ICDS (G)			ICDS (SN)		
	FR	EXP	RI	FR	EXP	RI	FR	EXP	RI	FR	EXP	RI	FR	EXP	RI	FR	EXP	RI
South	575.94	548.99	0.00	237.97	501.47	263.50	716.57	768.77	52.20	452.51	1336.76	884.25	19.63	28.59	100.00	47.41	62.49	70.20
North Poor	266.77	277.07	10.30	247.08	458.38	211.29	282.17	346.25	64.08	537.53	1019.90	482.38	5.46	19.98	83.93	54.03	55.06	56.20
North Rich	371.32	381.16	9.84	154.22	393.94	239.72	442.72	495.90	53.18	220.88	703.70	482.83	16.13	23.14	81.49	30.18	44.02	50.35
North Other	515.12	585.73	70.61	129.39	436.52	307.14	966.65	1100.57	133.92	532.05	966.18	434.13	46.71	46.78	47.28	75.68	54.82	29.25
North east	1147.44	681.86	0.00	305.19	672.78	367.59	1457.22	1216.24	0.00	1067.96	1031.32	0.00	21.26	43.94	-	71.42	34.77	-
Total	2876.59	2474.81	90.75	1073.86	2463.09	1389.23	3865.33	3927.72	303.38	2810.93	5057.87	2246.94	25.58	36.99	70.09	61.80	51.30	38.17

Note:
* FR - Funds Released by GoI
* EXP - Expenditure (GoI + Region)
* RI - Regional Investment

capita expenditure between 2006-07 and 2010-11 as compared to the other regions. This is of concern because the north poor had the largest number of beneficiaries in the ICDS programme in 2006-07 and has experienced one of the largest increments in the number of its beneficiaries between 2006-07 and 2010-11 (Table 5.3). Therefore it is likely that the north poor contributes a substantially high percentage of malnourished children in India. This will be discussed more in depth in the following sections.

Table 5.3

Number of Beneficiaries

# Beneficiaries	*2006-07*	*2010-11*
South	10,748,208.57	13,271,619.97
North Poor	35,300,758.48	53,988,273.48
North Rich	12,130,457.84	18,992,932.88
North Other	4,945,659.74	7,459,792.35
Northeast	2,918,505.90	4,233,881.92
Total	66,043,590.53	97,946,500.60

Note: * Calculated based on data from Government of India (2013).

ICDS (SN)

With regard to ICDS (SN), it was observed that there has been inconsistency between ICDS norms pertaining to financial allocation and the actual contribution by the Central government. This has been quite evident across most regions in the country. First, as per the ICDS policy with regard to the Supplementary Nutrition Programme, in 2006-07, all the regions in the country were to receive 50 per cent of the total expenditure on ICDS (SN) from the Central government.[6] This policy was changed in 2010-11 to account for a 90:10 provision to the northeastern region, while the other regions remained at 50:50.

It was found that funding for the regions of north rich and north other was not at par with the norms set for ICDS in 2006-07, where the Central government was responsible for contributing 50 per cent

6. As per the CAG Report, in 2006-07, states were to receive 50 per cent of the financial norms (based on per capita expenditure) or 50 per cent of expenditure incurred by the states. The amount contributed by the Central government would be based on lesser of the two.

of funds. It is worth noting that despite the Central government being responsible for contributing 50 per cent of expenditure, or 50 per cent of financial norms (funds to be disbursed per beneficiary), the regions on average are not allocating the amounts as per the per capita norms stated in the policy (please refer to Table 5.4 and Table 5.5 for an overview of ICDS's financial norms and how much each region is spending on average per beneficiary). Also, it can be observed that there has been an rise in the shortfall as observed in Table 5.5. Although this per cent rise in the shortfall is very small in the south region, that of north poor is of concern as the latter has a considerable presence of malnourished children. However, there has been an incremental increase in the per capita contribution by the Central and the state governments and consequently the total expenditure over time. On an average, there has been a 51.30 per cent increase in per capita expenditure from 2006-07 to 2010-11 (please

Table 5.4

Per Capita (in ₹) Financial Norms

Category	*2006-07 Rates*	*2010-11 Rates*
Children (6-72 Months)	2.00	4.00
Severely Malnourished Children (6-72 Months)	2.70	6.00
Pregnant Women and Nursing Mothers	2.30	5.00
Average Per Capita Expenditure	2.33	5.00

Note: * For the purposes of this report, the average per capita expenditure has been used.
Source: Ministry of Women and Child Development, Government of India (2008).

Table 5.5

Per Capita Expenditure (in ₹) Per Day 2006-07 and 2010-11

Region	*2006-07*		*2010-11*		
	Exp	*Shortfall to the norm*	*Exp*	*Shortfall to the norm*	*Percent increase in shortfall*
South	1.87	0.46	4.47	0.53	15.22
North Poor	1.58	0.75	3.10	1.9	153.33
North Rich	1.39	0.94	2.56	2.44	159.57
North Other	1.66	0.67	3.17	1.83	173.13
Northeast	2.22	0.11	3.66	1.34	1118.18

Source: Government of India (2013).

refer to Table 5.2). Nonetheless, the north rich and the south have experienced a decline in contributions from the Central government over time. These changes will be addressed in the following sections of the paper.

Physical Infrastructure and Human Capital

The AWC is where actual implementation of the ICDS programme takes place. It has been seen that the number of sanctioned AWCs have always been higher than that of operational ones, despite decrease in the shortfall over time (please refer to Table 5.6). As per the Budget Brief by Kapur (2013), although there has been a nearly 30 per cent increase in the number of operational AWCs across the country, that of AWCs that are opened continue to be less than what is sanctioned. This could imply that the number of functional AWCs are less than those actually required for effective implementation of the programme. This raises an additional concern as to whether the current norms as they relate to AWCs and programme placement are sufficient. For example, the norms of ICDS mandate one AWC per population of 400-800, while as compared to a neighbouring country like Thailand, it is 1 per 100 (Mohmand, 2012). As well, given that there is generally 1 Anganwadi worker (AWW) per AWC, it can be inferred that the human capital required to implement ICDS is also inadequate. Although the number of sanctioned posts for AWWs has been raised from 10.6 lakh in 2007-08 to 13.7 lakh in 2011-12, there are 9 per cent vacancies in these posts at an all-India level, as of 2012 (Kapur, 2013).

Ultimately, the infrastructural component of ICDS (physical infrastructure and human capital) is not sufficient to meet the demands of the programme. Although the gap between sanctioned and operational AWCs, as well as staff vacancies appear to be decreasing over time, the targets are not yet met. Furthermore, it can be seen from Table 5.6 that the less prosperous regions in the country, namely, north poor, north other and northeast, are experiencing the greatest percentage shortage in terms of physical infrastructure. This validates the claim made by Das Gupta *et al.* (2005) that programme placement is regressive across the country. More importantly, given the issues as they relate to coverage and overburdened human capital, it is perhaps necessary to re-evaluate the norms dictating programme placement. As it stands, the resources allocated for boosting the infrastructural component of ICDS appear to be inadequate, but this is quite possibly because the norms do not seem to adequately address the needs.

Table 5.6

Anganwadi Centres

Region	*2006-07*			*2010-11*		
	Sanctioned	*Operational*	*% Shortfall*	*Sanctioned*	*Operational*	*% Shortfall*
South	207584	186578	10.12%	242238	234315	3.27%
North Poor	432883	351926	18.70%	565931	526015	7.05%
North Rich	166407	144008	13.46%	213067	203824	4.34%
North Other	135883	80537	40.73%	164672	155553	5.54%
Northeast	64595	46623	27.82%	100344	92006	8.31%
Total	1007352	809672	19.62%	1286252	1211713	5.80%

Source: Government of India (2013).

ICDS and Nutrition Status

ICDS has often been touted as a controversial government scheme because it has not been directly linked with improving malnutrition rates across the country (Das Gupta *et al*., 2005). The programme is continuing to struggle post-universalisation and based on the data presented in the CAG Report that was released in January 2013, ICDS has failed to meet its own halfway performance targets. This was also reported by Maiorano (2013). However, there has been improvement in the levels of SNP beneficiaries that are receiving the benefits of this ICDS component. Across all regions with the exception of the northeast, there has been a substantial increase in the growth rate from 2006-07 to 2010-11 (refer Table 5.7).

With regard to changes in the nutrition status of ICDS beneficiaries over time, recent changes in Growth Monitoring Standards adopted by the GoI have altered how nutrition levels are

Table 5.7

Number of Eligible Beneficiaries (in Lakh) for Supplementary Nutrition

Region	2006-07			2010-11			Growth Rate (%)		
	Eligible	Actual	Shortfall	Eligible	Actual	Shortfall	Eligible	Actual	Shortfall
South	211.12	113.68	97.44	223.19	140.30	82.89	5.41	18.97	-162.37
North Poor	679.35	387.37	291.98	772.42	504.08	268.34	12.05	23.15	-740.47
North Rich	180.13	104.77	75.36	200.39	139.11	61.28	10.11	24.69	-146.43
North Other	101.47	44.82	56.65	115.45	70.87	44.58	12.11	36.76	-46.71
North east	60.07	26.33	33.74	81.52	49.94	31.58	26.31	47.28	12.90
Total	1232.14	676.97	555.17	1392.17	904.30	488.67	11.55	25.14	-1482.53

Note: * Data for West Bengal (2010-11) was not available in the CAG report. Therefore, data for West Bengal was used based on the earliest available year (2008-09).

reported. ICDS has adopted the WHO Child Growth Standards.[7] Therefore, for this paper, nutrition status will be examined over a 3, year time period between 2006-07 and 2008-09. During this time, all of the regions in India experienced a marginal increase in the percentage of children with normal nutrition status, with the exception of the northeast, which experienced a marginal drop in 2007-08 (refer Table 5.8a). However, the north rich region experienced the most significant change in its percentage of children with normal nutrition status. For moderately malnourished children, again there was a marginal fall across all regions over time, except for the northeast region that experienced an increase in the year 2007-08 (refer Table 5.8b). The analysis of severely malnourished children indicates a fluctuating trend over time, with some regions, such as the south and the northeast experiencing sharp rise in 2007-08, before falling back down again. Certain regions, namely, the north rich and north other have demonstrated a declining trend over time

7. The WHO Child Growth Standards, adopted by the Ministry of Women and Child Development on 15 August 2008, provides an international standard for assessing the physical growth, nutritional status and motor development of children 0-6 years of age. Significant implications of adopting these standards include both an increase in the proportion of children with normal nutrition status, as well as children suffering from severe malnutrition (Ministry of Women and Child Development, Government of India. *http://wcd.nic.in/icds/icds.aspx*). These implications can be verified in Appendix A-5.2 (please refer to the tables for depicting nutrition status in India, following the adoption of the WHO Child Growth Standards).

Table 5.8

a. Normal Nutrition Status (%): Pre-WHO Child Growth Standards

	2006-07	2007-08	2008-09
South	52.79	53.43	54.68
North Poor	47.15	48.16	50.14
North Rich	49.65	53.92	56.24
North Other	48.91	51.02	52.70
Northeast	69.11	67.61	69.85

b. Moderate Malnutrition (%): Pre-WHO Child Growth Standards

	2006-07	2007-08	2008-09
South	47.07	46.16	45.21
North Poor	51.99	51.15	49.01
North Rich	49.97	45.80	43.51
North Other	50.45	48.52	47.18
Northeast	30.05	31.36	29.77

c. Severe Malnutrition (%): Pre-WHO Child Growth Standards

	2006-07	2007-08	2008-09
South	0.14	0.40	0.11
North Poor	0.86	0.69	0.85
North Rich	0.38	0.28	0.25
North Other	0.65	0.46	0.12
Northeast	0.83	1.02	0.38

Source: Government of India (2013).

(refer Table 5.8c). However, there appears to be some inconsistency in the levels of severe malnutrition.

Discussion

Regional Highlights

Taking into consideration the funding patterns and levels of nutrition status across the regions, there is a concern that regions with the highest prevalence of malnutrition appear to have the least funding. This was also noted in previous research (Das Gupta *et al.*, 2005; Gragnolati *et al.,* 2006). In addition, this problem seems to persist over time. The north poor region is poorly funded, but has the highest number of beneficiaries; however the northeast region has the least number of beneficiaries, but is well funded. Although there is allowance in the policy for more funding for the northeast (due to terrain and high tribal population), the aforementioned point does shed light on the issues regarding funding patterns and expenditure for the ICDS programme. However, higher fund allocation does not imply efficient implementation of ICDS. Further research needs to be done to explore the technical efficiency of the ICDS programme.

Of particular concern is the north poor region because with over 40 per cent of the country's population and its large increment in the number of beneficiaries between 2006-07 and 2010-11, the north poor certainly contributes a substantially high percentage of malnourished children in India (Das Gupta *et al.,* 2005). In addition, as compared to the other regions, this region has the least number of children with normal nutrition status and the highest number of moderately and severely malnourished children. The issue at hand, as mentioned previously, is that the per capita expenditure in this region is not proportionate to the levels of malnourishment. Regional issues that have been found to persist across the states in the north poor region include low political prioritisation, ineffective financial allocation and gaps in staffing, and training and supervision of Anganwadi workers, thus inhibiting the ability of ICDS from assisting in improving health and nutrition (Nayak and Saxena, 2006).

For the northeast region, although the number of beneficiaries is the least, the per capita expenditure was the highest in 2006-07 and was the second highest in 2010-11. Also, as compared to other regions, the northeast region was characterised by the highest levels of children with normal nutrition status and the lowest levels of moderately malnourished children in 2006-07. This makes sense considering the fact that despite being a poorer region of the country, it is well developed as far as its social indicators are concerned. As well, as pointed out by Gragnoloti *et al.* (2006), there are two reasons for high levels of ICDS contribution. First, the northeast region has a large tribal population. This is beneficial because the ICDS policy accounts for the special needs of tribal groups. Instead of the norm of one AWC per 1000 people, there is a provision of one AWC per 700 people in the tribal areas. Second, although the Northeast maintains lower levels of malnutrition than all other regions, it maintains higher levels of enrolment in the programme. However, in the current study, it was found that there was an increase in the percentage shortfall of the number of beneficiaries that received SNP *versus* that beneficiaries that were eligible between 2006-07 and 2010-11.

As for the south and the north rich regions, there seemed to be an incremental increase over time as far as the funding patterns are concerned. These regions have experienced improvement in the levels of nutrition over time. As highlighted by Das Gupta *et al.* (2005), the coverage of ICDS was found to be regressive, in that funding was highest in regions where levels of malnutrition were the lowest. Based on the current study, this seems to hold true, especially in the south and the north rich, which are wealthier and are often considered to be progressive regions in the country, often characterised by their better infrastructure and governance for delivering the ICDS programme.

Implications

ICDS continues to struggle with a persistent gap between the ICDS policy and its implementation. In their study of the efficacy of ICDS, Das Gupta *et al.* (2005) also identified the prevalence of this policy-implementation gap. The mismatch between funds allocated by the Central government to some of the regions, particularly in regards to the SN Programme and the financial norms that dictate the funding that should be provided, can most certainly be considered a contributing factor to this problem. More importantly, the substantial increase in funding/expenditure towards the SN Programme, especially when compared with the provision for ICDS (G), indicates that the food bias still dominates the ICDS landscape. This is of concern for the simple reason that nutrition status has appeared to have only marginally increased in recent years, and with specific regard to severe malnutrition, the change over time has often been inconsistent. However, since 2009, ICDS has adopted the WHO Child Growth Standards for growth monitoring, which are recognised as an international standard for comparison across countries. Adopting these new standards has implications on how nutritional status is viewed and thus will alter levels of particular nutrition indicators. This standardisation in the measurement of nutrition compounds the existing problem by making it difficult to monitor the trends over time and evaluate the effectiveness of ICDS. This subject is beyond the scope of this paper, but has potential to impact how ICDS is funded and implemented, and thus would be useful to examine in future research.

The amount of funding provided for the SN Programme and the concern with the overemphasis on the programme is not a new area of contention, but it is worth highlighting once more that this focus on SNP will continue to pose challenges for the ICDS programme. The continued overemphasis on SNP gives weight to the idea that malnutrition is still largely viewed as an issue related to hunger and food distribution (Mohmand, 2012). This is problematic because it impacts the way the programme is run on a daily basis and the perception about ICDS. At present, AWWs spend the majority of their time focusing on the SN Programme, which invariably detracts from the other programmes being offered at the AWC (Gragnoloti *et al.*, 2006). The emphasis on SN is quite high across all regions, and funding for the programme continues to rise. It is important to remember that ICDS was designed to address the holistic needs of the child, and that nutrition services are not exclusive to SN (Drèze, 2011).

Unfortunately, despite the fact that SN programmes have been found to be limited in their effectiveness across large-scale interventions (Das Gupta *et al.*, 2005), significant resources, both financial and non-financial, continue to be put towards the programme. The incrementalist approach employed by the GoI in funding the ICDS programme is not necessarily the most effective way to plan for universalisation. Granted the programme will naturally require a substantial increase in the financial resources allocated towards it, but what needs to be kept in mind across all regions is that the effective implementation of ICDS depends upon the efficient utilisation of available funds and other resources

(Nayak *et al.*, 2006), and of resources is partially contingent upon prioritising high impact-low cost ICDS services (Gragnoloti *et al.*, 2006).

Ensuring Adequacy and Efficiency of Resources

The focus of the ICDS policy is broad based. There are regional disparities throughout the country that require further attention and greater assistance from a resource perspective (financial and infrastructural). The above analysis has shown that poorer regions in the country have lesser funding and higher levels of malnutrition. On a broader level, the policy needs to assume a greater element of "localisation", as also recommended by Das Gupta *et al.* (2005), in attempting to universalise the programme across the country and ensure effective implementation. More specifically, funding needs to be contingent upon regional need. As was accounted for with the northeastern region, it is perhaps necessary to employ a similar method of funding provision (i.e., region-specific norms) for lesser performing regions like the 'north poor'. This does not imply that an increase in funds is warranted, as there are issues beyond financial allocation affecting these regions, but it needs to be examined as to whether what is being provided is adequate and/or whether the Central-State contribution ratio is adequate.

Secondly, although there has been a considerable increase in the level of resources allocated towards the ICDS programme in recent years, it remains to be seen whether the resources provided are adequate for meeting the needs of ICDS beneficiaries and for the achievement of mandated universalisation targets. Considering the physical infrastructure and human capital components of ICDS, it is seen that there are gaps in operational AWCs and filled vacancies for AWWs. To go one step further, currently AWWs, as has been well established, are overburdened, undertrained and overworked (Gragnolati *et al.*, 2006; 2005). However, this is not the case across the entire country, as certain states, namely Tamil Nadu, have addressed infrastructural wekenesses of the programme effectively. For example, the state of Tamil Nadu, has adopted the "two worker model", wherein each AWC is managed by two AWWs and an Anganwadi Helper (AWH). This is an example of a localised intervention that has proven effective. Such a programmatic adjustment could be relevant across all regions.

Lastly, the overemphasis on the SN Programme has created a disconnect between what the ICDS policy actually is intended to do and what it actually does. Furthermore, it continues to be the component that requires the greatest amount of funding. As per the CAG audit in 2012-13, despite having norms that dictate greater allocations for this component, the expenditure was only 76 per cent of these norms, indicative of a massive deficit of 24 per cent. Lesser than allocated expenditure has led to lesser per capita expenditure, which as per the CAG report has implied that beneficiaries may be "receiving lesser nutrition". On further analysis, it was found that there were specific reasons for this shortfall in allocated expenditure: (1) an inadequate assessment of fund requirements, which resulted in lesser fund provision in the budget, (2) funds are often released at year end after the expenses have been incurred, (3) delays in fund disbursements from the ICDS centres, (4) delays in food procurement, and (5) the inability to identify the target population. These identified shortfalls have hindered the progress of ICDS and should be taken into consideration at the policy level and changes should be made accordingly.

Conclusion

There seems to be a gap in the funding patterns for the ICDS in India. Looking more closely at the sub-national context, it can be inferred that regions with a higher prevalence of child malnutrition do not seem to be receiving a proportionate level of financial support (from both Central and state governments) as the regions with a lower prevalence. While it has been established that funding is not contingent upon reducing the burden of malnutrition, it is indicative, to some extent, of the urgency with which this persistent problem is being addressed. The regional comparison showed that as far as nutrition indicators are concerned, the poorer regions in the country are not improving as much as the richer regions. The gap between the poorer and richer states seems to have increased over the years. Moreover, the nutrition levels across ICDS beneficiaries appear to have marginally improved over time. Accounting for the recent change in the growth monitoring standards, it is apparent that there is inconsistency in the reported levels of severe malnutrition. This issue could be addressed in future research.

Taking into consideration the GoI's incremental approach to financial provision for ICDS, its continued overemphasis on the SN component and an inconsistent improvement in the levels of severe malnutrition across the regions in the country, it is necessary to undertake further study of the ICDS scheme, with continued focus on resource adequacy and allocation. It is therefore imperative to understand and explore whether the scheme is technically efficient, and how well the government is using its resources to achieve its intended outputs and outcomes as they relate to ICDS, as well as, child and maternal health and nutrition.

References

Das Gupta, M., M. Lokshin, M. Gragnolati and O. Ivaschenko (2005). "Improving Child Nutrition Outcomes in India—Can the Integrated Child Development Services Program Be More Effective?" *The World Bank Policy Research Working Paper* 3647.

Drèze, J. (2006). "Universalisation with Quality: ICDS in a Rights Perspective", *Economic and Political Weekly* 41 (34): 3706-15.

Government of India, (2013).*Report of the Comptroller and Auditor General of India on Performance Audit of Integrated Child Development Services (ICDS).* New Delhi: Comptroller and Auditor General of India.

Gragnolati, M., C. Bredenkamp, M. Das Gupta, Y-K Lee and M. Sheka (2006). "ICDS and Persistent Undernutrition: Strategies to Enhance the Impact", *Economic and Political Weekly* 41 (12): 1193-201.

Kapur, A. (2013). *Budget Briefs: ICDS GOI, 2013-2014.* Centre for Policy Research, pp.1-8.

Maiorano, D. (2013). "Let the Country Grow", *Economic and Political Weekly* 68(22).

Mohmand, S.K. (2012). *Policies Without Politics: Analysing Nutrition Governance in India.* Institute of Development Studies.

Nayak, N., and N.C. Saxena (2006). "Implementation of ICDS in Bihar and Jharkhand", *Economic and Political Weekly* 34 (41): 3680-84.

Palmer, Stephen, and David J. Torgerson (1999). "Definitions of Efficiency", *Bmj* 318.7191: 1136.

The World Bank Group (2012). *Project Signing: Government of India and World Bank Sign $106 Million Agreement for Improving Nutrition Among Children in India. http://www.worldbank.org/en/news/press-release/2012/11/05/project-signing-government-of-india-and-world-bank-sign-106-million-agreement-for-improving-nutrition-among-children-in-india*

Wesites:

Ministry of Women and Child Development, Government of India, 2008. *http://wcd.nic.in/icds/icds.aspx*

Appendix A-5.1

Programmatic Deficiencies

Programmatic deficiencies impacting the performance of ICDS that have been identified in the existing research are inclusive of, but not limited to:

- An overemphasis on the SNP.
- Gaps in programme targeting:
  - o Children 0-3 years.
  - o Programme coverage.
- Inadequate human resources.

Supplementary Nutrition Programme

The issues as they relate to the SNP are rooted in the perception of the SNP component, the resources required in terms of finances and human capital and its effectiveness at reaching its target demographic. The SNP has come to dominate the ICDS landscape, and despite nutrition services extending beyond SNP, they are often restricted to it (Drèze, 2006). This is apparent based on the funding pattern for SNP, as it comprises the majority of spending towards the ICDS programme. As well, AWWs spend the majority of their time working on activities related to SNP (Gragnolati *et al.*, 2006). The aforementioned considered, the SNP runs inefficiently and frequently encounters issues relating to supply availability and leakages in food procurement. More importantly, the food supply is poorly targeted and leakages of SNP food often occur and are consumed by non-targeted and/or non-needy beneficiaries (Das Gupta *et al.*, 2005).

Programme Targeting

Children 0-3 Years

The ICDS programme has failed to appropriately focus on children under 3 years of age (Gragnolati *et al.*, 2006; Drèze, 2006; Das Gupta *et al.*, 2005). This is partially attributable to the fact that services provided by the ICDS programme and activities that take place at the Anganwadi Centre (AWC) tend to attract children 4-6 years of age. For example, the pre-school education component requires AWWs to devote much of their time to the children that receive these services (4-6 years), which detracts attention from the needs of children 0-3 years (Gragnolati *et al.,* 2006).

Programme Coverage

Historically, poor states with higher levels of undernutrition have received the least funding and were not adequately covered by the programme (Gragnolati *et al.,* 2006). Regressive programme placement has neglected situations where the need is the greatest (Das Gupta *et al.,* 2005), which could have influenced how the programme is governed and implemented.

Anganwadi Workers

The AWWs are often overworked, undertrained, improperly supervised and inadequately supported (Gragnolati *et al.,* 2006; Das Gupta *et al.,* 2005). Their duties require that they have knowledge and an understanding of nutrition, pre-school education and child and maternal health and nutrition as well as the tools, time and support to carry out their work both efficiently and effectively.

Appendix A-5.2

Nutrition Status Following the Adoption of the WHO Child Growth Standards

Normal Nutrition Status (%)

	2009-10	*2010-11*
South	55.56	58.86
North Poor	40.34	53.54
North Rich	58.30	68.08
North Other	52.15	64.74
Northeast	69.59	72.19

Moderate Malnutrition (%)

	2009-10	*2010-11*
South	44.34	40.43
North Poor	37.16	41.49
North Rich	41.45	29.53
North Other	47.37	33.61
Northeast	29.99	27.46

Severe Malnutrition (%)

	2009-10	*2010-11*
South	0.10	0.71
North Poor	22.50	4.96
North Rich	0.25	2.38
North Other	0.48	3.63
Northeast	0.42	0.35

Source: Government of India (2013).

6

SWADHIN MONDAL

Review of Equity in Health and Healthcare Financing in South East Asia

Introduction

Health equity has been conceptualised and defined in several ways, as its principles are derived from the fields of philosophy, ethics, economics, medicine, public health, and others. The WHO defines inequity as "differences in health status, which are unnecessary and avoidable, but in addition, are considered unfair and unjust" (Whitehead, 1992). The International Society for Equity in Health (ISEqH)[1] defines it as "the absence of potentially remediable, systematic differences in one or more aspects of health across socially, economically, demographically, or geographically defined population groups or subgroups." Braveman and Gruskin (2003) conclude that "equity in health is the absence of systematic disparities in health (or in the major social determinants of health) between groups with different levels of underlying social advantage/disadvantage—that is, wealth, power, or prestige." According to Macinko and Starfield (2002), the subsets of health inequalities that are judged unjust or unfair constitute health inequities.

The Commission on the Social Determinants of Health (CSDH) (WHO, 2008) has been an important and decisive participant in the discussions and debates around health equity and inequality. The importance of social causes of ill health and health inequalities received global recognition subsequent to the Commission's report. The Commission's report is said to be the first attempt to apply social epidemiological analysis to global health (Venkatapuram, 2010), instead of focusing on individual-level determinants relating

1. International Society for Equity in Health. Working definitions 2001. OpenURL

to environment and behaviour. The idea that ill health and health inequalities need to be viewed within the framework of ethics of justice is also an important contribution of the Commission.

The focus on avoidable health inequalities between groups of people within countries and between countries that emanate from social and economic conditions have an important corollary. Inequities can be addressed to a great extent if one tackles in the first instance, those that are accentuated because of existing anomalies in a variety of policies. Evidence exist that show that only addressing the needs of the better-off will accentuate the existing inequities (The Lancet, 2010). For example, a seminal study by UNICEF found that using an equity-focused strategy, a US$1 million investment to reduce deaths in children under 5 years in a low-income, high-mortality country would avert an estimated 60 per cent more deaths than the current approach (UNICEF, 2010). There is now a strong argument that efforts to reach the poorest would go a long way in meeting the Millennium Development Goals (MDGs) and reduce inequities significantly (The Lancet, 2010).

The report of SDH (social determinant of health) and subsequent extensions of the core messages have helped in gaining a deeper understanding of the areas where economy-wide policies can alleviate or accentuate health inequalities. The eight broad areas that contain within them major determinants of health and are integral to WHO's implementation strategy are the following (WHO, 2008): early child development, employment conditions, globalisation, social exclusion, health systems, priority public health conditions, women and gender equity, and urbanisation. A ninth one includes measurement and evidence, and nine knowledge networks have been established to assist the SDH Commission in its attempt to seriously address health inequities globally.

While all these themes impinge on the access and utilisation of healthcare in direct or indirect ways, the SDH Commission notes that:

> Access to and utilisation of healthcare is vital to good and equitable health. The health-care system is itself a social determinant of health, influenced by and influencing the effect

of other social determinants. Gender, education, occupation, income, ethnicity, and place of residence are all closely linked to people's access to, experiences of, and benefits from healthcare (WHO, 2008).

Clearly, policies of a wide variety directly or indirectly impact on the final outcome, including public and social policies not only on health and labour, but a much wider array sectors. For example, some have argued that food and nutrition security impact on health equity and are often a result of underlying social inequities requiring policies on the economic, agricultural, and social and health front (Friel and Baker, 2009). While there is a poor-rich divide among countries globally, evidence is mounting that even in relatively better-off regions, such as the WHO European region, there are visible social and economic inequalities within and between countries with accompanying health inequalities (Jakab and Marmot, 2012). A truly multi-pronged approach is clearly the most effective tool to deal with the wide range of issues that ultimately impact on social and economic inequalities (Dahlgren and Whitehead, 2007).

This paper takes a closer look at the situation in 11 countries[2] of South East Asia Region (SEAR) with respect to health equity and inequality. While inequality in health outcomes are measured using standard variables like IMR (infant mortality rate), the type of inequity discussed here mostly refers to the access to health services. Also, the attempt is to not analyse the reasons and all possible redressals of such inequities except to report on existing evidence, but rather examine the role of health protection as one of the tools for reducing inequities in access, both within the region as well as globally.

Social Determinants of Health in South East Asia Regional Office (SEARO): Some Evidence

Primary data on the social determinants of health is not easily available in a comparable format for the region. Thus, we use existing evidence from a variety of sources to confirm the presence

2. These countries are: Bangladesh, Bhutan, India, Indonesia, DPR Korea, Myanmar, Maldives, Nepal, Sri Lanka, Thailand and Timor-Leste.

of inequities and in health outcomes, as well as in the intervening variables like service use and health-seeking behaviour.

In Table 6.1, we present some selected statistics for countries for which data was available. While the data in the table is not current, it merely illustrates the point that health outcomes, service use and utilisation, all have a social gradient. The columns report ratio values for the lowest quintile to the highest quintile. Thus, for example, for Bangladesh, this ratio is 1.39 for IMR, indicating that lower-income households have a much higher IMR than those at the top end of the income distribution. Clearly, there are inequities in health outcomes for all the four countries. For service

Table 6.1

Inequities in Health Outcomes, Service Utilisation and Other Social Determinants in Four Countries

Sub-indicator	*Bangladesh*	*India*	*Indonesia*	*Nepal*
	R(L/H)	*R(L/H)*	*R(L/H)*	*R(L/H)*
Infant mortality rate	1.39	2.53	3.55	1.61
Under-5 mortality rate	1.69	3.11	3.51	1.92
Fertility rate	2.22	3.72	3.36	2.36
Children: severe stunting	3.97	3.56	na	2.57
Women: malnutrition	2.76	3.48	na	1.80
Immunisation coverage	0.66	0.33	0.57	0.66
Medical treatment of fever	0.23	0.71	0.55	0.57
Treatment in private facility	0.20	0.68	0.15	0.12
Multiple visits to a medically-trained person	0.17	0.26	0.76	0.21
School completion: Women	0.19	0.11	0.68	0.16
School completion: Men	0.21	0.38	0.73	0.42
School participation: Girls	0.87	0.60	0.85	0.59
School participation: Boys	0.79	0.72	0.85	0.79
Media exposure: Women	0.01	0.03	0.09	0.06
Media exposure: Men	0.14	na	0.11	0.12
Women's decision-making power for healthcare	0.97	0.71	0.83	0.81
Women's decision-making power for children healthcare	0.85	na	0.81	0.86

Source: Gwatkin *et al.* (2007).

utilisation like immunisation and treatment, the inequalities are also quite stark, with the lower-income groups showing much lower utilisation than the upper income groups. Similarly, for the other social determinants of health like education, there is significant inequity among the different income classes.

Table 6.2 presents data for Indonesia on selected service use variables for 1997-2007. Clearly, although there have been some improvements over the years in some parameters like safe delivery and institutional delivery, it is not across all the parameters, and substantial inequities remain in the system for immunisation, safe delivery and institutional deliveries. In another important piece of research (WHO, 2009), health inequities in selected countries of the SEAR of WHO were analysed. Five countries—Bangladesh, India, Nepal, Sri Lanka and Thailand—were considered in the analysis of inequity in health outcomes, health systems variables and key health determinants across and within these countries. Some of the selected results are presented in Table 6.2.

Table 6.2

Percentage Children Completely Immunised, Safe Delivery, Institutional Delivery, Underweight, 1997-2007, Indonesia

Variable	*Year*	*Lowest*	*Second*	*Middle*	*Forth*	*Highest*	*Ratio (L/H)*
Completely immunised	1997	42.9	47.2	46.5	58.0	72.1	0.60
	2003	37.1	46.6	52.2	58.1	64.7	0.57
	2007	39.4	53.0	58.1	68.0	74.9	0.53
Safe delivery	1997	21.3	34.9	48.1	64.5	89.2	0.24
	2003	38.8	56.0	68.7	80.6	63.6	0.61
	2007	43.8	66.3	78.8	87.2	95.5	0.46
Institutional Delivery	1997	3.9	8.4	17.8	29.8	52.6	0.07
	2003	10.8	24.7	37.9	53.4	81.3	0.13
	2007	13.6	31.7	47.9	61.7	83.3	0.16
Under weight children	2000	28.3	24.8	24.4	21.2	18.1	1.56
	2003	33.1	28.8	27.0	25.4	21.1	1.57
	2005	32.8	28.6	26.8	25.3	20.3	1.62

Source: Utomo *et al.* (2011).

Figure 6.1 shows that there are substantial inequities in use of modern contraceptive methods within and among these countries;

Nepal, for example, has the most inequity and Thailand the least. An analysis of the composition *vis-à-vis* reasons for inequities (Figure 6.2) for skill birth attendance, for example, indicates that socio-economic position in the society is the most important factor in all the four countries, followed by health system factors. A more detailed analysis of these determinants is given in Figure 6.3 that shows that wealth, geographic location, mother's biological characteristics and sanitation facilities are some of the important factors, in that order.

There are complex interplays among these groups of variables, in that the "socioeconomic" factors are often results of, and influenced by policy and politics. For examples, in India, evidence indicates that the marginalised sections such as SCs (scheduled castes)/STs (scheduled tribes) and the OBCs (other backward castes), make up a major part of the poor in India and also are at a disadvantage as far as health status and health services are concerned (Nayar, 2007).

Financial Protection and Health Inequity

While the SDH framework emphasises the multiple dimensions of health outcomes and service use that require a multi-sectoral approach (Dahlgren and Whitehead, 2007), it is also important to understand whether there are any policy options that can facilitate a faster reduction in inequities. Evidence is mounting that national

Figure 6.1

Inequities in Modern Contraception Between Poorest and Richest Wealth Quintiles by Countries

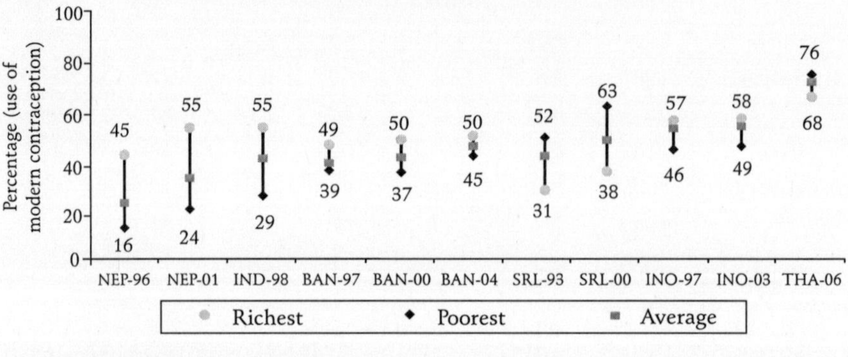

Source: WHO (2007).

Figure 6.2

Percentage Contribution to Inequities in Skilled Birth Attendance of Six of the Most Common Determinants

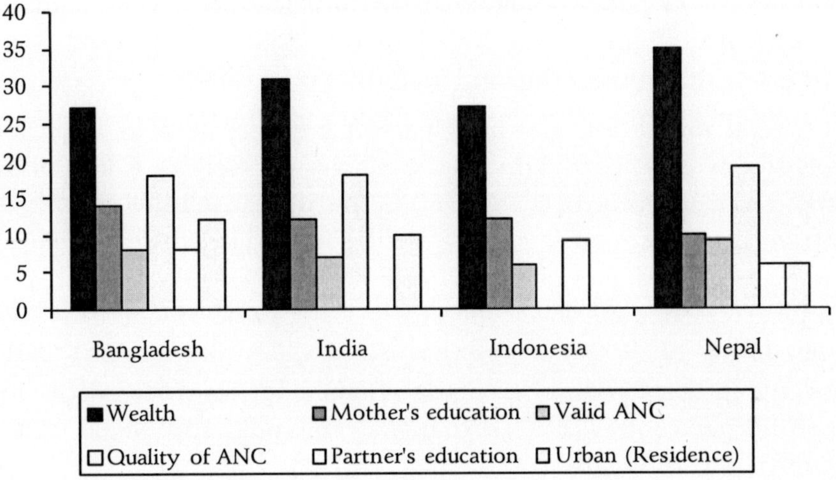

Note: ANC: Antenatal Care.

Source: Ismail *et al.* (2007).

Figure 6.3

Percentage Contribution to Inequities in Childhood Stunting of Six of the Most Common Determinants

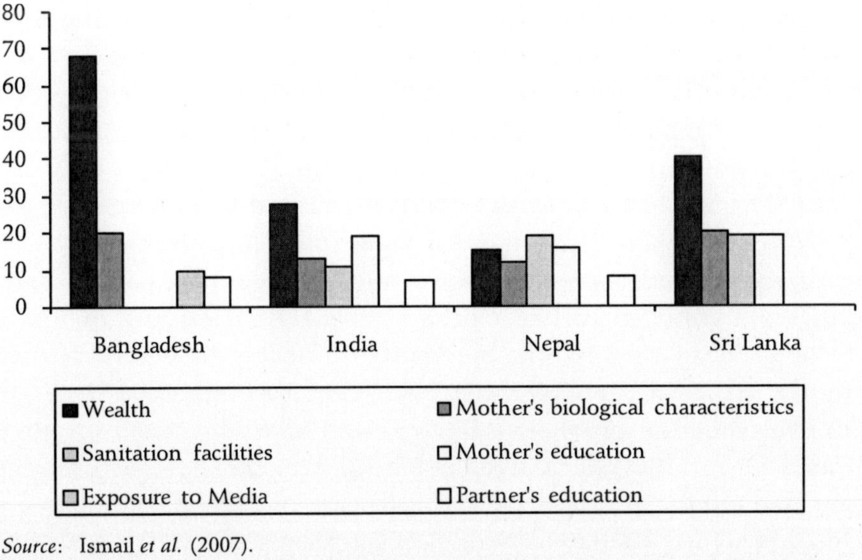

Source: Ismail *et al.* (2007).

governments as well as civil societies can play a major role in addressing such inequities. Government action is critical in three areas: as provider or guarantor of human rights and essential services; as facilitator of policy frameworks that provide the basis for equitable health improvement; and as a central agent that generates and gathers health information and data (Blas *et al.,* 2008).

Social protection and health cover are now seen as important both from a human rights perspective, as well as a key policy step, that can improve the well-being of households greatly by softening the economic impact of ill health. Literature around the impoverishing effects of out-of-pocket (OOP) spending (OOPS) has grown tremendously over the years. A study of 11 countries (van Doorslaer *et al.,* 2007) shows that if one takes into account OOPS, poverty in these countries is much higher; for countries with more than 60 per cent OOPS like Bangladesh, India and Nepal, rise in poverty was the highest.

Globally, evidence that inequalities in access have substantially reduced with systems of financial protection in place is mounting. Mexico, for example, has been able to reduce significantly the number of households with catastrophic and impoverishing health spending since it started its reform process (Knaul *et al.,* 2006; 2005). In Cuba, a government-run health system provides free, universal coverage, which has brought major improvements in the quality of care (Ugalde and Homedes, 2009). In contrast, in Costa Rica, there is a system of a single-payer managed by the social security organisation and financed by the employers, employees and the government, with the government subsidising care for the poor (Ugalde and Homedes, 2009). Brasil and Colombia have also pursued extensive reforms with significant improvements in the earlier years, but some mixed outcomes in the recent past (Esteves, 2012). A study on urban China shows that declining insurance coverage lead to a rise in inequality in access to health services (Gao *et al.,* 2001). In Cambodia, health equity funds have been used to overcome the problems of access and user fees, with improved outcome for the poor (Bigdeli, 2009). The presence of user fees lowered equity in utilisation of healthcare in Rwanda, compared to those who had insurance (Schneider and Hanson, 2005).

A World Bank study on Middle East and North African (MENA) countries indicate that OOP health expenditures tend to increase the poverty headcount in these countries from between 5 per cent and 14 per cent, with the exception of the West Bank and Gaza, where the difference was 80 per cent (Elgazzar *et al.,* 2010). The study documents those broad-based strategies that reduce the financial and administrative burden on the part of beneficiaries—as in the case of Iran and Tunisia where insurance coverage increased significantly—yielded the greatest gains in terms of improved healthcare access and outcomes.

The Universal Health Coverage Scheme (UHCS) in Thailand has not only increased accessibility and reduced the unmet need of healthcare, but also improved the equity of healthcare service (public and private) utilisation. The concentration index of overall healthcare service utilisation in 2001 (before UHCS) was -.090 and after 5 years of UHCS it was 0.177 (Evans *et al.*, 2012). The study also shows that with universal coverage scheme, the OOP payment has declined substantially and the gap between the poor and the rich in OOP expenditure has also reduced. Table 6.3 shows that the ratio of OOP expenditure to the total household income among the poor households has been reduced from 8.18 per cent to 2.23 per cent. The gap between poor and rich is close to 1.

Table 6.3

Household Out-of-pocket Spending

	1993	*2002*	*2004*
Poor	8.18	4.58	2.23
Middle	2.87	2.38	1.40
Rich	1.27	1.27	1.67
Ratio (Poor-Rich)	6.44	3.61	1.34

Source: Prakongsai *et al*. (2009).

Figure 6.4 shows that after introducing UHCS scheme, the poor are receiving twice the subsidies than that of the rich, with the result that a large number of households have been protected from financial impoverishments (Figure 6.5).

A calculation of benefit incidence of government spending shows that Sri Lanka has a very pro-poor public spending. Government

Figure 6.4

A Comparison of Percentage Distribution of Net Government Health Subsidies Among Different Income Quintiles in 2001 and 2003

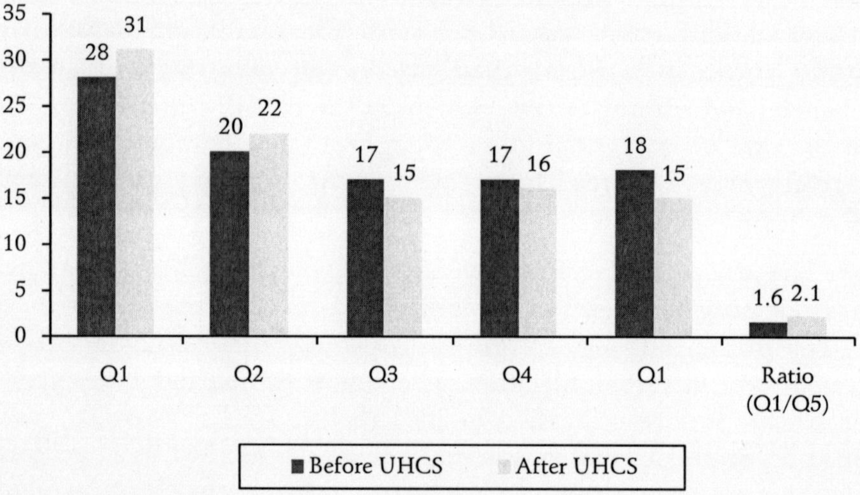

Source: Evans *et al.* (2012).

Figure 6.5

Number of Households (Per 1000 Households) Prevented from Impoverishment

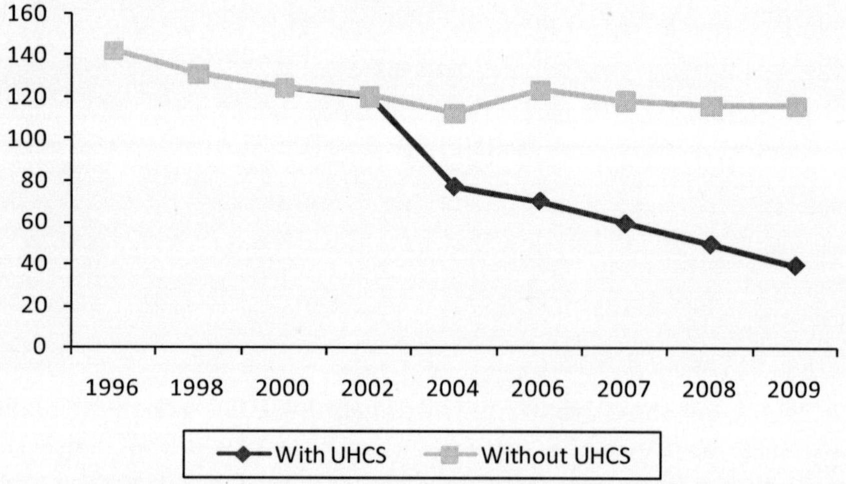

Source: Evans *et al.* (2012).

health expenditure has reached the poor quite effectively over the years due to a very good network of health facilities that make these accessible to the poor, lack of user charges, and the rich opting for the private sector (Ranan-Eliya and Sikurajapathy 2008). Sri Lanka is an often-cited example of good practices in health financing leading to equitable outcomes for the population and a distinct pro-poor reach.

Indonesia followed the trend of transformation of public healthcare system without increasing public spending or developing social health insurance (Thabrany *et al.,* 2003). As a result, access to healthcare particularly for poor people was very low.

The Government of Indonesia has initiated health sector reforms with a focus on the development of social health insurance, where a target was set to cover one-third of the poor by social health insurance by 2010 (Ministry of Health, 2010). The Jamkesmas programme (earlier called Askesin) provides health insurance to the poor and to the near-poor who are targeted through a means test. The programme is tax financed by the government and has no cost-sharing elements. The benefit packet also does not require any co-payments. The providers included in the Jamkesmas network are mainly government-owned facilities (World Bank, 2011) and are paid using a combination of capitation, fee-for-service, or Diagnostic Related Groups (DRGs), depending on the type of provider.

Figure 6.6 shows that during 2004-2009, the share of the poor in SHI (social health insurance) income group was almost half. Slightly more than 10 per cent went to the highest income group, with the remaining going to the middle income category. Apart from SHI, the government has started CCT (conditional cash transfer) schemes in 2007 to improve access to health services and basic education for the poor (Utomo *et al.,* 2011). Under this scheme, poor households receive conditional cash to pay for transportation and other related costs of using basic health and education services. These poor households also receive SHI and a basic education fellowship. An evaluation of CCT scheme shows that apart from cash transfer, 70 beneficiaries also received SHI and 20 per cent education fellowship (CHRUI 2010). In Indonesia, apart from SHI, the coverage of other health insurance is very limited (Utomo *et al.,* 2011). Clearly,

Figure 6.6

Coverage of Social Health Insurance (Jamkesmas) by Household Expenditure Deciles

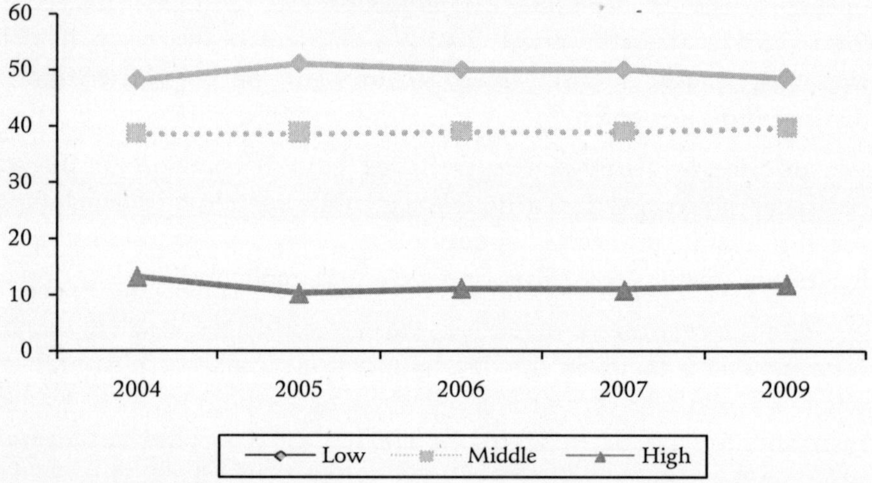

Source: Utomo *et al.* (2011).

Indonesia has taken a step in the right direction, but the coverage is still not wide enough to make a serious dent on inequities in access to health services.

Health Equity through Health Financing in SEARO

As discussed above, while Thailand and Sri Lanka seem to have addressed to a great extent inequities in access to services, other countries in the region have had less success in tackling health inequities.

In Bhutan, while the government continues to provide free access to basic health services and affordability is not a major constraint, opportunity costs such as time due to long distance travel, long waiting time, lack of transportation and ability to pay the same are some important deterrents to access. Bhutan does not have a problem with financial burden on households due to OOP payment to the extent other countries like India and Nepal in the region experience. However, accessibility remains a major issue for some of the rural and remotely-located communities due to the hilly terrain of Bhutan. Bhutan also has a shortage of doctors and other healthcare professionals, and combined with the burden of emerging and re-emerging diseases, the challenges in the health sector are significant, despite being different in nature from its neighbours.

In India, there is a significant overlap between social class and poverty, with concomitant inequality in a variety of social and economic indicators. These factors play out in the health sector too, resulting in multiple deprivations for the same class of individuals. While the evidence is mounting that the poorer sections of the population suffer worse health (Joe *et al.*, 2008), it is the composition of 'poor' that is of importance in the Indian context due to the complex social structure (Nayar, 2007). India remains a highly unequal society despite its impressive economic performance. In October 2010, the Planning Commission in India constituted a High Level Expert Group (HLEG) on Universal Health Coverage, which has submitted its report in late 2011 (Planning Commission 2011). However, there have been some concerns that the report does not have an operational vision (Rao, 2012) and it remains to be seen if and how the gulf between theory and practice will be bridged.

Nepal is in a similar situation with significant social and economic inequalities, more intensified due to its smaller size. Different races, castes and indigenous population live in three different ecological regions. Social inclusion of women, low castes and disadvantaged indigenous groups is poor, result in uneven access to resources and services, and make social cohesion and integration an important and on-going concern in Nepal (Government of Nepal, 2005).

Till recently, both India and Nepal have had poor success with health financing mechanisms that can protect people from impoverishment. India has been able to introduce the Rashtriya Swasthya Bima Yojana (RSBY) (National Health Insurance Scheme) in 2008 to provide health insurance coverage for BPL (below poverty line) families. The objective of this scheme is to provide protection to BPL households from financial liabilities arising out of health shocks that involve hospitalisation. The RSBY is also a good example of PPP (public-private partnership) and the innovative use by the government of a growing private insurance and health sector in India. Although definitely useful to those households that have taken this insurance, it is yet to cover all poor households for hospitalisation (Narayana, 2010) and touches only a small part of the high burden of treatment on households that emanate from outpatient treatment and purchase of drugs.

Bangladesh has been also struggling with high OOP expenses for health and has responded by initiating demand-side financing mechanisms in order to encourage use of maternal health services. Research indicates that the voucher program has been useful to target economically disadvantaged groups and therefore, helpful in improving equity of access to health services (Nguyen *et al.,* 2012). However, such approaches raise the question of efficiency of use of public resources; while-demand side financing may work on the target group, it raises the question of choice: should governments try to address inequities in health service utilisation using such schemes or think of larger initiatives like UHC that can cover more people and more services (Schmidt *et al.,* 2010).

Myanmar has high OOP spending on healthcare in a predominantly fee-for-service health sector. Government spending in total health spending is below 40 per cent (WHO, 2009a), and Myanmar is yet to move in any serious manner towards attaining UHC.

Timor-Leste has a more favourable health financing situation with OOP payment being around 25.6 per cent of total health spending, as given in the World Bank databank, although firm data is not available. The entire public health system is financed through the state budget and external resources, and the Timor-Leste government has given serious attention to the health sector and increased the expenditure on health substantially (WHO, 2009). However, the country continues to face major challenges. There is an acute shortage of healthcare personnel in the country, and an urgent need to add to and improve health infrastructure. In terms of inequity, there is a very significant gender imbalance in health outcomes (WHO, 2009), and coupled with high levels of poverty, inadequate availability of clean water and sanitation and inadequate coverage of health services in general (WHO, 2006), Timor-Leste requires serious health sector planning so as to make a dent in the current situation. In this environment, discussions on UHC seems a bit premature; the government's commitment to the health sector has been visible in the last few years, and whether or not the health system restructuring will improve equity remains to be seen.

To foreground an overview, Table 6.4 presents selected information for SEAR countries taken from an International Labour Organization (ILO) multi-country study on formal coverage and other related parameters (ILO, 2010). The last column of Table 6.4 is our assessment on the state of health coverage in these countries.

Bangladesh, India, Nepal and Myanmar have very low formal health coverage, high OOPS and less-than-optimal functioning of the public health infrastructure. Thailand has high coverage through SHI. Sri Lanka has low formal coverage but highly functional health infrastructure. The health sectors of Bhutan, Maldives and Timor-Leste are similar to Sri Lanka, in that these are being funded and visualised basically as a public-funded health infrastructure catering to the population without any formal health insurance. This is also true of DPR Korea, even though lesser data is available for this country. The differences in equity and health outcomes in these countries have to do with other determinants like efficiency, staffing and funding of such infrastructure.

There are sharp differences in the 11 countries in terms of their level of social and economic development, efficiency of health services, financing mechanisms and health equity. Clearly, health equity can be achieved by one of these three ways: (i) formal coverage through mainly one unified SHI programme, (ii) multiple schemes catering to different population groups and (iii) a well-functioning and efficient public healthcare infrastructure, with or without (i) and (ii) in place.

Countries in this region mostly do not have (i) or (ii) mentioned above, and a majority of countries cannot qualify to have a well-functioning health system with little or no problems of efficiency and equity—(iii) above. Thailand is the only country that is closest to this ideal, with a fairly well-functioning health system as well as publicly-funded health coverage. Sri Lanka is an example of one trying to achieve health equity through a strong focus on

Table 6.4

Percentage of Population Covered by Health Securities in SEAR Countries

	FHC (%)[1] Total	*SC*	*SHI*	*Deficit in FHC (%)[1]*	*OOPS as % of THE[2]*	*Not FHC Due to Financial Resources Deficit[3,4]*	*Comments*
Bangladesh	0.4	~ 0		100	55.8	91.3	Negligible formal coverage, substantial OOPS, low functionality of public health sector
Bhutan	...	...	...	...	31.4	79	Low OOPS, no formal insurance, functional public health sector
DPR Korea	na				0.4		Totally state-funded health infrastructure[5]
India	5.7	~ 0	5.2	94	75.6	92.4	Negligible formal coverage, high OOPS, low functionality of public sector, resources not a constraint
Indonesia	54.6	16.6	36.1	45	32.9	83.3	Moderate coverage by SHI, moderate gap in formal coverage, moderate level of OOPS, resources somewhat of a constraint
Maldives	...	...	...	...	...	...	No formal health coverage, mainly public-sector-oriented health services
Myanmar	...	...	...	...	80.4	...	No formal coverage, high OOPS, infrastructure not very functional

contd...

.Contd...

Nepal	0.1	~ 0		100	59.2	90.9	Negligible formal coverage, very high OOPS, low functionality of public health sector
Sri Lanka	0.1	~ 0		100	43.6	65.7	Negligible formal coverage, moderate OOPS, high functionality of public health system
Thailand	97.7	75.3	22.4	2	27.3	28.1	High formal and government coverage, low OOPS, low deficit in health coverage
Timor-Leste	...	...	...	...	4.2	53.7	No formal sector coverage, low OOPS, low functionality of public health sector

Note: 1. Latest available year. Detailed information is available in ILO (2008).
2. 2006 data.
3. Based on median value in low-vulnerability group of countries.
4. Percentage of total population NOT covered due to financial deficit (based on median value in low-vulnerability group of countries):
The ILO financial deficit indicator follows the same principle as the access deficit indicator regarding total health spending (in international $ PPP) except OOP payments. It uses the relative difference between the national health expenditure in international $ PPP (excluding OOP) and the median density observed in the country group with low levels of vulnerability as a benchmark for developing countries. This median value is just over 350 international$ PPP per capita.
5. WHO: *Source*: 11 health questions about the 11 SEAR countries.

public health services at reasonable cost. Bhutan and Maldives can probably strive to achieve (iii) but need a lot more planning and funding to achieve better results.

Discussions and Conclusion

Apart from Thailand and Sri Lanka, the countries that are most likely to improve their health equity status in the near future are Bhutan, Maldives, and Indonesia because of high levels of commitment from the government. While Bhutan and Maldives are much smaller countries with a predominantly public-sector financing and provision, Indonesia has started experimenting with expansion of SHI. All these three countries experience much less economic vulnerability in general, with lower poverty headcount ratios. It will not be too difficult for these countries to improve their health equity situation with proper planning and also a higher financial commitment to the health sector. Among these three countries, Indonesia has the most potential to make that leap to join Thailand as a country that has been able to tackle inequities in the health sector. While much less is known about DPR Korea, it is clear that the share of OOPS is very low in this country, and it probably will fit in the pattern of Sri Lanka and other such countries which rely mostly on the public health infrastructure for most of its services. However, not enough is known about the status of health equity in this country to make any predictions for the near future.

The countries that need to worry about not being able to reduce health inequities in the near future are India, Nepal and Bangladesh. These are countries where there is no legal framework yet on SHI that is broad enough to include the entire population. It has been contended that the lower the formal sector employment in a country, greater are the chances of most of the population to not have legal coverage in terms of social protection (ILO, 2010). Health financing that aims to give coverage to the vulnerable or to the entire population would first and foremost need a legal and administrative framework. While Indonesia has already put a similar framework in place, India, Nepal and Bangladesh have not done so yet. These are also countries that need to improve the efficiency of their public sector infrastructure in a major way, and have regulations for the private sector, which has grown tremendously in all three countries. India is in a position to improve its health financing situation, but is yet to take that major leap to a higher and sustainable level of funding. In a way, India is probably the only country in the South Asia region that can change its thinking on health coverage without worrying too much about growth and finances. While the other social determinants of health are quite adverse in these countries, there is scope to improve equity through health coverage as well.

Timor-Leste is in a different situation with huge issues of development and human-resource consistent growth patterns. Its overdependence on one sector—petroleum—has distorted the economy to a great extent, and SHI may not be its immediate priority. Improvement of the existing and damaged health infrastructure is the most important item on the government's health agenda.

Similarly, Myanmar is going through a serious political and administrative turmoil and the focus might not immediately be on UHC. Like Timor-Leste, it has to first rectify the damage done to the public health infrastructure to make the system more functional. While Timor-Leste has enough finances from its oil sector, Myanmar would continue to need internal as well as external resources for its economic restructuring and development. It currently spends very little on the health sector and its first priority should be increased funding for its health sector. Also, both Timor-Leste and Myanmar might be able to enhance health equity through an SDH approach by focusing on the other determinants of health as the first priority.

Clearly, while SHI and UHC are important tools of achieving health equity, an efficient and well-functioning health sector which is accessible and affordable to all population groups should be able to ensure the same health equity goals. The path that a country chooses will depend to a great extent on its political, legal and administrative framework on the one hand and political will on the other. Ultimately, covering the entire population with affordable and available healthcare for all requires first and foremost a vision of how current and future coverage would and commitment that could, include the ability to make difficult choices.

References

Bigdeli, M. and P. Annear (2009). "Barriers to Access and the Purchasing Function of Health Equity Funds: Lessons from Cambodia", *Bulletin World Health Organization* 87: 560–64.

Blas, E., L. Gilson, M. Kelly *et al.* (2008). "Addressing Social Determinants of Health Inequities: What can the State and Civil Society do?", *The Lancet* 372 (9650): 1684–89.

Braveman, P. and S. Gruskin (2003). "Defining Equity in Health", *Journal of Epidemiology.*

CHRUI (Center for Health Research University of Indonesia) (2010). *PKH Spot Check: Quantitative and Qualitative Assessments to Monitor Household Conditional Cash Transfers Operations*. Jakarta.

Dahlgren G, and M. Whitehead (2007). *European Strategies for Tackling Social Inequities in Health: Levelling up Part 2*. Copenhagen. WHO Regional Office for Europe (Studies on social and Economic Determinants of Population Health No. 3).

Doorslaer, E., O. O'Donnell, R.P. Rannan-Eliya et al. (2007). "Payments for Healthcare: Do They Aggravate Poverty?", *The National Medical Journal of India* 20(3): 139-41.

Elgazzar H., F. Raad, C. Arfa, A. Mataria, N. Salti, J. Chaaban, D. Salehi-Isfahani, S. Fesharaki and M. Majbouri (2010). *Out-of-Pocket Health Spending and Equity Implications in the Middle East and North Africa. Health, Nutrition and Population (HNP) Discussion Paper. The World Bank.*

Esteves, R. (2012). "The Quest for Equity in Latin America: a Comparative Analysis of the Healthcare Reforms in Brazil and Colombia", *International Journal for Equity in Health* 11: 6.

Evans, T.G., V. Tangcharoensathien, P. Jongudomsuk and S. Srithamrongsawat (2012). *An Independent Assessment of the First 10 years (2001-2010).* Presentation to Satellite Meeting of PMAC 24 January.

Friel, S. and I. Baker (2009). "Equity, Food Security and Health Equity in the Asia Pacific Region", *Asia Pacific Journal of Clinical Nutrition*18(4): 620-32.

Gao J., S. Tang, R. Tolhurst and K. Rao (2001). "Changing Access to Health Services in Urban China: Implications for Equity", *Health Policy and Planning* 16(3): 302-12.

Government of Nepal (2005). *Implementation of Brussels Programme of Action for the LDCs: Decade 2001-2010.* Progress Report Nepal.

Gwatkin, D., S. Rutstein, K. Jhonson, E. Suliman, A. Wagstaff and A. Amouzou (2007). *Socio-Economic Differences in Health, Nutrition and and Population Within Developing Countries*. Country report on HNP and poverty. The World Bank.

ILO (2008). *Social Health Protection: An ILO Strategy towards Universal Access to Healthcare.*

———. (2010). *World Social Security Report 2010/11: Providing Coverage in Times of Crisis and Beyond.* Geneva: ILO.

Ismail, F.S., R.R. Eliya and C.Perera (2007). *A Report on Inequities in Maternal and Child Health and their Determinants in South-East Asia Region (SEAR).* Institute for Health Policy.

Jakab, Z. and M. Marmot (2012). "Social Determinants of Health in Europe", *The Lancet* 379 (9811): 103-05.

Joe, W., U. Mishra, N. Navaneetham (2008). "Health Inequality in India: Evidence from NFHS 3", *Economic & Political Weekly.* August 2008. 41-47.

Knaul, M.F., H. Arreola-Omelas, Mendez-Canlado (2006). "Preventing Impoverishment, Promoting Equity and Protecting Households from Financial Crisis: Universal Health Coverage through Institutional Reforms in Mexico", *Working Paper Series: Innovation for Health Financing.* Mexican Health Foundation.

Knaul, F.M., H. Arreola-Ornelas, O. Mendez, M. Miranda (2005). "Preventing Impoverishment, Promoting Equity and Protecting Households from Financial Crisis: Universal Health

Insurance through Institutional Reform in Mexico", *Working Paper Series: Innovation for Health Financing*. Mexican Health Foundation.

Macinko, J.A., and B. Starfield (2002). "Annotated Bibliography on Equity in Health, 1980–2001", *International Journal for Equity in Health* 1: 1–20.

Ministry of Health (2010). *Pedoman Pelaksanaan Jaminan Pemeliharaan Kesehatan* (Guidelines for Social Health Insurance). Jakarta: Directorate General of Community Health.

Narayana, D. (2010). "Review of Rashtriya Swasthya Bima Yojana", *Economic and Political Weekly* XLV(9): 13-18.

Nayar, K.R. (2007). "Social Exclusion, Caste & Health: A Review based on the Social Determinants Framework", *Indian Journal of Medical Research* 12(6): 355-63.

Nguyen, H.T., L. Hatt, M. Islam, N.L. Sloan, J. Chowdhury, J.O. Schmidt, A. Hossain, H. Wang (2012). "Encouraging Maternal Health Service Utilisation: An Evaluation of the Bangladesh Voucher Program", *Scocial Science and Medicine*, Jan. 28.

Planning Commission of India (2011). *High Level Expert Group Report on Universal Health Coverage for India. http://planningcommission.nic.in/reports/genrep/rep_uhc0812.pdf*

Prakongsai, P., S. Limwattananon and V. Tangcharoensathien (2009). *The Equity Inpact of the Universal Coverage Policy: Lessons from Thailand*. Internationmal.

Rannan-Eliya, R. and S. Sikurajapathy (2008). "Sri Lanka: "Good Practice" in Expanding Healthcare Coverage", in Pablo Gottret, George J. Schieber and Hugh R. Waters (eds.), *Good Practices in Health Financing: Lessons from Reforms in Low- and Middle-Income Countries*. The World Bank.

Rao, S. (2012). "Long on Aspiration, Short on Detail: Report on Universal Health Coverage", *Economic and Political Weekly* XLVII (6): 12-16.

Schmidt, J.O., T. Ensor, A. Hossain and S. Khan (2010). "Vouchers as Demand Side Financing Instruments for Healthcare: A Review of the Bangladesh Maternal Voucher Scheme", *Health Policy* 96(2): 98-107.

Schneider, P. and K. Hanson (2005). "Horizontal Equity in Utilisation of Care and Fairness of Health Financing: A Comparison of Micro-health Insurance and User Fees in Rwanda", *Health Economics* 15(1): 19–31.

Sreshthaputra, N. and K. Indaratna (2001). *The Universal Coverage Policy of Thailand: An Introduction, Asia-Pacific Health Economics Network (APHEN), http://www.unescap.org/aphen/thailand_universal_coverage.htm*

Thabrany, H., A. Gani, Pujianto, L. Mayanda, Mahlil and Budi (2003). *Social Health Insurance in Indonesia: Current Status and the Plan for National Health Insurance.*

The Lancet (2010). "Equity as a Shared Vision for Health and Development", *The Lancet* 376 (9745): 929, 18 September 2010.

Ugalde, A. and N. Homedes (2009). "Health and Equity in Latin America", *Americas Quarterly.*

UNICEF (2010). *Progress for Children. Achieving the MDGs with Equity Number 9.* September.

Utomo, S., P. Sucahya and F. Utami (2011). "Priorities and Realities: Addressing the Rich-poorgaps in Health Status and Service Access in Indonesia", *Journal for Equity in Health* 10: 47.

van Doorslaer E, O. O'Donnell, R.P. Rannan-Eliya *et al.* (2007). "Payments for Healthcare: Do they Aggravate Poverty?" *The National Medical Journal of India* 20(3): 139-41.

Venkatapuram, S. (2010). "Global Justice and the Social Determinants of Health", *Ethics and International Affairs* 24(2) (Summer).

Whitehead, M. (1992). "The Concept and Principles of Equity and Health", *Int J Health Serv* 22: 429-45.

WHO (2006). *Timor-Leste Country Cooperation Strategy. (http://www.who.int/countryfocus/cooperation_strategy/ccsbrief_tls_en.pdf)*

——. (2009a). *Health Financing Strategy for the Asia Pacific Region (2010-2015). http://www.wpro.who.int/internet/resources.ashx/HCF/HCF+strategy+2010-2015.pdf*

——. (2007). *Health Inequities in the South-East Asia Region.*

——. (2008). *Closing the Gap in a Generation. Health Equity through Action on the Social Determinants of Health.*

——. (2009). *WHO Country Cooperation Strategy 2009-2013*: *Timor-Leste. http://www.searo.who.int/LinkFiles/WHO_Country_Cooperation_Strategy_-_Timor_Leste_2009-2013CountryHealth.pdf*

World Bank (2011). "Indonesia Health Sector Review. Does JAMKESMAS Protect the Population from Health Expenditure Shocks ?", *Policy and Discussion Notes. 60037.*

Others:

Country report–Bhutan: *http://www.seaphein.com/document/page/page_103.pdf*

Government of India. RSBY.

http://www.gdnet.org/ cms.php?id=research_paper_abstract& research_paper_id=10407

National Health Policy Programme, Presentation to the 3rd National Health Research Forum, 2009.

Social Security Policy Briefings, Paper 1 (Geneva).

The World Bank, *http://data.worldbank.org/indicator/SH.XPD.OOPC.ZS*

Part III

Health Delivery System: Personnel, Effectiveness and Gender Issues

7

SOBIN GEORGE

Does Social Profile of Healthcare Providers Matter?

Continuing Challenges of Inclusion in Healthcare Delivery System in India[1]

Introduction

The dominant discussions in public health in India often tended to sideline the questions of discrimination while examining the gap in health status among social groups, mainly due to the overinfluence of more visible issues such as unbalanced resource allocation and spending, poor coverage of services, infrastructure lacuna, human resource shortage, affordability and issues of governance. If not many, there is evidence that discrimination and resulting deprivation have an impact on health of the people in the Indian context. For instance, Borooah (2010) showed that people's health outcomes are significantly affected by their social group and there is a social gradient to health outcomes in India. Some studies highlighted the lower level of utilisation of health services among the Dalits as compared to the non-Dalits (Ram *et al.,* 1998; Kulkarni and Baraik, 2003; Baru *et al.,* 2010). Acharya (2007) drew attention to different levels of discrimination in Dalits accessing health services in the states of Gujarat and Rajasthan. Dasgupta and Thorat (2009) brought out the stark differentials in the rate of decline of IMR (infant mortality rate) and maternal health between SC (scheduled caste)/ST (scheduled tribe) and other social groups. Saroha *et al.* (2008), based on the study conducted among rural

1. An initial version of this article is published as working paper at Institute for Social and Economic Change, Bangalore.

Hindu women in Maitha in Uttar Pradesh (UP) noted that caste is a significant barrier to maternal healthcare service use among the rural women. The Indian health landscape thus is very complex due to the multiple deprivations that certain group of population face, which eventually lead to poor nutrition, poor hygienic environment and ecological conditions conducive to ill health and diseases. This paper attempts to situate this question in the analytical context that the inferior health outcomes of marginalised are to be seen in the context of existing intricacies of social exclusion that they experience and "graded discrimination" between and within various social groups. The following questions, subsequently, become important. Whether there are notable intergroup disparities in health outcomes and access to healthcare? If so, whether it could be understood by the discrimination in health service system? And finally if it is attributable to caste based discrimination, whether the present health service system has adequate personnel from discriminated groups to take care of the same? This paper draws from two official data sources including National Family Health Survey (NFHS 2 and 3) rounds in order to understand some of the health outcomes across social groups and National Sample Survey Organisation (NSSO) 68th round on employment and unemployment (2011-12) to present social group wise information of personnel in the healthcare delivery system. Apart from these data sets, the paper relies on published research on qualitative dimensions on healthcare access for marginalised social groups.

Marginalities and Inferior Health Outcomes

The linkages between group identity and health assume importance while we look at the level of deprivation of each group in comparison with other dominant communities and attempt to link with factors of discrimination and isolation. Some sets of studies have moderately attempted this task of bringing out the group-specific differentials of health. Barik and Kulkarni (2014), for instance, highlighted the intergroup differentials in health status of SCs and STs. The study showed that children from Dalit and Adivasi populations faced higher risks of mortality as compared to the non SC/STs. The disparities were noticeable in all states except a few including Assam, Haryana, Himachal Pradesh (HP), and Jammu and Kashmir (J&K). Similarly, the study revealed that the nutritional status of Dalit and adivasi women and children in India is relatively poor. Thorat (2007) discussed the disparities in health status and healthcare access of Dalit and Adivasi children as compared to other groups in various states. The study further attempted to link the disparities with practices of untouchability and discrimination against Dalits. Dasgupta and Thorat (2009) reiterated the persisting trend of inequalities in health status and healthcare access of Dalit and adivasi children that Barik and Kulkarni had brought out. The study noted that malnutrition, child mortality was the highest and immunisation remained the lowest for Adivasis, followed by Dalits during 2005-06. Borooah *et al.* (2012) brought out that morbidity and healthcare burden of Dalit women are higher than others due to their lower access to healthcare services. Studies have also explored how far group identity is associated with inferior health outcomes of STs.

Data from NFHS surveys also validates the inference that there are intergroup disparities in health outcomes, such as infant mortality, maternal mortality, nutritional status and institutional delivery unfavourable to SCs and STs. NFHS data for three rounds showed that the pace of reduction in IMR was low for SCs and STs between 1992 and 2006 as compared to non-SCs and STs. Similarly, under-five mortality remained the highest for adivasis during 1992-93, 1998-99 and 2006-07. NFHS data also showed that Dalit and adivasis children have the higher burden of malnutrition than others. States, where proportion of underweight Dalit children remained above the all-India average of Dalits in 2006, were Bihar and Madhya Pradesh (MP). Similarly, Bihar, MP and UP reported higher proportion of underweight adivasi children in 2006 as compared to all-India figures and that of other states (see Table 7.1). Access to ANC (antenatal care) was the lowest among adivasi women as compared to Dalits and other social groups. Institutional delivery was the lowest among Adivasis, followed by Dalits. States including Bihar, UP, Assam, Odisha, Rajasthan, HP and MP had lower access to skilled attendants for Dalits and adivasis (see Table 7.2).

Table 7.1

Percentage of Underweight Children (<3 years): Selected States

States	NFHS 2 (1998-99)				NFHS 3 (2005-06)			
	Non SC/ST	SC	ST	Total	Non SC/ST	SC	ST	Total
Andhra Pradesh	36.3	43.5	46.4	38.4	30.3	37.7	41.3	32.6
Assam	41.8	32	20.5	36.2	31.8	42.6	20.8	32.1
Bihar	53.2	58.8	60.7	54.8	53.3	66.7	62.9	56.6
Gujarat	41.9	46	57.4	45.7	42.5	43.6	63	44.7
Haryana	53.2	40	NA	34.8	37	47.4	NA	40
Himachal Pradesh	42.3	52.6	42.9	44.5	33.3	43.1	34.1	35.9
Jammu & Kashmir	31.5	55.1	40	34.9	25.3	47.1	34.8	31.6
Karnataka	40.5	52.7	57.1	43.9	35.8	42	46.7	37.6
Kerala	25.6	42.9	57.1	27.2	20.6	34	56.5	23.4
Madhya Pradesh	51.4	57.5	64.6	55.4	51.0	58.5	64.2	55.8
Maharashtra	47.6	51.4	65.3	50.1	31.1	41.3	55.7	36
Odisha	51	59.9	59.9	54.9	32.5	44.9	54	40.5
Punjab	23.4	39.1	NA	29.2	17.3	34.7	NA	24.2
Rajasthan	47.5	56.5	59.4	51	37.3	46.2	45.6	40.4
Tamil Nadu	32.8	49.2	55.6	37.1	25.4	40.1	35.7	29.5
West Bengal	45.8	56.6	57.7	49.4	34.4	41.5	57.7	38.1
Uttar Pradesh	49.2	60.2	59.3	51.9	39.6	46.7	61.2	41.7
New Delhi	32.7	40.9	50	34.6	26.5	29	33.3	27.1
All India	44.1	53.3	56.3	47.1	39.4	47.8	54.4	42.6

Source: NFHS 2 and NFHS 3, estimated.

Social Profile of Caregivers and the Question of Discrimination

The data presented from NFHS surveys and available published literature showed that even though the health outcomes and access to health marginally improved for all social groups, marginal positions of people continue to be a factor that reproduces and widens disparities, especially in the context of Dalits. As a result, there is a substantial social gap in terms of health status and access to health services existing for these social groups.

Table 7.2

Births Attended by Skilled Personnel: Selected States

State	NFHS 2 (1998-99)				NFHS 3 (2005-06)			
	Non SC/ST	SC	ST	Total	Non SC/ST	SC	ST	Total
Andhra Pradesh	69.8	60.3	28.4	65.3	77.6	79.5	44.7	75.2
Assam	21.6	24.6	20	21.6	36.8	30.3	33.5	35.1
Bihar	27.1	18	6.7	23.6	33.6	17.6	16.3	28.8
Gujarat	60.8	50.7	33.9	53.5	68.1	62.9	31	63.2
Haryana	45.8	31	N.A	42	50.7	44.4	NA	49
Himachal Pradesh	41.3	36.5	33.3	40.2	51.8	38.3	40.8	47.8
Jammu & Kashmir	45.8	27.1	24.3	42.8	51.8	45.3	35.3	47.1
Karnataka	64.1	47.6	38.3	59.2	74.9	55.9	53.7	69.7
Kerala	95.3	96.4	57.1	95	100	99	88.5	99.5
Madhya Pradesh	37.5	25.9	14	29.8	44.9	37.0	15.1	35.6
Maharashtra	62.3	65.3	36.7	59.6	76	68.6	31.6	69.1
Odisha	43.3	28.1	14.8	33.5	59	40.8	17.6	44.1
Punjab	69.8	50.5	N.A	62.6	77.5	55.4	N.A	69
Rajasthan	40.9	26.9	23.7	35.7	45.6	35.2	30.2	41
Tamil Nadu	87.1	74.8	44.4	83.8	93.9	82.6	92.9	90.7
West Bengal	45.7	46.5	25.3	44.5	54.4	53.3	25.6	52
Uttar Pradesh	24.8	17.1	13.3	22.8	32.1	20.5	12.8	28.8
New Delhi	71.2	51.7	50	66.6	69.2	47.3	44.4	64.1
All India	47.2	37	23	42.8	51.8	40.5	25.6	46.8

Source: NFHS 2 and NFHS 3, estimated.

The literature shows that much of this also could be attributed to the group-specific indicators of social exclusion such as discrimination and isolation for Dalits and adivasis. Identified forms of discrimination in the sphere of health services against Dalits included separate standing lines, being ignored and kept waiting for long, discrimination in health check-up and treatment, including the avoidance of physical touch, discrimination in the delivery of the medicine and avoidance of house visits by public and private doctors and medical practitioners (Acharya, 2010). The study by

Acharya (2010: 218) revealed that 94 per cent of children in the studied village experienced discrimination from grass-root level workers in the form of 'ANMs (Auxilliary Nurse Midwifery) not entering the house'; 92 per cent in the form of 'ANMs spend less time'; 69 per cent in the form of 'ANMs do not speak gently'; and 55 per cent in the form of 'ANMs do not touch while dispensing medicine' in the villages of Gujarat and Rajasthan. The study brings out both subtle and active practices of discrimination against Dalits by healthcare providers as follows:

> During diagnosis, doctors are sometimes less probing regarding the health problem, and adopt unsympathetic attitude and rude behaviour towards Dalits. The pharmacist, while dispensing of medicine, often keep it on the window still, without explaining the doses properly. The lab technician does not touch the Dalit children during the conduct of a test, and often tests are not conducted properly; the patient is told that the 'time for rest is over', and demeaning words are used as well. While applying medicine, or putting the bandage on to a Dalit user, nurses show lack of any concern or sympathy. They do not explain to the Dalits how to take care of the wound/dressing. The ANM/LHV/VHW often do not visit the Dalit quarters for counselling or dispensing medicine, or for dissemination of information regarding a health programme, a camp, except in the case of target based programmes like immunisation, particularly polio (Acharya 2010: 221)

Shah *et al.* (2006) in a study conducted in 17 districts from Andhra Pradesh (AP), Bihar, Tamil Nadu (TN), and UP revealed the discrimination faced by Dalit women in health services in government hospitals. Five hundred Dalit women who were interviewed described their experiences of discrimination in public sphere. This study foregrounded the discriminatory practices against Dalit women and children in various spheres by doctors, nurses and village health nurses when they entered government hospital or contacted medical staff inside and outside these institutions. This study also discussed the consequences of discriminatory treatment in access to health services on Dalit women and their families. The study specifically showed that out of 375 villages surveyed, untouchability, which is prevented by law, was found to be practiced in PHCs (primary health centres) against Dalits in 68 villages (Shah *et al., 2006*: 70). Similarly, discriminatory treatment in PHCs was reported from 37 villages. Most striking practice of discrimination in the health service against Dalits that the study highlighted is the unwillingness of health workers to visit Dalit households. This was found to be prevailing in 142 out of 434 villages covered. (Shah *et al., 2006*: 72). It bears greater significance in the context that household visit by health workers is a vital part of health service system in ensuring childhood vaccination, nutrition and treatment for communicable diseases, above all health education in the rural areas. Irudayam *et al.* (2006) highlighted the discriminatory practices against Dalit women and children while accessing health services in public and private centres in the villages of AP, TN, Bihar and UP. The study shows that discrimination predominantly is reflected in the form of medical negligence. The study quotes several instances of medical negligence from these states. The narrations given in the study provide a fair account on how taboos, like untouchability, can multiply casualties for a Dalit woman at the time of prenatal, delivery and antenatal care when 'touch' by care providers is very significant. The study reports 15 such cases from these states. In some circumstances, negligence by the practitioners in the public hospital made them vulnerable to the exploitations in the private hospital, which in turn put them in to debt trap. Major types of medical negligence from public health providers that the study revealed include ignoring the patients or keeping them waiting for long, indifferent and verbal response, refusal of medical treatment and substandard medical treatment (Irudayam *et al.,* 2006: 363-66). Although Dalit women and children sought medical treatment in private clinics and hospitals out of desperation, they had to face different sets of discriminatory treatments there. It included omission of professional expertise, commission of error in exercising professional expertise, and commission of error in exercising professional expertise, alongside commercial motivation (Irudayam *et al.,* 2006: 367-68). Deshpande (2007) in a study conducted in the villages of Manvi block, Raichur district in Karnataka delineates how the status of Dalit women as an equal citizen is at stake while accessing public health services, which are supposedly universal and inclusive. Her study highlighted discriminations with regard to 'reluctance to touch', 'long waiting' and 'different treatments' for Dalits and non-Dalits in PHCs. Some studies also highlighted the discriminatory practices in associated sectors like Mid-day Meal Scheme (MDMS). For instance, Thorat and Lee (2006) brought out the practices of caste and untouchability-based discrimination and exclusion in the MDMS and the PDS (public distribution system) in selected states in India. This study, which covered 531 villages from 30 districts in Rajasthan, UP, Bihar, AP and TN, brought out various forms of discrimination and caste prejudices that operate in the functioning of these programmes and its negative implications on access to this scheme for Dalits and Adivasi children. They identified five types of discrimination against Dalit children including separate seating, separate meal, resistance of higher caste to eat the food prepared by Dalit cooks, and inferior or insufficient food in the Mid-day Meal schemes in these states (Thorat and Lee, 2006: 293). Similarly Drèze and Goyal (2003) highlighted the discrimination faced by Dalit children in accessing the service of mid-day meal.

Some studies have shown that caste can hinder an individual's health-seeking. Navaneetham and Dharmalingam (2002) reveal that proportion of lower caste women who received maternal healthcare services, such as antenatal care, iron folic acid supplements, having a trained attendant present at birth, contraceptive service, curative health services from qualified providers, and gynaecologic services, are less when compared to upper-caste women. Saroha *et al.* (2008) found that the use of maternal healthcare services, such as antenatal care, tetanus toxoid, iron folic acid supplement, trained birth attendants, and contraceptives among Hindu Dalit women in UP was very low. In certain cases, discrimination in health services and financial un-affordability determined the decisions of treatment seeking in context of Dalit families. Dalip (2005) showed that the proportion of untreated patients among Dalits and adivasis living in rural areas was higher as compared to other groups. He notes that while proportion of untreated patients among Dalits and adivasis in rural India was 18.1 per cent and 21.5 per cent respectively, it was 16.8 per cent for 'others'.

Table 7.3

Distribution of Various Healthcare and Related Occupations Across Social Groups, All India, (2011-12)

Personnel		*Rural*					*Urban*				
		ST	*SC*	*OBC*	*OTH*	*TOTAL*	*ST*	*SC*	*OBC*	*OTH*	*TOTAL*
Health professionals except nursing	Number (%)	15104 (1.3)	194008 (16.5)	493319 (41.9)	473561 (40.3)	1175992 (100)	26861 (1.5)	97344 (5.50)	548002 (30.8)	1108548 (62.3)	1780755 (100)
	Ratio to population	0.02	0.12	0.14	0.26	0.15	0.25	0.22	0.42	0.86	0.57
Nursing professional	Number (%)	2270 (1.9)	12433 (10.7)	19775 (17)	81948 (70)	116426 (100)	15169 (12.1)	34667 (27.8)	38498 (30.8)	36524 (29.3)	124858 (100)
	Ratio to population	0.00	0.01	0.01	0.05	0.02	0.14	0.08	0.03	0.03	0.04
Health Associate professional except nursing	Number (%)	63507 (8.7)	137331 (18.8)	279724 (38.3)	249457 (34.2)	730019 (100)	26646 (2.7)	240321 (24.0)	357508 (35.7)	377779 (37.7)	1002254 (100)
	Ratio to population	0.08	0.09	0.08	0.14	0.09	0.25	0.53	0.27	0.29	0.32
Nursing and midwifery associate professionals	Number (%)	23255 (4.0)	98168 (16.8)	309857 (52.9)	154378 (26.4)	585658 (100)	48101 (7.7)	118357 (19.0)	189694 (30.5)	266307 (42.8)	622459 (100)
	Ratio to population	0.03	0.06	0.09	0.09	0.08	0.45	0.26	0.15	0.21	0.20

Source: NSSO 68th round, employment and unemployment (2011-12), unit level data.

Since the literature validates discrimination by healthcare providers while delivering services, it is important to understand the social profile of caregivers in the health service system. There is no direct data available on the social profile of personnel including doctors, technicians, nurses, assistants, Accredited Social Health Activists (ASHA), etc., across the public and private sectors. However, we can get some indications from the NSSO employment and unemployment data, which provide information on health and related occupations as under the National Classification of Occupation 2004. It should be mentioned that the data does not give an absolute picture on the social group wise distribution of healthcare personnel; however is indicative of the social distribution. As Table 7.3 shows, except associate professionals of nursing, midwifery, ASHA, etc., the share of Dalits in the occupation of healthcare sector is far below as compared to other social groups and is notably under-represented as a proportion to their total population in both rural and urban India. The health-worker population ratio across social groups (Table 7.3) shows that only the 'others' group, which includes the middle and upper level castes, have adequate/over-representation among all health-related professionals including general medical practitioners, specialists doctors, trained nurses, technician and associated health staff. While this group constitutes a little less than 24 per cent of the population in rural India, their share is 40 per cent in the occupational category of health professionals, 70 per cent in nursing professionals, 34 per cent in health associate professionals and 26 per cent in nursing and midwifery associate professional. Since the data do not portray distribution across private and public sectors, one cannot argue that upper and middle level caste groups are dominant in the healthcare delivery system in the public sector. However, the overall pattern of their dominance in the sector is indicative of their strong presence in the public health delivery system as well. The over-representation of health professionals from upper and middle caste groups is starker in urban India, except in the category of nursing professionals.

Other side of the story is under-representation of certain social groups, especially SCs and STs. While STs and SCs have a population share of 11 and 21 per cent respectively in rural India, their corresponding shares in the category of health professional are 1.3 and 16.5 per cents. In rural India, the under-representation of SCs is found to be the highest in nursing profession, the most crucial group of caregivers who need to closely interact with patients in a hospital setting. Urban India also followed the similar trend of under-representation of STs in all categories. For SCs, it was pronounced most in the category of general and specialist doctors in urban areas. While the population share of SCs in urban India stands at a little less than 15 per cent, their share in the category of general doctors and specialist doctors is 5.5 per cent. In short, the data indicate that there is visible over-representation of middle and upper caste groups and under-representation of lower castes and STs in the most important sections of care providers such as doctors and nurses. The dominance of upper and middle level caste groups in the key positions of health service system hence falls in line with the argument of discrimination in hospitals by personnel from these castes.

Do such under and over-representations have meanings for the inferior health outcomes of the discriminated groups? It is difficult to completely answer this question with the limitation of data and methodology used in this paper. However, some prospective could be gained towards answering this question with the data on some of the health outcomes across social groups in various states. We would like to take data on births attended by skilled personnel as an example, which could directly explain the issue of accessibility to health services. Table 7.2 presents data on births attended by skilled personnel across social groups in some of the Indian states. The top ones among the better performing states are Kerala, TN, AP and Karnataka (The National Rural Health Mission indeed has added more states to this group by 2014) and the bottom performers among the least performing states are Bihar and UP. Kerala, being an exception, has only negligible intergroup disparity in access to skilled personnel for child birth. Similarly, the difference between SCs and non-SCs in AP is low, but stark between STs and non-STs. What is more important is the common pattern of higher level of intergroup disparity among the other top performing states

(TN and Karnataka) and the least performing states (Bihar and UP). While the differences in percentage point of access to skilled personnel at delivery between SCs and non-SCs in TN, an overall better performing state, was 10.7 in 2005-06, it was 11.6 in UP, one of the overall least performing states. This opens up the question of social profile of caregivers beyond mere issues of physical and financial access.

Let us examine an assumption to understand this linkage of discrimination and inferior health outcomes of SCs. The assumption is that adequate representation of personnel from discriminated groups in the healthcare delivery system do not completely validate the argument of the existence of a favourable environment for discrimination in health services. The social profile of caregiver in the states with higher levels of intergroup disparities despite the achievements in health outcomes and the states with negligible levels of disparities would be apt for examining this assumption. We take Bihar from the poor performer's group and TN from the better performing group. We also take AP, which showed both better performance and lower disparities between SCs and non-SCs. The social profile of healthcare personnel in Bihar and TN shows some common features (see Tables 8.4 and 8.5). Firstly, the share of health professionals including general doctors, specialists and associated health personnel from SC communities in rural Bihar and TN is far below their population share. While urban TN has relatively better representation of SCs in the category of general and specialist doctors; SCs in this category is notably underrepresented in rural areas. Secondly, there is a sweeping presence of health personnel from OBC (other backward classes) community, which is the dominant social group (politically, educationally and economically) in rural Bihar and TN due to the changed caste equations with the relocation of middle and upper caste to urban areas. The urban healthcare landscape of these states is also dominated by non-SC groups, except the category of general and specialist doctors in TN. What is more striking in these states is the very low representation of SCs as compared to the all India averages at the lower end of healthcare delivery system, which includes health workers and ASHAs. These health personnel play a critical role in the preventive and promotive healthcare such as vaccination, nutrition and pre- and post-natal care. They are also pillars of the ambitious National Rural Health Mission (NRHM), which has a special focus on direct contact with people and communities through house visits. The social profile of healthcare professionals in Bihar and TN shows that SCs are notably underrepresented in rural areas and hence validates the argument that there is a conducive environment of discrimination existing based on the lines of purity and pollution of caste system.

Table 7.4

Distribution of Various Healthcare and Related Occupations Across Social Groups, Bihar (2011-12)

Personnel	*Rural*				*Urban*				
	SC	*OBC*	*OTH*	*Total*	*ST*	*SC*	*OBC*	*OTH*	*Total*
Health professionals except nursing	2088	105035	11176	118299	1019	831	11060	3971	16881
%	1.77	88.79	9.45	100	6.04	4.92	65.52	23.52	10
Health associate professional except nursing		11870	68679	80549		27406	26573	15120	69099
%		14.74	85.26	100		39.66	38.46	21.88	100
Nursing and midwifery associate professionals	602	7989		8591			12287	4605	16892
%	7.01	92.99		100			72.74	27.26	100

Source: NSSO 68th round, employment and unemployment (2011-12), unit-level data.

It is important to examine the social profile of health personnel in AP, which showed both better health outcomes and less disparity between SCs and non-SCs. Although AP and TN are in the group of better performing states, the former has better distribution of personnel from SC community in all sections of healthcare personnel in the rural areas (see Table 7.6), which could in turn explain the low intergroup difference in health outcomes to an extent. Most importantly, the state has a better representation from SC community in the category of nursing and midwifery associate personnel, which is an important part of preventive and promotive care. Similarly, SCs are adequately represented in the diagnostic and therapeutic services both rural and urban areas, although representation of general and specialist doctors are not adequate for SCs in urban areas.

Table 7.5

Distribution of Various Healthcare and Related Occupations Across Social Groups, Tamil Nadu (2011-12)

Personnel	*Rural*			*Urban*				
	SC	*OBC*	*Total*	*ST*	*SC*	*OBC*	*OTH*	*Total*
Health professionals except nursing		36096 (100)	36096 (100)		47871 (37.14)	57458 (44.57)	23576 (18.29)	128905 (100)
Health associate professional except nursing	874 (1.95)	44027 (98.05)	44901 (100)	2169 (2.51)		84197 (97.49)		86366 (100)
Nursing and midwifery associate professionals		42436 (100)	42436 (100)		10632 (13.56)	63399 (80.87)	4362 (5.56)	78393 (100)

Note: Figure is parentheses are in per cent.

Source: NSSO 68th round, Employment and Unemployment (2011-12), unit-level data.

Concluding Remarks

Denial of access to health services for marginalised groups occurs primarily due to two reasons. First is the physical and financial inaccessibility to services both in public and private sectors. Second is the practice of discrimination by health service providers with regard to denial of admission in the PHCs in villages and/or through discriminatory access to public and private health centres. The published studies presented in the paper have highlighted the discrimination in public health services. It should also be noted that public health services are the only options for poor Dalits to seek healthcare as far as financial affordability is concerned. This paper, drawing from data on healthcare personnel across social group, substantiates the argument of discrimination in hospitals. It indicates that dominance of caregivers from upper and middle level caste groups creates an environment that supports discrimination.

Table 7.6

Distribution of Various Healthcare and Related Occupations Across Social Groups, Andhra Pradesh (2011-12)

Personnel	*Rural*					*Urban*			
	ST	*SC*	*OBC*	*OTH*	*Total*	*SC*	*OBC*	*OTH*	*Total*
Health professionals except nursing		4861	38725	31866	75452		24146	28367	52513
%		6.44	51.32	42.23	100		45.98	54.02	100
Health Associate professional except nursing	2743	46876	55294	46459	151372	19400	28705	12963	61068
%	1.81	30.97	36.53	30.69	100	31.77	47.00	21.23	100
Nursing and midwifery associate professionals	258	1764	10081		12103	18814	77682		96496
%	2.13	14.57	83.29		100	19.50	80.50		100

Source: NSSO 68th round, Employment and Unemployment (2011-12), unit-level data.

The similarities in social profile of healthcare personnel, which is unfavourable to SCs in Bihar, a less performing state and TN, a better performing state, is indicative of the facilitative environment for discrimination of SCs in the rural areas. This is further verified by the example of AP, which is a better performing state with less intergroup disparities and relatively adequate distribution of health personnel from SCs at all levels of healthcare delivery system in rural areas. Since discrimination has a strong dimension of personal experience, one cannot argue that such dominance is an absolute condition for discrimination. It is contextual and also varies from places to places and person to person. However, one cannot discount the possibility of exclusion with this lop sided distribution unfavourable to SCs taking the pervasive nature of caste system and its continuity in one form or another and above all its potential to recreate itself in any context without losing the original forms and contents. The Indian health service system at present is not equipped with addressing this issue. This is a challenge to the agenda of inclusion in the health services.

The possible way to overcome this is to ensure adequate representation of healthcare personnel at all levels of the health delivery system. It is debatable whether such practices would further reinforce the existing caste relations in the villages. However, health being an area of urgent attention, immediate strategy should be to ensure adequate representation of healthcare personnel from excluded communities. Lower access to healthcare services is a complex problem and discrimination is only a part of it. The data on health-worker population ratio given in the paper showed that there is significant shortage of doctors, specialists, qualified nurses, health workers and ASHAs in India. Therefore, it is incorrect to assume that inclusion of members of excluded communities would help increase overall access. However, it will undoubtedly reduce discrimination. Since prejudices based on caste are intense in the Indian society, there should also be adequate legal safeguards to check discrimination. Flagship programmes, like NRHM must have a special focus on social inclusion. This should be reflected in resource allocation since localities where Dalits and Adivasis reside still have severe shortage of health facilities, personnel and resources. Further, the inclusion agenda needs to be integrated in the written-down roles of duty-bearers such as ASHA, ANM, Panchayati Raj Institutions (PRIs), NGOs (non-governmental organisations), district administration and the state.

References

Acharya, S. Sanghmitra (2007). *Healthcare Utilisation Among Dalit Children: Understanding Social Discrimination and Exclusion: A Study in Selected Villages of Gujarat and Rajasthan.* UNICEF-IIDS Study. New Delhi: Indian Institute of Dalit Studies.

———. (2010). "Caste and Patterns of Discrimination in Rural Public Healthcare Services", in Sukhadeo Thorat and Katherine Newman (ed.), *Blocked by Caste: Economic Discrimination in Modern India*. New Delhi: Oxford University Press. pp.208-29.

Baraik, V.K. and P.M. Kulkarni (2014). "Health and Nutritional Status", in S. Thorat and N.S. Sabharwal (eds.), *Bridging the Social Gaps: Perspectives on Dalit Empowerment*. New Delhi: Sage. pp.155-68.

Baru, R., A. Acharya, S. Acharya, A.K. Shivkumar and K. Nagaraj (2010). "Inequities in Access to Health Services in India: Caste, Class and Region", *Economic & Political Weekly* 45(38): 49-58. 24 September.

Borooah, V.K. (2010). "Inequality in Health Outcomes in India: The Role of Caste and Religion", in Sukhadeo Thorat and Katherine Newman (eds.), *Blocked by Caste: Economic Discrimination in Modern India*. New Delhi: Oxford University Press. pp.179-207.

Borooah, V.K., N.S. Sabharwal and S. Thorat (2012). "Gender and Caste Based Inequality in Health Outcomes in India", *IIDS Working Paper Series* 6(3). New Delhi.

Das, B.M., Soumya Kapoor, Denis Nikitin (2010). "A Closer Look at Child Mortality among Adivasis in India", *Policy Research Working Paper No* 5231. The World Bank South Asia Region.

Dasgupta, Purnamita and S.K. Thorat (2009). "Will India's Attainment of MDGs be an Inclusive Process?", *IIDS Working Paper Series* III(02). New Delhi.

Deshpande, Mita (2007). *Through the Lens of Universality: Dignity, Trust and Exclusion in the Era of Health Sector Reforms, Social Policy in a Globalising World: Developing a North-South Dialogue.* Paper presented at University of Florence, Italy. 6-8 September.

Dilip, T.R. (2005). "Extent of Inequality in Access to Health Services in India", in L.V. Gangolly, R. Duggal and A. Shulka (eds.), *Review of Healthcare in India, Centre for Enquiry into Health and Allied Themes*. Mumbai. pp.247-68.

Drèze, Jean and Aparajita Goyal (2003). "Future of Mid-Day Meals", *Economic and Political Weekly* 38(44): 4673-83.

Irudayam, A., J.P. Mangubhai and J.G. Lee (2006). *Dalit Women Speak Out: Violence against Dalit Women in India.* Volume I and II. New Delhi: National Council for Dalit Human Rights.

Kulkarni, P.M. and V.K. Baraik (2003). "Utilisation of Healthcare Services by Scheduled Castes in India", *Working Paper* No. *39*. New Delhi: Indian Institute of Dalit Studies (IIDS).

Ram, F, K.B. Pathak and K.I. Annamma (1998). "Utilisation of Healthcare Services by the Underprivileged Section of Population in India- Results from NFHS", *Demography India* 30(2): 128-47.

Navaneetham, K. and A. Dharmalingam (2002). "Utilisation of Maternal Healthcare Services in Southern India", *Social Science & Medicine* 55(10): 1849-69.

Saroha, E., M. Altarac, L. Sibley (2008). "Caste and Maternal Healthcare Service Use Among Rural Hindu Women in Maitha, Uttar Pradesh, India", *Journal of Midwifery & Women's Health* 53(5): 41-47.

Shah, Ghanshyam, Harsh Mander, Sukhadeo Thorat, Satish Deshpande and Amita Baviskar (2006). *Untouchability in Rural India*. New Delhi: Sage Publications.

Thorat, Sukhadeo (2007). "Human Poverty and Socially Disadvantaged Groups in India", *Discussion Paper Series*, 18. New Delhi: Human Development Resource Centre, UNDP.

Thorat, Sukhadeo and Joel Lee (2006). "Food Security Schemes and Caste Discrimination", *IIDS Working Paper* 1(3).

Others:

National Family Health Survey, Round 2 (1998-99) and Round 3 (2005-06). Mumbai: International Institute for Population Sciences.

National Sample Survey Organisation (2011-12). "Employment and Unemployment", 68th Round. New Delhi- Ministry of Statistics and Programme Implementation, Government of India.

8

RAM KUMAR MISHRA, GEETA POTARAJU and PRANAV GARIMELLA

Monitoring Health System Improvements through a Results Framework Document Mechanism

A Case Study of India

Introduction

The issues confronting healthcare systems are often very challenging and complex especially in the context of public sector. Delivering effective healthcare to citizens with heterogeneous needs becomes a major challenge for any government. This coupled with the declining socio-economic factors puts further pressure on the fragile and fragmented health service delivery systems. Many developing and developed countries have set their focus on establishing robust healthcare systems, thereby making it a part of their governance reform agenda.

The World Health Organization (WHO) has been, in accordance with its mandate, been putting out statistical data of health and health system of all its 194 member states. For this part of the article, however, we will concern ourselves with only health infrastructure and health personnel and try to discern where India stands among its peers not only in its own neighbourhood, but across the globe as well. Health infrastructure and personnel are the cornerstones of a good health system. Infrastructure like hospitals, beds, doctors, nurses, and pharmacists are essential for ensuring good health service delivery. The WHO in its 2013 statistical report focuses on the 'health gap' between the developed and developing countries around the globe. To show this is in greater contrast, we will look at a selection of developed and developing countries from across different continents.

We want to see India's health infrastructure and expenditure in the context of its neighbours, its global competitors and developed economies in Europe and North America. This could potentially lead us to an understanding on where we are and what needs to be done henceforth. This could also shed light on where we must critically focus our efforts in the health sector.

Health Personnel and Infrastructure

Healthcare personnel are an essential element in the healthcare system of any country. Adequate numbers of doctors and nurse have to be available in both urban and rural areas, working with proper infrastructure to deliver healthcare appropriately. Failing which, outcomes from the health system are impossible. We will look at the growth of the health sector in India, in terms of infrastructure and personnel.

Health service delivery in India is done through different systems in both rural and urban India. At the rural level, a network of sub-centres, PHCs (Primary Health Centres) and CHCs (Community Health Centres) provide health services. While in urban areas, hospitals and dispensaries, etc., provide health services.

There are three kinds of healthcare service units at the rural level in India,[1] namely,

1. *Sub-Centres*: These centres provide the first level of health service at the community level in rural areas. The sub-centres are manned by one ANM (Auxiliary Nurse Midwife) and one MHW (Male Health Worker). Along with this, one LHW (Lady Health Worker) is in charge of six sub-centres. The centres are responsible for interpersonal communication to bring about behavioural change at the community level. These centres are also responsible for providing services related to maternal and child health, family welfare, nutrition, immunisation, diarrhoea control

1. *Health and Family Welfare Statistics in India, 2013* (https://nrhm-mis.nic.in/PubFWStatistics%20 2013/Executive%20Summary%20and%20Overview.pdf)

and control of communicable diseases programmemes. Men, women and children go to these centres for drugs for minor ailments and other essential health needs.

2. *PHCs:* These centres are the first point of contact between the village communities and the Medical Officer (MO). The medical officer is assisted by 14 other staff and the centres are referral centres to six sub-centres, with 4-6 beds for patients. It is responsible for curative, preventive, promotive and family welfare services. PHCs are essential cogs in the health service machinery in rural India. The government is proposing massive expansion of capacity and volume of PHCs in the coming years.
3. *CHCs:* These centres are established and maintained by the state governments and as per standards it is supposed to be manned by four medical specialists i.e., surgeon, physician, gynaecologist and pediatrician, supported by 21 paramedical and other staff. It has 30 in-door beds with one OT (operation theatre), X-ray, and labour room and laboratory facilities and serves as a referral centre for four PHCs. It provides facilities for emergency obstetrics care and specialist consultations. Indian public health (IPH) standards lays down that this CHC is to be manned by six medical specialists, including anaesthetics and an eye surgeon (for 5 CHCs), supported by 24 paramedical and other staff including two nurse midwives in the present system of seven nurse midwives.

In 2005,[2] all over India there were 23,236 PHCs according to the Ministry of Health and Family Welfare (MoHFW). This number grew to 24,448 in 2013, which is an increase of 5.22 per cent over the nine-year period. While the numbers of operational PHCs have increased since 2005, the centres have faced challenges with vacancy and shortfall of personnel. In 2005, the sanctioned strength of doctors in PHCs was 24,476; the same in PHCs, in 2013, increased by 36.9 per cent to 33,515 doctors. However, there were 4,282 vacancies in 2005, which is a vacancy rate of 17

2. *Health and Family Welfare Statistics in India, 2013 (https://nrhm-mis.nic.in/PubFWStatistics%20 2013/Section%20G%20-%20Infrastructure.pdf)*

per cent for that year. Vacancies increased to 7,467 vacancies in 2013, an increase of nearly 75 per cent. The same is the case with shortfalls in requirement of doctors. The numbers indicate an ever increasing trend in terms of the shortfall of doctors in the PHCs. The required strength of doctors in PHCs in 2005 stood at 23,236, which increased to 24,448 in 2013, but it is interesting to note that the shortfall in 2005 was 1,004 and the same number increased to 2,225 in 2013, meaning that the shortfall of doctors for PHCs more than doubled in 9 years. This is a serious concern as the vacancies are showing an upward trend.

According to the Ministry's data there were 146,026 sub-centres in 2005 which grew to 151,684 in 2013, an increase of 3.87 per cent; and 3,346 CHCs were operating in 2005 which grew to 5,187 in 2013, an increase of 55 per cent over the nine-year period.

Global Context

The figures in terms of infrastructure and personnel in the health sector are a mixed bag in India. There are some encouraging signs and some not so. An international comparison will set the context for where India stands among its international peers. We begin with our immediate neighbours, moving on to our global competitors and finally to the developed nations.

South Asian Association for Regional Co-operation (SAARC) and Health Sector Personnel

In our immediate neighbourhood, the SAARC region, India is doing reasonably well in terms of health sector personnel. For the purpose of this paper, we have taken the following countries for the comparison, namely, Pakistan, Sri Lanka, Bangladesh and Bhutan. The data we used is the statistical data brought out by the WHO in 2013 for the years 2005-2012. The figures are calculated per 10,000 people from the respective countries. India is ranked second among the countries chosen above, in terms of physicians per 10,000 people. Pakistan leads the group with regard to the number of physicians. Pakistan recorded 8.1 physicians for every 10,000 people between 2005 and 2012, while India recorded 6.5 physicians for every 10,000 people, according to the data. Sri Lanka, Bangladesh and Bhutan followed in the same order.

With reference to nursing and midwife personnel, India again comes in behind Sri Lanka, which has 19.3 nursing and midwife personnel for every 10,000 people. India has 10 nursing and midwife personnel per 10,000 population. The rest of the countries in this group have significantly lesser nursing and midwife personnel in comparison to India and mainly Sri Lanka. While the data on pharmacists is not available for Pakistan, India has the highest number of pharmacists in this group with 5.4 pharmacists for every 10,000 people. Bangladesh, Sri Lanka and Bhutan follow in the same order.

Figure 8.1

Health System Personnel in SAARC Countries (2005-2012)[3]

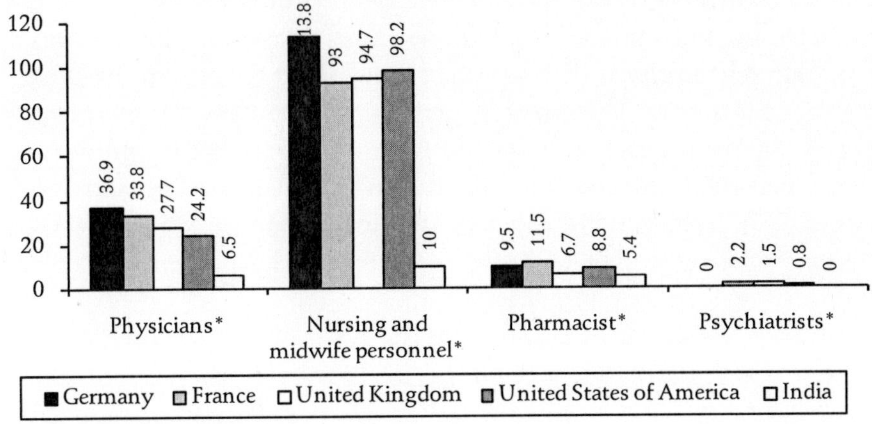

Note: * Per 10,000 population.
Source: *World Health Statistics 2013*, WHO.

BRICS and Health Sector Personnel

India is doing reasonably well in the context of the Indian subcontinent in terms of healthcare personnel, but India is a big nation and is competing on the global stage with other developing countries like China, Russia, Brazil and South Africa, a group that is now commonly referred to as the BRICS. The BRICS comprises the developing economies with similar potential and who are vying for the same resources and goals; they also find themselves facing similar problems internally. Hence, it is essential to know how we

3. *World Health Statistics 2013 (http://www.who.int/gho/publications/world_health_statistics/EN_WHS2013_Full.pdf)*

are doing in the context of these nations. According to the WHO data, India ranked the lowest among the BRICS countries in terms of physicians. Russia had the highest number of physicians with 43.1 physicians per 10,000 people, followed by Brazil (17.6), China (14.6), South Africa (7.6) and then India (6.5).

With reference to nursing and midwife personnel again, India finds itself at the bottom while Russia tops the list. There are 85.2 nursing and midwife personnel in Russia for every 10,000 people, while in India the same number is 10. China is closer to India than Russia in terms of nursing personnel with 15.1 nurses and midwives for every 10,000 people, while Brazil is closer to Russia than India with 64.2 nurses and midwives per 10,000 people. The figures for South Africa are not available for nursing and midwife personnel. However, the scenario is very different in terms of pharmacists. India and Brazil lead the BRICS countries in terms of pharmacist per capita. There are 5.4 pharmacists per 10,000 people each in India and Brazil. This number is significantly more than the other countries like Russia (0.8), China (2.6), and South Africa (2.5). India is not doing very well in comparison with the BRICS nations when it comes to healthcare personnel, but there is a silver lining in the form of pharmacists.

Figure 8.2

Health System Personnel in BRICS Countries (2005-2012)[4]

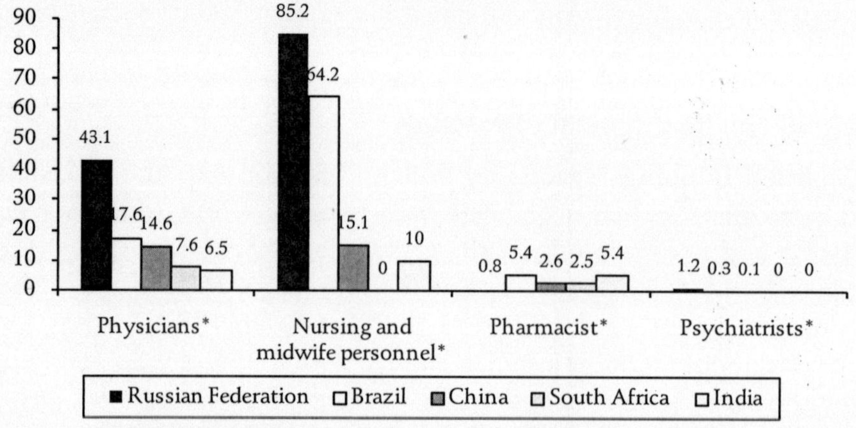

*Note:** Per 10 000 population.
Source: *World Health Statistics 2013*, WHO.

4. Ibid.

Developed Countries and Health Sector Personnel

India is found wanting in this group of nations. The developed economies show remarkable figures in terms of healthcare personnel. Germany leads the pack with an astounding 36.7 physicians for every 10,000 people, followed by France (33.8), UK (27.7), USA (24.2) and India (6.5) in that order. It's easy to see the stark difference in the figures in terms of nursing as well, Germany again leads with 113.8 nursing staff per 10,000 people; the other developed countries have figures similar to Germany. We saw India leading the SAARC and BRICS countries in the numbers of pharmacists; here too India manages to hold its ground with the other developed countries. India has 5.4 pharmacists per 10,000 people, while the other countries recorded figures like: France (11.5), Germany (9.5), USA (8.8) and UK (6.7). Significant steps need to be taken to ensure the improvement of health systems in India in terms of personnel and monitor improvement of the systems.

Figure 8.3

Health System Personnel in Developed Countries (2005-2012)[5]

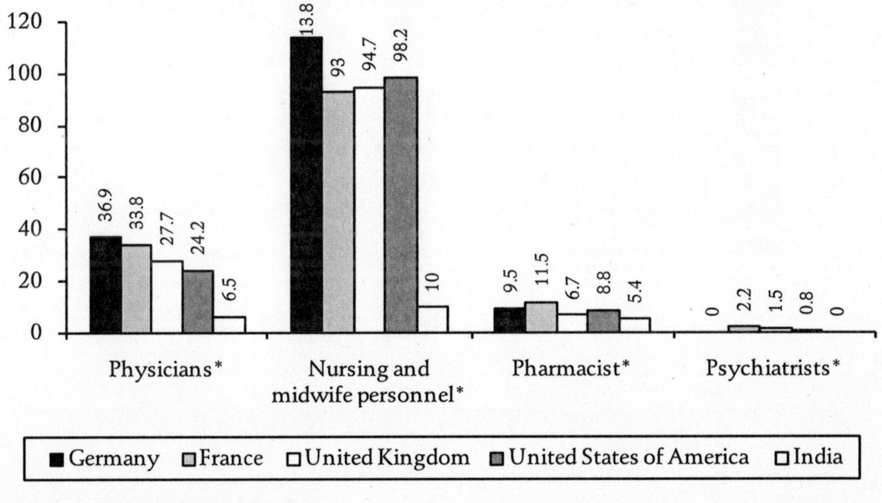

Note:* Per 10,000 population.

Source: *World Health Statistics 2013*, WHO.

---

5. Ibid.

Health System Infrastructure

The next important step towards building a robust healthcare system is infrastructure. In a country with a large population, adequate number of hospitals and hospital beds, along with healthcare technology like radiotherapy units, are essential. This section deals with the progress of India in terms of infrastructure in the global context.

SAARC and Health System Infrastructure

Among its immediate neighbours, India is placed in the middle. Sri Lanka has the highest number of hospital beds per 10,000 people between 2005-2012, followed by Bhutan (18), India (9), Bangladesh and Pakistan (6). Psychiatric beds and radiotherapy units per capita are very small figures in these countries.

Figure 8.4

Health System Infrastructure in SAARC[6]

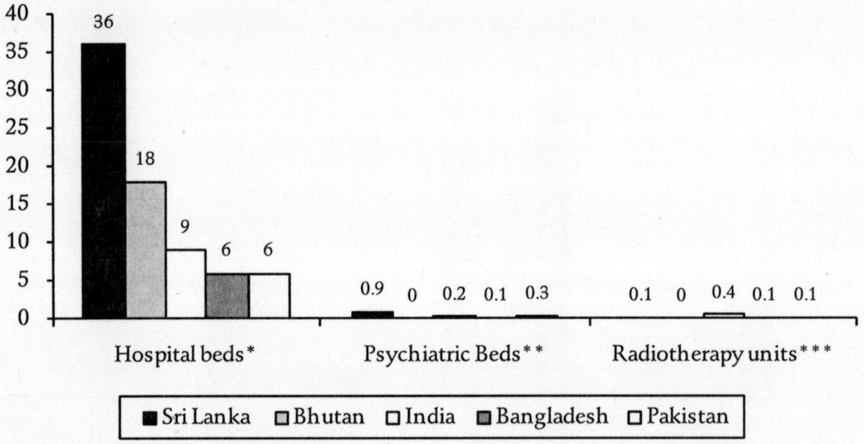

Note: *: Per 10000 population (2005-2012); **: Per 100000 population (2005-2012); ***: units per million population 2010.

Source: *World Health Statistics 2013*, WHO.

BRICS and Health System Infrastructure

The BRICS nations are doing much better than India in terms of hospital beds with Russia topping the list with 97 hospital

6. Ibid.

beds for every 10,000 people, while China was next in this group with 39 beds per 10,000 people. The numbers for South Africa are not available. In this grouping too, psychiatric beds do not have significant figures, except for Russia, which is way ahead of the other countries in this category.

Figure 8.5

Health System Infrastructure in BRICS[7]

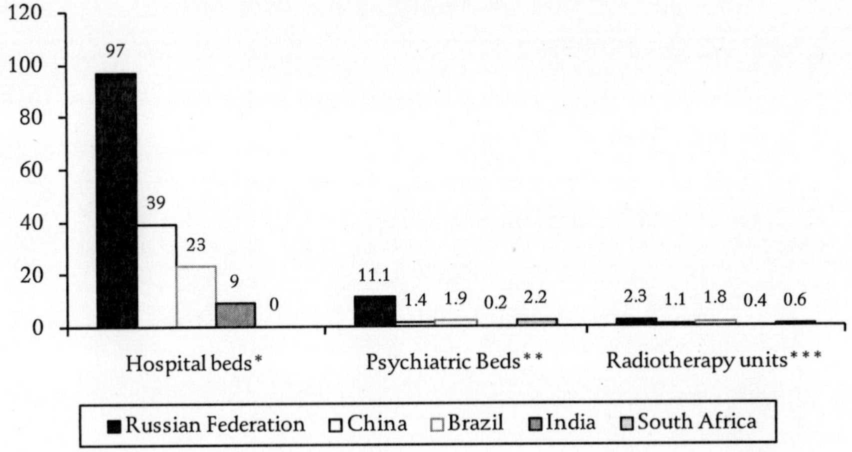

Note: *: Per 10000 population (2005-2012); **: Per 100000 population (2005-2012); ***: units per million population 2010.

Source: *World Health Statistics 2013,* WHO.

Developed Countries and Health System Infrastructure

This group of countries is a little surprising since we see France and Germany with relatively high numbers of hospital beds, but US and UK show low numbers compared to even developing countries. In terms of psychiatric beds and radiotherapy, each of these developed nations recorded significant numbers showing probably indicating the maturity of their healthcare systems.

Health Expenditure

Health expenditure is another critical link for an effective healthcare delivery system. Health expenditure typically gets diverted towards infrastructure and personnel. In the earlier section,

7. Ibid.

we examined the shortfalls and problems area in terms of health infrastructure and personnel. The way to fill the existing gaps in the present system, capital must be invested where needed. The private sector as well as the government spends on health. For this paper, in order to examine the state of health expenditure in India, among its neighbours, international rivals and finally the developed economies, we will be considering the following data points:

a. Total expenditure on health as per cent of the GDP (gross domestic product.

b. Private expenditure on health as a percentage of total expenditure on health.

c. General government expenditure on health as percentage of total government expenditure.

Figure 8.6

Health System Infrastructure in Developed Countries[8]

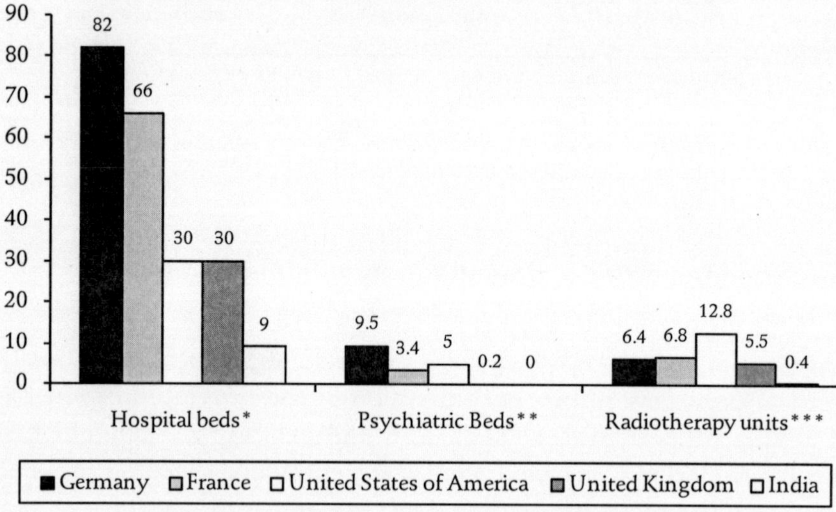

Note: *: Per 10000 population (2005-2012); **: Per 100000 population (2005-2012); ***: units per million population 2010.

Source: *World Health Statistics 2013,* WHO.

These statistics should give us a rough idea of how the different nations are looking at health expenditure and their outlook towards

8. Ibid.

healthcare. The WHO in its 2013 statistical data published the health expenditure among the member states in the decade from 2000 to 2010. This gives us a rough trend on the issue.

Health Expenditure in the SAARC Region

First we take a look at India and its immediate neighbours, the SAARC countries, which consist of all developing nations and note how the developing economies of the region are spending on health.

In this group of nations we can immediately see that with the exception of Bangladesh, all the other countries have experienced a decline in the total expenditure on health as a part of the GDP. While Sri Lanka and Pakistan have only seen a slight decline in the health expenditure as a per cent of the GDP, India and Bhutan have underone noticeable drops in health expenditure.

Private expenditure on health as per cent of the total health expenditure also reveals a very interesting picture. Excepting Bhutan, expenditure in other countries on health by the private sector is quite high. But there seems to be a declining trend of private expenditure in India and Pakistan, while Sri Lanka is showing an upward trend of health expenditure by the private sector.

A similar analysis, when done to the BRICS nations, shows a different picture. Among the BRICS nations, India is the only country where the expenditure on health as a percentage of its GDP has reduced over the decade between 2000 and 2010. Every other country has seen a steady rise in health expenditure by their governments as a percentage of the total government expenditure, except India. The private sector expenditure on health, however, is a mixed bag with some countries such as China, Brazil, India and South Africa experiencing decreasing trend of expenditure.

Among the developed nations again, we find an increasing trend of expenditure on health as a percentage of the country's GDP; India is an exception here too. We see the same increasing trend of government spending on health increasing as a percentage of its total government expenditure. The governments of all the developed nations are moving towards increased health expenditure.

Table 8.1

Health Expenditure in the SAARC Region

Member States	Total Expenditure on Health as per cent of Gross Domestic Product		Private Expenditure on Health as per cent of Total Expenditure on Health		General Government Expenditure on Health as per cent of Total Government Expenditure	
Year	2000	2010	2000	2010	2000	2010
Sri Lanka	3.7	3.5	51.6	54.4	6.8	6.9
Bhutan	6.9	4.3	20.7	15.4	12.2	8.4
India	4.3	3.7	74	71.8	7.4	6.8
Bangladesh	2.8	3.7	61	63.5	7.6	8.9
Pakistan	1.1	1	41.3	23.4	2.4	3.4

Source: *World Health Statistics 2013*, WHO.

Table 8.2

Health Expenditure in the BRICS Countries

Member States	Total Expenditure on Helath as per cent of Gross Domestic Product		Private Expenditure on Health as per cent of Total Expenditure on Health		General Governemnt Expenditure on Health as per cent of Total Government Expenditure	
Year	2000	2010	2000	2010	2000	2010
Russian Federation	5.4	6.5	40.1	41.3	12.7	9.7
China	4.6	5	61.7	45.7	10.9	12.1
Brazil	7.2	9	59.7	53	4.1	10.7
India	4.3	3.7	74	71.8	7.4	6.8
South Africa	8.1	8.7	57.7	53.4	10.9	12.4

Source: *World Health Statistics 2013*, WHO.

What is interesting to note in this particular grouping is that the private sector expenditure on health is quite low in all the European countries, below 50 per cent of the total expenditure on health. The US and India are the only countries which have high private sector spending on health. However, even in these two nations, namely, US and India where the private sector spending on health is high, there is a decreasing trend of the same. This is a cause for worry in India as not only is the health expenditure as a percentage of GDP lower than the developed nations, but the figure is falling too.

Systemic Challenges in Health System: Indian Context

A study by WHO (2007-08) ranks India in 171 position out of 175 in public health spending, which is even lower than some of the sub-Saharan African countries. The spending on healthcare is about 5.2 per cent of the GDP in a country with around 1 billion population. The private sector spends 4.3 per cent while the share of the public sector is only 0.9 per cent on public health.

The Tenth Plan document clearly indicates barriers in terms of governance systems, governance structures, roles, functions, capacities, and mindset issues. Some of the critical elements indicated in the document which have direct effect on the service delivery are lack of sensitivity, transparency and accountability in many facets of the working of state machinery, particularly those that have an interface with the public; lack of credibility—the gap between the intent and the actions of some institutions in society; inadequate system of incentives/disincentives for people (particularly for a civil servant); and existence of a significant number of voiceless poor with little opportunities for participating even in institutions of local self-governance.[9]

Table 8.3

Health Expenditure in the Developed Countries

Member States	*Total Expenditure on Health as Per cent of Gross Domestic Product*		*Private Expenditure on Health as Per cent of Total Expenditure on Health*		*General Government Expenditure on Health as Per cent of Total Government Expenditure*	
Year	*2000*	*2010*	*2000*	*2010*	*2000*	*2010*
Germany	10.4	11.5	20.5	23.2	18.3	18.5
France	10.1	11.7	20.6	23.1	15.5	15.9
United States of America	13.4	17.6	56.8	51.8	17.1	19.9
United Kingdom	7	9.6	21.2	16.8	15.1	15.9
India	4.3	3.7	74	71.8	7.4	6.8

Source: *World Health Statistics 2013*, WHO.

9. *Tenth Five Year Plan 2002-2007*, Planning Commission. *(http://planningcommission.nic.in/plans/planrel/fiveyr/10th/10defaultchap.htm).*

The National Health Policy (NHP) 2002 of Government of India (GoI) spells out the critical aspects of healthcare in India. There is a clear mention about the issue of poor access to the public health system for the more vulnerable sections of society in comparison with the advantaged sections of the society. This is particularly true for women, children and the socially disadvantaged sections of society. The statistics given in Table 8.4 highlights the handicap suffered in the health sector on account of socio-economic inequity in India.[10]

Table 8.4

Differentials in Health Status among Socio-Economic Groups

Indicator	*Infant Mortality/1000*	*Under-5 Mortality/1000*	*Per cent Children Underweight*
India	70	94.9	47
Social Inequity			
Scheduled Castes	83	119.3	53.5
Scheduled Tribes	84.2	126.6	55.9
Other Disadvantaged Group	76	103.1	47.3
Others	61.8	82.6	41.1

Source: *National Health Policy*, Government of India, 2002.

The focus of the NHP 2002 is to evolve an inclusive framework for delivery of health services by strengthening healthcare and improving accessibility to all sections, thus reducing inequities and allowing the disadvantaged sections of society a fairer access to public health services. The NHP 2002 also focuses on generating beneficiary interest in the public health system, which will ensure a more effective supervision of the public health personnel through community monitoring, along with the regular administrative line of control.

The National Rural Health Mission, the flagship programmeme of GoI highlights some of the key barriers and challenges in public health systems. These include lack of spending capacity in the system, lack of synergy between vertical health and family

10. *National Health Policy 2002*, Ministry of Health and Family Welfare. *(http://www.MoHFW.nic.in/showfile.php?lid=2325).*

welfare programmemes at operational levels, lack of community ownership of public health programmemes impacting levels of efficiency, accountability and effectiveness, and lack of integration of sanitation, hygiene, nutrition and drinking water issues, needed in the overall sectoral approach for health and striking regional inequalities.

In the service delivery aspect, there are always two sides to the problem that needs to be examined—the supply side and the demand side. The supply side aspect includes the institutions that are involved in the delivery of services to the common man and are primarily the provider side. The demand side includes the citizens/common man who accesses these services. In the case of India, there are a number of problems both in terms of the supply side and demand side. On the supply side, certain glaring issues create barriers for efficient health service delivery. Various studies highlight certain glaring problems with the health systems. The primary healthcare facility, which is the first point of contact for the poor at the field level, is often not located at an appropriate place for the poor to reach as and when required. There is no proper road connectivity in many places which is coupled by lack of proper means of transport to reach the health facility. Poor HR (human resource) systems and practices have been identified as a major concern plaguing the health systems. Lack of motivation is noticed among the medical personnel to provide timely and effective services in the backward and tribal areas, due to lack of adequate monetary incentives, lack of adequate skill and training, poor monitoring, and lack of convergence and coordination among various departments. These collectively create a major concern for effective functioning of the health system.

System Improvement Initiatives in India

India, has taken major strides to cope with the problems related to systems in public service delivery, especially in the past few decades which has impacted the administration and has brought about considerable pressure on the systems to change and perform to ensure satisfaction of the stakeholders. Major changes have been witnessed with the Chief Secretaries Conference (1997) and the First and the Second Administrative Reforms Commission (1966;

2005) that has suggested recommendations for revamping the public administration systems in the country. The major agenda set by GoI under the reform programme is to streamline service delivery, especially to the poor, by ensuring effective administration at the state level, district level and sub-district levels, by overhauling the delivery systems and making them more responsive and citizen friendly.[11]

The primary objective of NRHM which was launched by GoI in 2005, has been to provide effective healthcare to the rural population, along with the disadvantaged groups including women and children, by improving access, enabling community ownership, strengthening public health systems for efficient service delivery, enhancing equity and accountability and promoting decentralisation. Health system strengthening is an integral part of the health revamping plan by the GoI for improving health service delivery to the poorest and the remotest corners of the country, as indicated in the Preamble.

There are many novel experiments undertaken by various state governments in the country in order to streamline and strengthen health service delivery especially to the disadvantaged groups. In India, several states have adopted critical initiatives to streamline and strengthen health service delivery, with special focus on disadvantaged groups, such as Emergency Response Management System (108 Ambulance Service), community-centric approach to responsive healthcare, etc.

In the Indian context, strengthening of the healthcare system systems has been a critical governance reform agenda for more than two decades accounting for the steep rise in population. This has posed a tremendous challenge for the government to improve health service delivery system which is still inaccessible to a majority of the population. The Tenth Plan identifies the need to empower marginalised groups in India who live in remote or hilly areas and the felt need to identify a system to ascertain whether these targeted populations have the necessary awareness about

11. Second Administrative Reforms Commission, Department of Administrative Reforms and Public Grievances, Ministry of Personnel, PG & Pensions, GoI. *(http://arc.gov.in/)*

the available health care facilities. Capacity building of individuals through human development strategies, involving access to education, basic healthcare facilities and opportunities of livelihood is of utmost importance where, media and the voluntary sector have a very important role in exposing and bringing the issue to the fore-front.

Government Performance Monitoring Tool Adopted by India

To effectively establish performance culture, the GoI established a Performance Management Division (PMD) in the Cabinet Secretariat in January 2009. The key mandate of the PMD is to establish mechanisms for performance monitoring and performance evaluation in government departments on a regular basis. It involves preparation of a Results Framework Document (RFD) by each department every year. The RFD highlights the departmental objectives and priorities for the current financial year as well as the achievements of the department against those pre-specified targets indicated in the RFD at the end of the year.

Thus, RFD works as an accountability tool and provides the required focus by government departments to deliver effectively and efficiently. It helps in bringing about objectivity to the working of government departments and facilitates measurement of performance of the government agencies so as to make necessary improvements wherever required. RFD as a tool also provides an opportunity to the agencies to demonstrate to the citizens at large the efforts being taken up by them for improving their service delivery and in the bargain enhancing their credibility and developing citizen perception on government services.

A RFD is essentially a record of understanding between a minister representing the people's mandate, and the secretary of a department responsible for implementing this mandate. This document contains not only the agreed objectives, policies, programmes and projects, but also success indicators and targets to measure progress in their implementation. To ensure the successful implementation of agreed actions, RFD may also include necessary operational autonomy. RFD seeks to address three basic questions: (a) What are ministry's/department's main objectives for the year?

(b) Which are the actions proposed by the department to achieve these objectives? (c) How would someone know at the end of the year the degree of progress made in implementing these actions? That is, what are the relevant success indicators and their targets that can be monitored?

The GoI categorised all the Central government departments/ministries into six syndicates and the health ministry has five departments including AYUSH, Health and Family Welfare, Health Research, AIDS Control and Ministry of Women and Child Development (Annexure A-8.1). In the sections below, the RFD developed by MoHFW, GoI has been discussed in detail (also see, Annexure A-8.2). RFD primarily focuses on bringing about system enhancement by identifying critical areas for improvements and during the financial year focusing on improving these aspects. RFD has two main purposes: (a) move the focus of the department from process-orientation to result-orientation, and (b) provide an objective and fair basis to evaluate department's overall performance at the year end. This helps the department to monitor system delivery efficiency and make necessary corrections for enhancing efficiency. The six sections contained in the RFD are detailed as below.

Section 1: Ministry's/Department's Vision, Mission, Objectives and Functions

This section provides the context and the background for the RFD. Creating a vision and mission for a department is a significant enterprise. Ideally, vision and mission should be a by-product of the strategic planning exercise undertaken by the department. Both concepts are interrelated and much has been written about them in the management literature. We will look at the RFD for the Department of Health and Family Welfare (2014-15) as an example of how vision and mission is framed in the RFD.

Department of Health and Family Welfare

Vision

According to the latest RFD, the department envisions ensuring the availability of equitable, accessible and affordable health services across regions and communities with special focus on under-served population and marginalised groups. Through a vision statement, the department states its priorities clearly and moves firmly on the set direction.

Mission

The department's Mission is the nuts and bolts of the vision. For example, for the year 2014-15, the Department of Health and Family Welfare set out six points in its mission statement, such as:

a. Establishing comprehensive primary healthcare delivery system and well-functioning linkages with secondary and tertiary healthcare delivery system

b. Improvement of maternal and child health outcomes.

c. Reduction in the incidence of communicable diseases and formulation of strategy to reduce the burden of non-communicable diseases.

d. Achieving population stabilisation through reduction in population growth rate.

e. Development of training capacity to improve quality of human resources for health with adequate skill mix at all levels.

f. Regulation of health service delivery and promotion of rational use of pharmaceuticals in the country.

It is clear from the above points that the mission statement in the RFD is a more specific statement compared to the vision statement and is set to be achieved at the medium term. The mission statement is a set of deliverables which the department sets for itself but at the same time, the mission statement differs from specific indicators (success indicators) in the RFD which are short-term goals and annually set and keep on changing.

Objectives

Objectives represent the developmental requirements to be achieved by the department in a particular sector through a selected set of policies and programmes over a specific period of time (short, medium long).

For example, the objectives of the MoHFW states that: (a) universal access to primary healthcare for all sections of society with effective linkages to secondary and tertiary healthcare. (b) improving maternal and child health. (c) reducing overall disease burden of the society.

Functions

The functions of the department as envisaged under the law are to be listed in this section and these functions must be consistent with the allocation of business rules for the department/ministry. This section represents the legal/administrative reality of the department and should not be a list of functions that the department aspires to carry out.

For example, the MoHFW in its RFD for the year 2014-15 lists out the following functions:

a. Policy formulation on issues relating to health and family welfare sectors.
b. Reduction of the burden of communicable and non-communicable diseases.
c. Focus on development of human resources through appropriate medical and public health education.
d. Providing regulatory framework for matters in the concurrent list of the Constitution *viz.*, medical, nursing and paramedical education, pharmaceuticals, etc.

Section 2: *Inter se* Priorities Among Key Objectives, Success Indicators and Targets

The heart of the RFD is section 2 of the document (provided in Annexure A-8.2 and A-9.3). Annexure A-8.2 in section 2 has 7 columns, which are objectives, weight, action, success indicators, unit, weight, and target/criteria value. The broad objectives of the department/ministry are assigned weights, and are further linked to actions and success indicators and finally to evaluation targets in the RFD.

For example, in the 2014-15 RFD for the MoHFW, universal access to primary healthcare services for all sections of society with effective linkages to secondary and tertiary health is the first objective for that RFD annual cycle. There are three actions to be carried out with respect to this objective such as: (a) strengthening of health infrastructure; (b) augmentation of availability of human resources in identified high priority districts; and (c) capacity building.

Further, these actions have several success indicators linked to each action. For example for the first action, namely, strengthening of health infrastructure—the success indicators that are to be achieved are as follows: (a) operationalisation of 24x7 facility at PHC level out of the total number of 24,000 PHCs; (b) operationalisation of CHCs and SDHs (sub-divisional hospitals) into First Referral Units (FRU) out of the total number of 5,800 CHCs and SDHs; (c) Increase in the number of patients transported over the baseline figure for 2013-14; (d) Establishment of special new born care units in the remaining district hospitals.

The other actions linked to the objectives have similar success indicators linked to them with assigned weightages; all weightages assigned to the success indicators add up to the total weightage of the RFD objectives.

The RFD targets should be aligned with Plan priorities and be consistent with departmental budget as well as the outcome budget. A well-framed RFD document should be able to account for a majority of the budget. Towards this end, departments must ensure that all major schemes, relevant mission mode projects and Prime Minister's Flagship Programmes are reflected in the RFD.

Evaluation Methodology

At the end of the year, achievements of the government department is compared with the set targets, and composite score is determined. Annexure A-8.3 provides an example from the health sector. Only one objective has been chosen to show the evaluation method and calculation of score under the RFD system.

The Raw Score for Achievement in column 6 is obtained by comparing the achievement with the agreed target values. For example, the achievement for first success indicator (percentage increase in PHCs) is 15 per cent. This achievement is between 80 per cent (Good) and 70 per cent (Fair) and hence the Raw Score is 75 per cent (Table 8.5). The Weighted Raw Score for Achievement in Column 6 is obtained by multiplying the Raw Score with the relative weights. Thus for the first success indicator, the Weighted Raw Score is obtained by multiplying 75 per cent by 0.50. This gives us a Weighted Raw Score of 37.5 per cent. Finally, the Composite Score is calculated by adding up all the Weighted Raw Scores for achievements. The Composite Score is calculated to be 84.5 per cent. The Composite Score shows the degree to which the government department in question was able to meet its objectives. The fact that it got a score of 84.5 per cent in our hypothetical example implies that the department's performance *vis-à-vis* this objective was rated as 'Very Good.'

The methodology outlined above is transcendental in its application. Various government departments will have a diverse set of objectives and corresponding success indicators. Yet at the end of the year, every department will be able to compute its Composite Score for the past year. This Composite Score will reflect the degree to which the department was able to achieve the promised results.

Table 8.5

Composite Scores

Departmental Rating	*Value of Composite Score*
Excellent	100-96%
Very Good	95-86%
Good	85–76%
Fair	75-66%
Poor	65% and below

RFD Process and Timelines

A. Beginning of the Year

- At the beginning of each financial year, with the approval of the Minister concerned, each Department prepares a RFD consistent with these guidelines.

- To achieve results commensurate with the priorities listed in the RFD, the Minister in-charge approves the proposed activities and schemes for the ministry/department. The Minister In-charge also approves the corresponding success indicators (key result areas—KRAs, and success indicators) and time-bound targets to measure progress in achieving these objectives.
- Based on the proposed budgetary allocations for the year in question, the drafts of RFDs should be submitted to PMD by 5 March every year. The RFD should be aligned to the Plan priorities and outcome budget. To ensure uniformity, consistency and coordinated action across various departments, the Cabinet Secretariat reviews these drafts and provides feedback to the ministries/departments concerned.
- These draft RFDs are then reviewed by an independent group of non-government experts. This group is called the Ad-hoc Task Force (ATF) and consists of former secretaries to GoI, distinguished academicians, former CEOs (Chief Executive Officers) of public enterprises, and private sector domain experts.
- After the review by ATF, the RFDs are sent for approval of the High Power Committee (HPC) on government performance consisting of the Cabinet Secretary (Chair), Finance Secretary, Expenditure Secretary, Secretary (Planning Commission), and Secretary (Performance Management).
- The final versions of all RFDs, approved by HPC, should be put up on the websites of the respective Ministries by 15 April each year.
- The revised RFD of each department/ministry should be submitted to the Cabinet Secretariat, by the 15 April, each year.

B. During the Year

After six months, the RFD, as well as the achievements of each ministry/department against the performance goals laid down at the beginning of the year, is reviewed by the HPC on government performance and, if required, the Secretary of the department concerned could be invited for resolving any disagreements. At this stage, the RFD may have to be reviewed and the goals reset, taking into account the priorities at that point of time. This enables us to factor in unforeseen or *force majeure* circumstances such as drought conditions, natural calamities or epidemics. The report of the HPC on government performance is to be submitted to the Prime Minister, through the concerned minister, for further action as deemed necessary.

C. End of the Year

- At the end of the year, all ministries/departments will review and prepare a report listing the achievements of their ministry/department against the agreed results in the prescribed format. This report will be required to be finalised by the 1 May, each year.
- After scrutiny by the Cabinet Secretariat, these results will be placed before the Cabinet for information by 1 June, each year.

RFD Submission Process

All RFDs must be submitted to the Performance Management Division, Cabinet Secretariat, by 5:30 pm. RFD data should be entered in the Results Framework Management System (RFMS) and to be locked at 5:30 pm. To avoid last minute computer glitches, early entry of the relevant RFD is much appreciated.

Conclusion

To conclude, the system of RFD has provided a comprehensive performance evaluation tool to the departments for constant monitoring and providing scope for performance improvement.

Apart from identifying success indicators by departments and monitoring them on a regular basis, the PMD has identified areas for strengthening the processes in the departments. Three key initiatives have been undertaken by the GoI for the central government departments/ministries, like ISO 9001 certification by departments in a phased manner. In the initial phase, departments have been advised to pick up part of their overall functions and work on standardising them.

The second big initiative taken up by GoI is the development of corruption action plan by government departments, wherein a general understanding is developed on the key processes thereby giving rise to malpractices in the system and initiatives necessary to plug these malpractices.

The third big system improvement initiative is the development of innovation action plan. The departments are encouraged to identify key areas for innovation and improvements, and are also exposed to various initiatives taken by other departments for learning and replication.

Annexure A-8.1

Categorisation of Departments

Syndicate	*S. No.*	*Ministry/Department*
Syndicate 1 (Agriculture & Rural Development)	1	D/o Agriculture & Cooperation
	2	D/o Agricultural Research & Education
	3	D/o Animal Husbandry, Dairying & Fisheries
	4	M/o Food Processing Industries
	5	D/o Rural Development
	6	M/o Panchayati Raj
	7	M/o Environment & Forests
	8	D/o Land Resources
	9	M/o Drinking Water & Sanitation
	10	M/o Earth Sciences
	11	D/o Official Language
Syndicate 2 (Human Development)	1	D/o Health & Family Welfare
	2	D/o AYUSH
	3	D/o Health Research
	4	D/o AIDS Control
	5	D/o School Education & Literacy
	6	D/o Higher Education
	7	M/o Women & Child Development
	8	D/o Sports
	9	D/o Youth Affairs
	10	M/o Statistics & Programmeme Implementation
	11	D/o Justice
	12	D/o Legal Affairs
	13	Legislative Department
Syndicate 3 (Resosurce Management)	1	D/o Chemicals and Petrochemicals
	2	D/o Fertilisers
	3	D/o Pharmaceuticals
	4	M/o Coal
	5	M/o Mines
	6	M/o New & Renewable Energy
	7	M/o Petroleum & Natural Gas
	8	M/o Power
	9	M/o Steel
	10	M/o Water Resources
	11	D/o Disinvestment

Syndicate 4 (Trade, Industry & Services)	1	D/o Commerce
	2	M/o Textiles
	3	D/o Industrial Policy & Promotion
	4	M/o Corporate Affairs
	5	D/o Heavy Industries
	6	D/o Public Enterprises
	7	M/o Micro, Small & Medium Enterprises
	8	M/o Tourism
	9	M/o Culture
	10	M/o Information & Broadcasting
	11	D/o Personnel & Training
	12	D/o Defense Production
	13	D/o Defense Research & Development
Syndicate 5 (Infrastructure Management)	1	M/o Civil Aviation
	2	D/o Telecommunications
	3	D/o Posts
	4	D/o Information & Technology
	5	M/o Dev. of North-Eastern Region
	6	M/o Road Transport & Highways
	7	M/o Shipping
	8	D/o Science & Technology
	9	D/o Scientific & Industrial Research
	10	D/o Bio-Tech
	11	D/o Space
	12	M/o Railways
Syndicate 6 (Social Welfare)	1	D/o Food & Public Distribution
	2	D/o Consumer Affairs
	3	M/o Housing and Urban Poverty Alleviation
	4	M/o Labor & Employment
	5	M/o Minority Affairs
	6	M/o Overseas Indian Affairs
	7	M/o Social Justice & Empowerment
	8	M/o Tribal Affairs
	9	M/o Urban Development
	10	D/o Administrative Reforms & Public Grievances
	11	D/o Pension & Pensioners Welfare
	12	D/o Ex-Servicemen Welfare
	13	D/o Disability Affairs

Health Ministry has following departments under the RFD system:

Syndicate 2 (Human Development)	1	D/o Health & Family Welfare
	2	D/o AYUSH
	3	D/o Health Research
	4	D/o AIDS Control
	5	M/o Women & Child Development

Annexure A-8.2

Inter se Priorities among Key Objectives, Success Indicators and Targets

Objective	Weight	Action	Success Indicator	Unit	Weight	Target/Criteria Value				
						Excellent	Very Good	Good	Fair	Poor
						100%	90%	80%	70%	60%
(1) Universal access to primary health care services for all sections of society with effective linkages to secondary and tertiary health care	30.00	(1.1) Strengthening of health infrastructure	(1.1.1) Operationalisation of 24x7 facility at PHC level out of the total number of 24000 PHCs	%	5.00	39	38.5	38	37.5	37
			(1.1.2) Operationalisation of CHCs and SDHs into First Referral Units (FRU) out of the total number of 5800 CHCs and SDHs	%	5.00	37	36.5	36	36.5	35
			(1.1.3) Increase in the number of patients transported over the baseline figure for 2013-14	%	5.00	5	4	3	2	1
			(1.1.4) Establishment of speical new born care units in remaining District Hospitals	%	3.00	45	40	35	30	25
		(1.2) Augmentation of availability of Human Resources in identified High Priority Districts	(1.2.1) Deployment of new ANMs	Number	3.00	450	400	350	300	250
			(1.2.2) Deployment of new doctors/specialists	Numbers	3.00	250	200	150	100	70
			(1.2.3) Deployment of new staff nurses	Number	4.00	450	400	350	300	250
		(1.3) Capacity building	(1.3.1) ASHA Trained (up to Module VI & VII)	Number	2.00	150000	130000	110000	90000	70000

contd...

Objective	Weight	Action	Success Indicator	Unit	Weight	Target/Criteria Value				
						Excellent	Very Good	Good	Fair	Poor
						100%	*90%*	*80%*	*70%*	*60%*
(2) Improving maternal and child health	8.00	(2.1) Promoting institutional deliveries	(2.1.1) Percentage point increase in institutional Deliveries over the baseline of 31 March 2014 in high priority districts	%	3.00	12	10	8	6	4
		(2.2) Targeting full immunisation (age group of 0-12 months)	(2.2.1) Target children immunised	%	3.00	88	87	86	85	84
			(2.2.2) Percentage point increase in targeted children immunised over the baseline of 31 March 2014 in high priority districts	%	2.00	12	10	8	6	4
(3) Focusing on population stabilisation in the country	8.00	(3.1) Promoting post partum IUCD	(3.1.1) Increase in IUCD insertions over previous financial year	%	2.00	16	15	14	13	12
		(3.2) Registration of pregnancy in first trimester	(3.2.1) Increase in the registration over the previous finanial year	%	2.00	11	10	9	8	7
			(3.2.2) Increase in the registration over the previous financial year in high priority districts	%	2.00	11	10	9	8	7
		(3.3) National Inspection & Monitoring Committee (PCPNDT Act) visits	(3.3.1) Increase in number of visits over previous financial year	%	2.00	300	270	240	210	180

Objective	Weight	Action	Success Indicator	Unit	Weight	Target/Criteria Value				
						Excellent	Very Good	Good	Fair	Poor
						100%	90%	80%	70%	60%
(4) Developing human resources for health to achieve health goals.	9.00	(4.1) Strengthening and upgradation of government medical colleges	(4.1.1) Completion of upgradation of identified medical colleges (post graduation)	Number	3.00	26	25	19	18	17
		(4.2) Upgradation of government medical college for increase in MBBS seats	(4.2.1) Completion of upgradation of identified medical colleges (MBBS)	Number	1.00	10	8	6	4	2
		(4.3) Establishment of new medical colleges attached with district/referral hospital	(4.3.1) MoU with state governments for establishment of new medical colleges in 58 identified districts	Number	1.00	58	55	52	49	45
		(4.4) Setting up 1 National Institute of Paramedical Sciences (NIPS) and 8 Regional Institutes of Paramedical Sciences (RIPS)	(4.4.1) Commencement of work for NIPS	Date	1.00	31/12/2014	31/12/2014	31/12/2014	31/12/2014	31/12/2014
			(4.4.2) Commencement of work for RIPS	Number	1.00	5	4	3	2	1
		(4.5) Establishment of Nursing institutes at various levels	(4.5.1) Commencement of teaching in new ANM/GNM institutes	Number	1.00	35	30	25	20	15

contd...

Objective	Weight	Action	Success Indicator	Unit	Weight	Target/Criteria Value				
						Excellent	Very Good	Good	Fair	Poor
						100%	*90%*	*80%*	*70%*	*60%*
			(4.5.2) Increase in number of nurses completing the course	Number	1.00	810	729	648	576	486
(5) Reducing overall disease burden of the society	20.00	(5.1) Reduce incidence of malaria cases	(5.1.1) Annual Parasile incidence (API)	Per 1000 population	2.00	0.6	0.7	0.8	0.9	1.0
		(5.2) Reduce incidence of Filariasis	(5.2.1) Endemic districts (250) achieving micro filaria rate of <1%	Number	2.50	230	225	220	215	210
		(5.3) Reduce incidence of *Kala-azar*	(5.3.1) BPHCs reporting less than 1 case of *Kala-azar* per 10000 population	Number	2.50	500	495	490	485	480
		(5.4) Reduce incidence of Leprosy	(5.4.1) High burden districts having annual new case defection rate of more than 10 per lakh population (cumulative)	Number	2.00	55	50	44	39	33
			(5.4.2) Reconstructive surgeries conducted	Number	1.00	2800	2500	2240	1960	1680
		(5.5) Control of tuberculosis (TB)	(5.5.1) New Sputum Positive (NSP) success rate	%	1.00	90	88	85	75	70
			(5.5.2) Default rate amongst CAT-II patients	%	1.00	125	13	13.5	14	15
			(5.5.3) MDR TB cases notified put on treatment	%	1.00	90	85	80	75	70

Objective	Weight	Action		Success Indicator		Unit	Weight	Target/Criteria Value				
								Excellent	Very Good	Good	Fair	Poor
								100%	90%	80%	70%	60%
		(5.6)	Reduction in prevalence of blindness	(5.6.1)	Cataract surgeries performed (in lakhs)	Number	0.50	70	65	60	55	50
				(5.6.2)	Spectacles to school children screened with refractive error (in lakhs)	Number	0.50	9	8	7	6	5
		(5.7)	Facilities for diagnosis and treatment of cancer	(5.7.1)	Strengthening operationalisation of Tertiary Cancer Centres	Number	1.00	8	6	4	2	1
		(5.8)	Ensure availability of minimum mental health care services	(5.8.1)	Starting academic session in Centres of Excellence	Number	1.00	4	3	2	1	0
				(5.8.2)	Approval for starting up of PG courses in mental health specialities	Number	1.00	25	20	15	10	5
		(5.9)	Opportunistic screening, diagnosis and management of diabetes, cardiovascular diseases and stroke	(5.9.1)	Set up additional NCD clinics and Cardiac Care Units in district hospitals	Number	1.00	170	150	130	100	80
		(5.10)	Provide health care to the elderly population	(5.10.1)	Establishment of Regional Geristric Centres	Number	1.00	4	3	2	1	0

contd...

Objective	Weight	Action	Success Indicator	Unit	Weight	Target/Criteria Value				
						Excellent	Very Good	Good	Fair	Poor
						100%	90%	80%	70%	60%
			(5.10.2) Establishment of National Institute of Aging, AIIMS Delhi & MMC, Chennai	Number	1.00	2	1	0.75	0.50	0.00
(6) Strengthening secondary and tertiary health care	10.00	(6.1) Setting up of AIIMS	(6.1.1) Make hospitals at new AIIMS functional for the purpose of MBBS teaching	Number	6.00	6	5	4	3	2
		(6.2) Upgradation of government medical colleges (Phase I & II)	(6.2.1) Completion of construction work	Number	2.00	6	5	4	3	2
		(6.3) Upgradation of 39 medical colleges in third phase of PMSSY	(6.3.1) Award/start of work	Number	2.00	9	8	6	4	3
* Efficient functioning of the RFD System	3.00	Timely submission of RFD Draft for 2015-16 for approval	On-time submission	Date	2.0	05/03/2015	06/03/2015	09/03/2015	10/03/2015	11/03/2015
		Timely submission of results for 2013-14	On-time submission	Date	1.0	01/05/2014	02/05/2014	03/05/2014	06/05/2014	07/05/2014

	Objective	Weight	Action	Success Indicator	Unit	Weight	Target/Criteria Value				
							Excellent	Very Good	Good	Fair	Poor
							100%	90%	80%	70%	60%
*	Enhanced transparency/ improved service delivery of ministry/ department	3.00	Rating from independent audit of implementation of Citizens'/Clients' Charter (CCC)	Degree of implementation of commitments in CCC	%	2.0	100	95	90	85	80
			Independent audit of implementation of Grievance Redress Management (GRM) system	Degree of success in implementing GRM	%	1.0	100	95	90	85	80
*	Reforming administration	8.00	Update departmental strategy to allign with revised priorities	Date	Date	2.0	01/11/2014	02/11/2014	03/11/2014	04/11/201	05/11/2014
			Implement agreed milestones of approved mitigating strategies for reduction of potential risk of corruption (MSC)	% of implementation	%	1.0	100	90	80	70	60
			Implement agreed milestones for implementation of ISO 9001	% of implementation	%	2.0	100	95	90	85	80
			% of responsibility centres with RFD in RFMS	Responsibility centres covered	%	1.0	100	95	90	85	80

contd...

Objective	*Weight*	*Action*	*Success Indicator*	*Unit*	*Weight*	*Target/Criteria Value*				
						Excellent	*Very Good*	*Good*	*Fair*	*Poor*
						100%	*90%*	*80%*	*70%*	*60%*
		Implement agreed milestones of approved innovation Action Plans (IAPs)	% of implementation	%	2.0	100	90	80	70	60
* Improve compliance with the financial accountability framework	1.00	Timely submission of ATNs on Audit paras of C&AG	Percentage of ATNs submitted within due date (4 months) from date of presentation of report to Parliament by CAG during the year.	%	0.25	100	90	80	70	60
		Timely submission of ATRs to the PAC Sectt. on PAC Reports.	Percentage of ATRS submitted within due date (6 months) from date of presentation of report to Parliament by PAC during the year.	%	0.25	100	90	80	70	60
		Early disposal of pending ATNs on Audit paras of C&AG reports presented to Parliament before 31/3/2014	Percentage of outstanding ATNs disposed off during the year.	%	0.25	100	90	80	70	60
		Early disposal of pending ATRs on PAC reports presented to Parliament before 31/3/2014	Percentage of outstanding ATRS disposed off during the year	%	0.25	100	90	80	70	60

Note: * Mandatory Objective(s).

Annexure A-8.3

Examples of Performance Indicators: Department of Health and Family Welfare

S. No.	*Objective*	*Action*	*S. No.*	*Success Indicators*
1	Universal access to primary healthcare services for all sections of society with effective linkages to secondary and tertiary healthcare	Strengthening of health infrastructure	1	Operationalisation of 24×7 facility at PHC level
			2	Equipping districts with mobile medical units
			3	Operationalisation of CHCs into First Referral Units (FRUs)
			4	Establishment of Special New Born Care Units
			5	Establishment of stabilisation units for new borns
			6	Establishment of New Born care corners in PHCs
			7	Operationalisation of 108 Emergency Referral Transport Ambulance
			8	Construction of new sub-centre building
		Strengthening of community Involvement	1	Holding village health and nutrition days
			2	Preparation of annual District Health Action Plan (DHAP)
		Augmentation of availability of human resources	1	Deployment of new ANMs
			2	Depolyment of new doctors/ specialists
			3	Deployment of new staff nurses
			4	Deployment of new paramedical staff

.contd...

		Capacity building	1	ASHA Training (up to Module V)
			2	Personnel trained on IMNCI
			3	Doctors trained on LSAS
			4	Doctors trained on EMoC
			5	ANMs/SNs/LHVs trained as SBA
			6	Navjat Shishu Suraksha Karyakram (NSSK)
2	Improving maternal and child health	Promote institutional deliveries		Institutional deliveries as a percentage of total deliveries
		Support through Janani Suraksha Yojana (JSY)		JSY beneficiaries
		Tageting full immunisation (age group of 0-12 months)		Target children immunised
3	Focusing on population stabilisation in the country	Female sterilisation		Female sterilisation acceptors
		Male sterilisation		Male sterilisation acceptors
		Intra Uterine Device (IUD) insertion		IUD insertion
4	Developing human resources for health to achieve health goals.	Strengthening and upgradation of government medical colleges	1	Number of medical colleges approved for upgradation
		Setting up 1 National Institute of Paramedical Sciences (NIPS) and 8 Regional Institutes of Paramedical Sciences (RIPS)	2	Finalisation of land and approval of DPR for NIPS
			3	Approval of DPR for RIPS
		Establishment of nursing institutes at various levels	4	Approval for DPRs for new ANM schools
			5	Approval for DPRs for new GNM schools

5	Reducing overall disease burden of the society	To reduce incidence of malaria cases		Annual Parasite Incidence (API)
		To reduce incidence of Filariasis		Coverage of eligible people under Mass Drug Administration (MDA)
		To reduce incidence of *kala-azar*		Number of BPHCs reporting less than 1 case of *Kala-azar* per 10000 population out of 514 such BPHCs
		To reduce incidence of leprosy		Annual New Case Detection Rate (ANCDR)
				Reconstructive surgeries conducted
		Control of tuberculosis		New Sputum Positive (NSP) success rate
				New Sputum Positive (NSP) case detection rate
		Reduction in prevalence of blindness		Cataract surgeries performed
				Number of spectacles to school children screened with refractive error
				Collection of donated eyes for corneal transplantation
		Strengthening facilities for diagnosis and treatment of cancer		Development of district cancer facilities
				Strengthening of tertiary centres
		Establishment of tobacco testing laboratories		Operationalisation of tobacco testing labs
		Ensure availability of minimum mental healthcare services	1	Establishment of Centres of Excellence
			2	Approval for starting up of PG courses in mental health specialities
		Opportunistic screening, diagnosis and management of diabetes, cardiovascular diseases and stroke		Set up NCD clinics and Cardiac Care Units in district hospitals

.contd...

				Screening of NCDs at CHCs and below initiated in districts
				NCD risk factor surveillance in selected districts
		Provide healthcare to the elderly population		Set up Geriatric OPD and ward at district hospitals
				Strengthening of regional geriatric centres
6	Strengthening secondary and tertiary healthcare	Setting up of 6 AIIMS like institutions	1	Completion of construction work in medical colleges
			2	Completion of work in hospitals
		Upgradation of 13 government medical colleges	3	Upgraded facilities at government medical colleges made functional
		Up-gradation of 6 government medical colleges in Phase II	4	Start of construction of work in 5 medical colleges

Annexure A-8.4

Example of Performance Evaluation at the End of the Year

Column 1	*Column 2*	*Column 3*		*Column 4*		*Column 5*					*Column 6*		
						Target/Criteria Values							
Objective	*Action*	*Criteria/ Success Indicators*		*Unit*	*Weight*	*Excellent*	*Very Good*	*Good*	*Fair*	*Poor*	*Achievement*	*Raw Score*	*Weighted Raw Score*
						100%	90%	80%	70%	60%			
Better rural health	Improve Access to primary health care	1	% Increase in number of primary health care centers	%	.50	30	25	20	10	5	15	75%	37.5%
		2	% Increase in number of people with access to a primary health center within 20 kms	%	.30	20	18	16	14	12	18	90%	27%
		3	Number of hospitals with ISO 9000 certification by 31 December 2009	%	.20	500	450	400	300	250	600	100%	20%
Composite Score =													84.5%

Annexure A-8.5

Mandatory Success Indicators for 2014-15

	Objective	*Actions*	*Success Indicator*
1	Efficient functioning of RFD system	Timely submission of results for 2013-2014	On-time submission
2	Enhanced transparency/ improved service delivery of ministry/ department	Rating from independent audit of implementation of Citizens'/ Clients' Charter (CCC)	Degree of implementation of commitments in CCC
		Independent audit of implementation of Grievance Redress Management (GRM) system	Degree of success in implementing GRM
3	Reforming administration	Update departmental strategy to align with revised priorities	Date
		Implement agreed milestones of approved mitigating strategies for reduction of potential risk of corruption (MSC).	% of Implementation
		Implement agreed milestones for implementation of ISO 9001	% of implementation
		% of responsibility centres with RFD in RFMS	Responsibility centres covered
		Implement agreed milestones of approved Innovation Action Plans (IAPs).	% of implementation
4	Improve compliance with the Financial Accountability Framework	Timely submission of ATNs on audit paras of C&AG	Percentage of ATNs submitted within due date (4 months) from date of presentation of the report to Parliament by CAG during the year.
		Timely submission of ATRs to the PAC Sectt. on PAC reports.	Percentage of ATRS submitted within due date (6 months) from date of presentation of report to Parliament by PAC during the year.
		Early disposal of pending ATNs on audit paras of C&AG reports presented to Parliament before 31/3/2014.	Percentage of outstanding ATNs disposed off during the year.
		Early disposal of pending ATRs on PAC reports presented to Parliament before 31/3/2014	Percentage of outstanding ATRS disposed off during the year.

9

SUBODH KANDAMUTHAN

Incentives to Retain Health Staff in Rural Areas in India

Introduction

One of the major problems of lower health status in countries like India is the lack of dedicated manpower in the rural areas (Sundararaman and Gupta, 2010; Rao and Ramani, 2011, Rao *et al.*, 2010). Any improvement in health status can happen mostly with the presence and dedicated work of the health officials in the rural areas where the poor and marginal groups reside. According to the Global Health Work Force Guidelines:

> The growing gap between the supply of healthcare professionals and the demand for their services is a critical issue facing governments, managers and professionals seeking to improve international health and development. There are a number of complex and interrelated factors that contribute to the ongoing workforce shortage globally, including poorly resourced health systems, unsatisfactory working conditions and inadequate human resources management.

Inequitable distribution of doctors and other staff with high concentration in urban cities negatively affects the public health objective of health for all. Thus, it is one of the main concerns for most health policymakers, particularly in developing countries (Wibulpolprasert and Pengpaibon, 2002).

The shortage of health staff in rural areas is an area of concern not just in India but in all countries of the world. According to World Health Organization (WHO) (2006) and Caldwell and Kingma (2007), there are complex and interrelated factors that contribute to the ongoing workforce shortage globally. These include:

a. Insufficiently resourced and neglected health systems.

b. Poor HR (human resources) planning and management practices and structures.

c. Unsatisfactory working conditions characterised by:

- heavy workloads;
- lack of professional autonomy;
- poor supervision and support;
- long working hours;
- unsafe workplaces;
- inadequate career structures;
- poor remuneration/unfair pay;
- poor access to needed supplies, tools and information; and
- limited or no access to professional development opportunities.

Various countries use different strategies to overcome certain manpower issues in the health sector. Wilson *et al.* (2009) have looked into retaining health staff strategies in rural areas in South Africa and found that short-term benefits of many coercive measures to retain health staff, like compulsory rural service, making rural practice compulsory for registration, limiting foreign nationals to rural practice, etc., are there, but very few evidence of long-term benefits and its positive impact are noticed. However the study highlights that there is merit in implementation of well-defined selection and education policies, along with incentive and support schemes that may have value.

Rural Health West, an NGO (non-governmental orgainisation)in Australia, in 2013, looked into the various ways to retain health staff for primary healthcare in rural Australia. The study found that:

> Recruitment and retention are a result of a complex interaction between many factors. Overall, health workforce shortages in rural areas require an integrated, sustained and evidence-based approach by universities, governments and civil society

to address educational, organisational, financial, social and other factors associated with recruitment and retention of health professionals in rural areas. Although much has been learned from the research into medical workforce, the focus needs to move beyond the medical profession to cover dental, nursing, allied health and associated professions, with more integration across disciplines. Improved study designs should be implemented for the evaluation of interventions to increase the rural health workforce.

Henderson and Tulloch (2008) have noted in the review on Pacific and Asian countries that severe shortage of health workers is a critical issue that must be addressed as an integral part of strengthening health systems. They found that the factors that contributed to the shortage of skilled health workers included lack of effective planning, limited health budgets, migration of health workers, inadequate numbers of students entering and/or completing professional training, limited employment opportunities, poor working conditions, weak support and supervision, and limited opportunities for professional development.

Lehmann *et al.* (2008) looked at issues of appointing health staff in remote and rural areas in middle and low income countries. The study found complex factors that influence attraction and retention of health staff, but there is a need to greatly emphasise on living environments, working conditions and development opportunities. The study also noted that there are no set answers to the problem of attraction and retention and is only through learning about what works in terms of fit between problem analysis and strategy and effective navigation through the politics of implementation that any headway will be made against the almost universal challenge of staffing health service in remote rural areas.

Mbemba *et al.* (2013) did a review of nurse retention at the global level by reviewing existing literature. The study aim was to synthesise the current evidence on effectiveness of the interventions to promote nurse retention in rural or remote areas and thereafter to present taxonomy of potential strategies in order to improve nurse retention in those regions. The study identified four types of retention strategies for nurses in rural and remote areas that included: a) education and continuous professional development interventions, b) regulatory interventions, c) financial incentives, and d) personal and professional support. The study highlighted the need for rigorous evaluation of all retention strategies

Daniels *et al.* (2007) looked into the factors associated with rural retaining of health staff in the United States (US) among the graduates in various health professional programmes. The important factors that led to retention of graduates in rural areas are rural training programme, financial incentives, professional opportunity and desirability of rural locations.

Incentives in India

In India, under the National Rural Health Mission (NRHM) of the Government of India (GoI), different measures have been initiated by the Centre and state governments to retain health staff in rural areas (Sundararaman and Gupta, 2010). They include:

1. Appointment of staff on contractual basis under the NRHM.
2. Reorganisation of human resources from state cadre to district cadre.
3. Provision of incentives to health staff in rural areas.
4. Compulsory rural service for medical doctors.
5. Rotational transfer policy from rural to urban areas, and
6. Having Indian systems of medicine doctors to work in rural primary health centres (PHCs).

Table 9.1 presents the various strategies undertaken by different states in order to retain health staff in rural areas.

Providing incentives to retain health staff in rural areas is one of the most important ways followed all over the world, including India. Incentives are used to improve recruitment, motivation and retention of healthcare professionals. Mathauer and Imhoff (2006) define an incentive as "an available means applied with the intention to influence the willingness of physicians and nurses to exert and maintain an effort towards attaining organisational goals." More tightly defined, an incentive is "an explicit or implicit financial or non-financial reward for performing a particular act" (Zurn *et al.*, 2005). Incentives are thus a good means of attracting, retaining, motivating, satisfying, and improving performance. Incentives help to encourage and motivate health staff to stay in their jobs, in their profession and in their countries. Incentives are provided to health professionals in rural and remote areas as: a) they encourage providers to furnish specific services, b) support staff recruitment and retention, c) enhance the productivity and quality of services, and d) allows for effective management.

Table 9.1

Strategies to Retain Health Staff in Rural Areas in India

Sl. No.	*Strategy Adopted*	*States*
1	Appointment of Staff on contractual basis	Gujarat, Himachal Pradesh, Karnataka, Madhya Pradesh, Odisha, Uttaranchal, Tamil Nadu
2	Reorganisation of human resources from state cadre to district cadre	Himachal Pradesh, Odisha, West Bengal, Haryana
3	Provision of incentives to rural doctors	Nagaland, Tamil Nadu, Uttaranchal and Madhya Pradesh
4	Compulsory rural service for medical doctors	Odisha, West Bengal, Andhra Pradesh, Nagaland
5	Human resource development/ training policy and personal management database	West Bengal, Chattisgarh, Kerala, Haryana, Odisha, Madhya Pradesh
6	Rotational transfer policy	Uttaranchal, Tamil Nadu, West Bengal
7	Integration of ISM medical officers in national programmes	Madhya Pradesh, Uttaranchal, Haryana,

Source: Author's compilation.

There are two types of incentives provided to retain staff in rural areas. They can be classified as financial and non-financial incentives.

Financial incentives are provided to health workers wherein the incentives are made in monetary terms. According to Langenbrunner and Liu (2004), financial incentives are provided to health workers in terms of three main categories:

a. Basic wages.
b. Additional payments or bonuses that are linked to the achievement of performance outcomes.

c. Additional financial incentives that are not directly related to the performance of a person's duties, such as access to financial services or fellowships.

Henderson and Tulloch (2008) have highlighted that various countries used different types of financial incentives to counter the low remuneration of the health staff. These included rural location/hardship allowance, the public sector retention allowance and the accommodation allowance. Other financial benefits included overtime allowance, pension benefits, health/life insurance and transportation allowance. The study also noted that in Thailand, there are special hardship allowances provided as incentives to doctors and other health staff in rural areas. As part of financial incentive, many doctors get salaries three times more than their basic salary.

Chimbari *et al.* (2008) in their study on the incentives to retain health staff in rural areas in Zimbabwe have noted that financial incentives to doctors equalled almost 70 per cent additional salary at par with civil servants. The nurses with experience in mid-wifery were provided 65 per cent of the basic salary as incentives. Other health staff received almost 20 per cent of their basic salary as incentives.

Table 9.2 presents some of the financial incentives that could be provided to retain health staff in rural areas in India.

Non-financial incentives are incentives that do not have a monetary component, but is a benefit provided as a means by which employing organisations can recognise and acknowledge employees' contributions and commitment, as well as the challenges they face in daily lives. Non-financial incentives are usually given when countries find a budget constraint to provide financial incentives.

Many countries have adopted non-financial incentives as a way of retaining health staff in rural areas. According to a study by Munga and Mgilinyi (2008) in Tanzania, promotions and continued education opportunities are the best non-financial incentives.

Table 9.2

Potential Financial Incentives for Retaining Staff in Rural Areas in India

Additional salary, Pension	*Tax rebates/reduced interest rates on loans*
Illness, Health, Accident and life insurance premium	Bonus (festivals)
Travel and transport allowances	Performance based incentives
Child Care allowance	Allowing Private Practice
Rural location allowance	Marriage allowance
Retention and Professional allowance	Reimbursement of medical bills
Subsidised meals, clothing and accommodation	Subsidies on daily goods; subsidies in purchase of land, vehicle.

Source: Author's compilation.

Table 9.3 presents a list of potential non-financial incentives that could be provided to retain health staff in rural areas in India.

Table 9.3

Non-Financial Incentives

Guaranteed promotion	*Vacation days*
Choice of future posting	Flexible working hours
Quota for higher education	Access to training and education/fellowships abroad
Residential and conveyance facilities	Sabbatical and study leave, planned career breaks
Servant facilities	Occupational health
Help in looking after relatives in urban areas	Functional and professional autonomy
Free education for children	Reward Systems/awards
Good school in rural areas for children	Safe and clear workplace
24×7 water and electricity facilities	Coaching and mentoring structures, feedback from supervisor
Good markets nearby	Counselling services
Internet and telephone facilities	Recreational facilities
Job for spouse nearby	Festival gifts

Source: Author's compilation.

Table 9.4 provides details of the incentives prevalent in various countries to retain health staff in rural areas.

Table 9.4

Incentives Provided in Different Countries

Sl. No.	*Incentives*	*Financial/ Non-financial Incentive*	*Country*
1	Providing training and promotion opportunities for nurses and medical auxiliaries; resulted in successful retention of staff in rural areas	Non-financial	Nepal
2	Allowing after hours private practice in public institutions	Financial	Bahrain
3	Providing higher salaries as premium payments for working in rural areas	Financial	Thailand, Vietnam, Papua New Guinea, Uganda, Cambodia, South Africa, Zimbabwe, Kenya, Sri Lanka
4	Providing opportunities for government-sponsored further education	Non-financial	Ghana, Zimbabwe, Kenya
5	Provide housing and good quality educational opportunities for health workers' families	Non-financial	Nepal, Australia, Kenya

Source: Author's compilation.

Incentives Provided in Indian States

Providing incentives has become more prominent in the health sector especially after the launch of NRHM in 2005 through Janani Suraksha Yojana (JSY) and incentives to Accredited Social Health Activists (ASHA) for immunisation and even earlier to NGOs as part of blindness control programme. Different states in India have adopted different types of incentives to retain staff in rural areas. (Sundararaman and Gupta, 2010; Rao and Ramani, 2011; Rao *et al.*, 2010). While many states have gone for financial incentives like increased salary, pension, rural allowances, performance-based payments, etc., there are also that which have gone for non-financial incentives like additional marks for higher education in case of doctors, quota for higher education, preferential postings after working in rural areas, awards and other recognition, schools for children, better housing facilities and working conditions, etc. The additional salary or rural allowance is the most prominent financial incentive in most Indian states. The best non-financial incentive that has worked is awards and recognition for well-performing staff in rural areas.

Issues in Providing Incentives

There is however certain concerns while providing incentives to retain staff in rural areas. The beneficiary of the incentive package should be clear from the beginning. For example, if a doctor in a PHC is only provided an incentive, the other staff like nurses, Auxiliary Nurse Midfifery (ANM) etc., who would have contributed to the performance may feel let down; this can bring in competition among team members and ultimately spoil working environment and performance. Monitoring of the incentive scheme thus becomes a major challenge. Financial incentives have a bigger problem as budget becomes a major concern in India. Even if its solved, the irregularity of payment of incentives could demotivate the staff working in rural areas. Another issue with financial incentive is that regular receipt of incentives would no longer be able to motivate staff as they feel it is part of their salary in the long run.

Conclusion and Strategies in Providing Incentives

There is no doubt that incentives are required to retain health staff in rural areas in India. But it is important to carry out regular and systematic reviews and evaluate impact of the incentive schemes. There is need to consult all the major stakeholders before finalising the incentives. It is also ideal to plan the incentives in a proper manner; otherwise costs associated could be shooting up. The incentives according to WHO whether financial or non-financial should have the following major characteristics—clear objectives; realistic and deliverable; reflect health professionals' needs and preferences; well-designed, strategic and fit-for-purpose and are contextually appropriate; fair, equitable and transparent and measurable. Lastly international research shows that mere financial incentives cannot be a sustaining mechanism; a combination of financial and non-financial incentives could lead to better retention of health staff in rural areas in a sustainable way. Asante *et al.* (2014) in their study in rural Timor-Leste argues that in order to retain health staff in rural areas, adequate budget should be there for financial incentives along with non-financial incentives, such as career development opportunities, supporting and supervision structures in rural areas. Financial and non-financial incentives are one of the tools by which governments can retain staff in rural areas as effective health manpower for strengthening our health system.

References

Asante, Augustine D., Nelson Martin, Michael E. Otim and John Dewdney (2014). "Retaining Doctors in Rural Timor-Leste: A Critical Appraisal of the Opportunities and Challenges", *Bulletin of the World Health Organization* 92: 277-82.

Caldwell, P. and M. Kingma (2007). "Incentives and the Recruitment/Retention of Nurses", Paper presented at *National Experiences in Assessing and Reducing Shortcomings and Negative Trends Affecting Human Resources of the Health System: An International Symposium on Health Workforce.* Lisbon, Portugal. 10-12 October. ICN-International Centre for Human Resources in Nursing.

Chimbari, M.J., D. Madhina, F. Nyamangara, H. Mtandwa and V. Damba (2008). "Retention Incentives for Health Workers in Zimbabwe", *Discussion Paper* 65.Regional Network for Equity in Health in East and Southern Africa,

Langenbrunner, J. and Xingzhu Liu (2004). *How to Pay? Understanding and Using Incentives.* Washington: World Bank.

Lyn, N. Henderson and Jim Tulloch (2008). "Incentives for Retaining and Motivating Health Workers in Pacific and Asian Countries", *Human Resources for Health.* Bio Med Central.

Mathauer, I. and I. Imhoff (2006). "Health Worker Motivation in Africa: The Role of Nonfinancial Incentives and Human Resource Management Tools", *Human Resources for Health* 4(24).

Mbemba, Gisèle, Marie-Pierre Gagnon, Guy Pare and Jose Cote (2013). "Interventions for Supporting Nurse Retention in Rural and Remote Areas: An Umbrella Review", *Human Resources for Health Guidelines: Incentives for Health Professionals by International Council of Nurses.* International Pharmaceutical Federation, World Dental Federation, World Medical Association, International Hospital Federation, World Confederation for Physical Therapy, 2008.

Munga, Michael A. and Deogratius R. Mbilinyi (2008). "Non-Financial Incentives and Retention of Health Workers in Tanzania", *Discussion paper* 61. Regional Network for Equity in health in East and Southern Africa.

Rao, Krishna and Sudha Ramani (2011). *What Works, Where and How Well? Lessons from a Comparative Assessment of Current Rural Retention Strategies for Doctors in India.* Human Resources Background paper. Public Health Foundation of India

Rao, Krishna D., Sudha Ramani, Seema Murthy, Indrajit Hazarika, Neha Khandpur, Maulik Chokshi, Saujanya Khanna, Marko Vujicic, Peter Berman, and Mandy Ryan (2010). Health Worker Attitudes toward Rural Service in India: results from Qualitative Analysis; HNP Discussion Paper; November.

Rural Health West (2013). *Critical Success Factors for Recruiting and Retaining Health Professionals to Primary Healthcare in Rural and Remote Locations: Contemporary Review of the Literature.* August.

Suwit Wibulpolprasert and Paichit Pengpaibon (2003). *Integrated Strategies to Tackle the Inequitable Distribution of Doctors in Thailand: Four Decades of Experience.* Human Resources for Health Biomed Central.

Sundararaman, Thiagarajan and Garima Gupta (2010). "Indian Approaches to Retaining Skilled Health Workers in Rural Areas", *Bull World Health Organ* 89: 73–77 (2011).

Uta, Lehmann, Marjolein Dieleman and Tim Martineau (2008). *Staffing Remote Rural Areas in Middle- and Low-income Countries: A Literature Review of Attraction and Retention.* BMC Health Services Research.

Wilson, N.W., I.D. Couper, E. De Vries, S. Reid, T. Fish, B.J. Marais (2009). "A Critical Review of Interventions to Redress the Inequitable Distribution of Healthcare Professionals to Rural and Remote Areas", *Rural and Remote Health* 9: 1060.

World Health Organization (2006). "The Global Shortage of Health Workers and Its Impact", *Fact Sheet* no. 302. Geneva.

Zina, M. Daniels, Betsy J. VanLeit, Betty J. Skipper, Margaret L. Sanders and Robert L. Rhyne (2007). *Factors in Recruiting and Retaining Health Professionals for Rural Practice.* National Rural Health Association.

Zurn P., Dolea L. and Stilwell, B. (2005). *Nurse Retention and Recruitment: Developing a Motivated Workforce.* Geneva: ICN.

10

R. MUTHARAYAPPA and BIBPLAB DHAK

Gender Differetials of Morbidity and Disease Pattern

Introduction

In general, it can be presumed that morbidity or burden of disease would accentuate mortality of any individual. People with higher burden of diseases are likely to experience higher risk of mortality. However, the presumption that higher level of mortality is the result of higher level of morbidity is not always the reality. One of the most talked about evidence, observed mostly in developed nations, is that females' survival chances are greater despite their heavier burden of diseases compared to males. A similar scenario was observed for India recently. There was a mismatch between the level of mortality and morbidity while analysing gender differentials in health. Females in India gained mortality advantage even with a higher level of disease burden or morbidity, particularly from the age of 30 years (NSSO, 2006; Registrar General of India, 2007).

The observed paradox regarding gender differential in health in developed nations is that females with health disadvantage end up with a mortality advantage. There was keen interest among researches to recognise clues behind the paradox. Researchers like Nathanson (1984), Verbrugge (1982), and others suggested, after analysing US data, that the gender differential in disease pattern played an important role in explaining the paradox. It has been observed that females experienced higher levels of morbidity with diseases that are not life threatening. On the other hand, males experienced higher level of mortality with life-threatening diseases.

Nevertheless, studies based on developed countries have not spilled over to India since the paradox were regarding gender differential in health appeared very recently. Therefore, it remains an important and interesting task to look into that aspect for some clues behind the paradox of gender differential in health. With the aim of finding clues behind the paradox in India, this paper examines the gender differential in disease pattern, severity in illness and distribution of the causes of death. Finally, this paper explains some probable causes for the gender differential in disease pattern through healthcare utilisation, food consumption and risk behaviour in terms of smoking, drinking alcohol and chewing tobacco. Considering the availability of data sets, this study examines two hypotheses through which gender differential in health might have occurred—acquired risk by considering risk taking behaviours, and food consumption and health-seeking behaviour.

Objectives of the Study

The objectives of the study are:

- To examine the gender differential of morbidity and type of illness.
- To understand factors affecting morbidity and risk behaviour.

Data and Methodology

Data for this study has been taken from National Sample Survey (NSS), 60th Round, National Family and Health Survey-1998-99 (NFHS-2) and National Family and Health Survey-2005-06 (NFHS-3). The NSS 60th Round was conducted in 2004 and covered nationally representative sample of 73,868 households consisting 3,83,338 household members (NSS report no. 507 of NSSO, 2006). NFHS-2 was conducted in 1998-99 and covered nationally representative sample of 91,196 households consisting of 89,199 eligible women in the age group of 15-49 years. NFHS-3 was conducted during 2005-06 and with 109,041 households, 124,385 women aged 15-49 years, and 74,369 men aged 15-54 years.

The NSS collected information on morbidity prevalence and nature of illness. In this study, data have been analysed to examine gender differentials in the prevalence of short-term and long-term morbidity for different diseases. NFHS-2 collected information on socioeconomic and reproductive health status, as well as risk behaviour of each individual in terms of smoking, alcoholism, chewing tobacco etc., and about four diseases—tuberculosis, malaria, jaundice, and asthma. This study uses information of all household members relating to risk behaviour and two diseases—tuberculosis and asthma. These two diseases have been taken to test how gender differential in risk behaviour shapes that in life-threatening diseases. The study uses NHFS-3 data to understand only the gender differential in nutritional status since this survey provides information on food consumption and height-weight of males and females.

Analysis

The analysis of this study comprises two parts: bi-variant analysis and multivariate analysis. The bi-variant analysis has been used to estimate the disease-specific prevalence rates, severity in illness, percentage of seeking healthcare, exposure to risk behaviour, etc. The multivariate analysis—logistic regression model—have been carried out to understand the impact of gender differentials in risk behaviour on gender differential in the prevalence of two life-threatening diseases—tuberculosis and asthma. For k explanatory variables and n number of individuals, the model expression is:

$$\text{Log}\,[P_i\,/1\text{-}P_i] = \alpha + \beta_1 X_{i1} + \beta_2 X_{i2} + \ldots + \beta_k X_{ik}$$

Where, P_i is the probability of reporting tuberculosis or reporting asthma (in another model). In this model, output is coded upon two categories, 1= reporting tuberculosis or reporting asthma and 0 = not reporting tuberculosis or not reporting asthma. For both the outcome variables, four separate models have been executed. Model 1 has been applied to understand the impact of every risk-behaviour—chewing tobacco, drinking and smoking—on reporting tuberculosis and asthma. Models 2-4 have tried to understand how gender differentials in risk behaviour influence gender differential in these two diseases. In each model, confounding factors like caste, place of residence, marital status, literacy, work status and household condition have been considered as controlled.

Gender Differential in Disease Pattern

The NSS has collected information on the status of health as well as disease pattern, if any individual had been ill during 15 days prior to the date of survey. As many as 41 diseases were reported in the survey. All diseases reported in NSS are classified into three groups following the international classification of disease patterns given by the World Health Organization (WHO) (1992) as communicable diseases, non-communicable diseases and injuries. Table 10.1 presents prevalence rates for all major diseases, and in aggregate for all communicable and non-communicable diseases and by injury. The disease-specific prevalence rate is defined as the ratio of number of persons experiencing a specific disease and the population exposed to the risk of that disease. The rate has been expressed per 1000 individuals.

As the Table shows, the leading communicable diseases are diarrhoea, fever, respiratory illness, eye ailments and tuberculosis (TB). In general, it has been observed that communicable diseases were more prevalent during the childhood period and non-communicable diseases were more prevalent during the old age period. In other words, the prevalence rate of non-communicable diseases increased with age. However, communicable diseases like diarrhoea, fever, respiratory illness, tuberculosis, etc., had higher prevalence rate during the old age period too.

As for gender differential in the prevalence rate of all communicable diseases, females experienced a higher prevalence rate compared to males in most of the age groups. Only exception is the childhood period when female children experienced lower prevalence rate compared to males, and the old age period showed almost equal prevalence rate for both males and females. Diseases showing gender differential in prevalence rate for the childhood period were diarrhoea and respiratory illness where male children were at a disadvantage. For the age group 15-29 years, gender differential against females was found for fever only. Other age groups like 30-44 years, 45-59 years and old age, showed gender differential in three diseases—eye ailments, fever and TB. Among these diseases, prevalence of TB was higher for males compared to females. On the other hand, prevalence rates for eye ailment and fever were higher for females.

For non-communicable diseases, the prevalence rate among females was greater for most of the age groups. In childhood and early adulthood period, the prevalence rate was higher for males compared to females as far as all non-communicable diseases were concerned. Nevertheless, gender differential in the prevalence rate of any particular non-communicable disease became prominent from the age 30 itself. For all adult and old age groups, females had higher prevalence rate from diseases like gastritis, bone disorder and cancer. On the other hand, males had excess prevalence rate for cardiovascular diseases, asthma, disorder of kidney, tuberculosis, respiratory diseases, etc.

Significant gender gap against males in the prevalence rate of injury was found in most of the age groups. Only for the old age period, gender gap in the prevalence rate of injury was not seen. The greater rate of incidence of injury for males across age groups seems to be the result of males' greater exposure to health hazards from risky jobs, adventurous activity, sports, etc.

Gender Differential in Severity of Illness by Age Groups

Severity of illness is an important aspect that has to be looked into while searching the underlying paradox in gender differentials in health. It is expected that severity of illness would lead to high mortality. Therefore, gender differential in severity of illness would be an important factor to explain gender differentials in mortality. With the intention of finding clues behind the apparent paradox in gender differential in health, this section does detail analyses on gender differential in severity of illness by age groups. To judge severity of illness, three indicators have been considered in this study: duration of illness, duration of restricted activity days and duration of bedridden days due to illness.

Table 10.1

Prevalence Rates (Per 1000) of Some Leading Diseases by Gender and Age Groups

Name of Diseases	Age groups											
	0-14		15-29		30-44		45-59		60+		Total	
	M	F	M	F	M	F	M	F	M	F	M	F
Communicable Diseases												
Diarrhoea	10	7*	2	2	2	3	3	4	6	5	4	4
Malaria	2	2	1	1	1	1	1	2	2	1	1	1
Jaundice	0.5	1	1	0.5	1	0.5	1	0.5	0.5	0.5	1	0.5
Whooping cough	3	3	1	1	1	1	2	2	5	4	2	2
Fever	24	23	8	10**	8	12**	9	15**	13	15**	14	16*
Respiratory infection	9	7*	4	4	4	5	7	7	12	11	7	6
Eye ailments	-	-	-	-	-	-	2	4*	15	18**	2	2
Tuberculosis	-	-	1	1	3	1**	5	2**	6	3**	2	1**
All	46	42**	18	20*	21	25**	30	35**	59	59	30	33*

.contd...

.contd...

Name of Diseases	Age groups											
	0-14		15-29		30-44		45-59		60+		Total	
	M	F	M	F	M	F	M	F	M	F	M	F
Non-Communicable Diseases												
Gastritis	-	-	2	2	3	6**	6	8*	13	11	3	4*
Cardiovascular												
Diseases	-	-	1	1	7	4**	22	20	59	50*	10	8
Asthma	-	-	-	-	2	2	8	5**	30	18**	4	3*
Disorders of bones	-	-	1	1	3	5	6	14**	31	47**	5	7*
Diseases of kidney	-	-	1	1	2	1	3	2*	6	3**	2	1**
Neurological	1	1	2	1*	2	3*	4	4	9	9	2	3
Diseases of skin	2	2	1	1	1	2	2	2	5	3**	2	2
Diabetes	-	-	-	-	2	1	9	10	23	20	3	4
Blindness	-	-	-	-	-	-	1	1	6	9*	1	1
Hearing	-	-	-	-	-	-	-	-	5	5	1	1
Cancer	-	-	-	-	1	2**	2	3*	3	4*	1	1
All	9	6**	12	10*	26	31**	69	74	191	196	36	38
Injuries	2	1**	3	1**	6	2**	6	3**	7	7	4	2**

Note: ** denotes $p<0.01$, * denotes $p<0.05$.
Source: NSS 60th round data (2004).

Data provided in Table 10.2 shows that there was a gender differential in severity of illness across almost all age groups. Particularly, gender differential appeared for restricted activity days and duration of bedridden days. In both the cases, males were at a disadvantage compared to females. Greater duration of restricted activity of males over females varied from 3 per cent for the old age period to 14 per cent for the age group 15-29 years. For bedridden days, the gender differential varied from 5 per cent for the childhood period to 22 per cent for the age group 30-44 years. The general observation is that although gender differential in restricted activity days and bedridden days remained minimal at the childhood period, it became widest for the adult age groups and narrowed down at the old age period. In case of illness episode, gender differential was negligible; gender differential appeared to be marginal for age groups 0-14 years and 45-59 years with greater duration for males.

Table 10.2

Duration of Illness, Restricted Activity Days and Duration of Bedridden Days by Age Groups and Gender

Age Groups	*Illness Episode*			*Restricted Activity Days*			*Bedridden Days*		
	M	F	F/M	M	F	F/M	M	F	F/M
0-14	6.78	6.52	0.96*	4.57	4.34	0.95	3.01	2.86	0.95
15-29	9.07	9.02	0.99	6.65	5.72	0.86**	4.03	3.01	0.75**
30-44	10.48	10.50	1.00	7.26	6.32	0.87**	4.11	3.21	0.78**
45-59	12.01	11.71	0.98*	7.76	7.10	0.91**	4.26	3.46	0.81**
60+	13.04	13.07	1.00	8.69	8.46	0.97	4.68	4.29	0.92¬*
Total	10.46	10.58	1.01	7.12	6.70	0.94**	4.02	3.49	0.87**

Note: **< 0.01, b denotes *<0.05

Source: NSS 60th round data, 2004

As far as the duration of illness episode, restricted activity days and bedridden days are concerned, there is a strong relationship with the age of an individual. The duration of each mentioned episode increased with the increase in age for both males and females. The illness episode increased from around 6.5 days during the childhood period to 13 days for the old age period. Restricted activity days increased from around 4.5 days for the childhood period to 8.5 days for the old age period, and bedridden days increased from around 3 days for the childhood period to 4.5 days for the old age period.

Major Causes of Death in Rural India

In India, there is scarcity of data on the causes of death. Although there are few community-based surveys, as cited in the literature review, information on causes of death pertaining to whole India is scarce. The only one accessible source available to us to understand the causes of death is the survey report entitled "Annual Report of Survey of Causes of Death (Rural India)" conducted in 1998 by Registrar of India. Although the survey is based on rural India, information presented here can give some idea about the pattern of causes of death in India since the majority of Indian people live in rural areas (around 70%). The percentage distribution of diseases by causes of deaths in rural India is given in Table 10.3. It can be seen that diarrhoea, respiratory infection and injury were three main major causes of diseases for the childhood period. For adult age groups, tuberculosis, cardiovascular diseases, injury, and cancer were the main diseases that caused the majority of deaths. At the old age period, along with adult age groups' diseases, there were few more prevailing diseases like respiratory infections, diabetes, digestive disorders, etc., which caused death. However, it can be seen that cardiovascular diseases accounted for around 50 per cent deaths and cancer accounted for around 10 per cent of all deaths in the old age period.

Comparing Health and Mortality by Age Groups

After analysing gender differential in disease prevalence rate, severity of illness in terms of restricted activity days, bed disability days and gender differential in percentage distribution of major causes of death in rural India, this section tries to give some probable explanation for the newly appeared paradox in India that males die but women become sicker, particularly after the childhood period. For each stage of life, explanations for the mismatch between morbidity and mortality have been discussed below.

Age Group 0-14 Years

This age group is characterised by excess male morbidity rate with marginally excess female mortality compared to males. At the same time, males experienced more severe illness in terms of restricted activity days and bedridden days than females. Looking at the gender differential in disease pattern and major causes of deaths in rural India, it can also be seen that morbidity prevalence rate for males was higher from diseases like respiratory illness and diarrhoea that caused majority of deaths in the childhood period. Therefore, given the biological superiority of females, one can expect that males should have ended with higher level of mortality compared to females. Nevertheless, the expected picture of higher male mortality during the childhood period did not appear in India. At this point, it can only be assumed that there were some hidden disadvantages in female children causing some deaths, despite lower prevalence rate of life-threatening diseases and less severity in illness. Those disadvantages probably stemmed from gender discrimination in terms of inadequate nutritious food, quality healthcare or negligence to take females to doctor for some minor illness. Discrimination against the female child in intra-household resource allocation, in terms of food and quality of health, was an inevitable and widely accepted phenomenon causing excess female mortality in India (Das Gupta, 1987; Amin, 1990).

Age Group 15-29 Years

Females in the age group 15-29 years experienced higher level of morbidity with almost equal level of mortality with males. This picture of equal mortality rate for both male and female, despite higher level of morbidity of females, can be justified mainly through gender differential in injuries. Injury was the leading cause of death for both males and females for this age group and males experienced much higher injury than females. Other leading causes of death for this age group were tuberculosis and cardiovascular diseases, but no significant gender differential from these diseases has been observed in our analysis. Apart from higher prevalence from injury, greater severity in illness for males compared to females might have caused some excess male mortality from each disease. Therefore, it can be concluded that females suffered greater morbidity, but because of greater injury among males and severity in illness, females and males ended with almost equal mortality rate.

Table 10.3

Percentage Distribution of Deaths by Major Causes, Sex and Age Groups in Rural India, 1998

	Age Groups											
	0-14		*15-29*		*30-44*		*45-59*		*60+*		*Total*	
	M	*F*	*M*	*F*	*M*	*F*	*M*	*F*	*M*	*F*	*M*	*F*
Diarrhoea	16.3	14.3	0.4	0.2	0.6	0.4	0.4	0.5	0.8	0.9	5.1	5.1
Malaria	1.3	1.4	0.2	0.2	0.1	0.2	0.0	0.1	0.0	0.0	0.3	0.5
Jaundice	0.0	0.0	0.8	0.6	0.9	0.4	0.9	0.4	0.3	0.1	0.5	0.2
Respiratory infection	21.3	21.0	1.9	1.6	1.6	1.0	1.4	1.4	9.0	5.7	10.1	11.1
Tuberculosis	0.5	0.5	10.1	9.6	14.1	12.7	10.6	7.1	3.8	2.0	5.4	3.5
Nutritional deficiency	1.6	2.4	1.0	0.6	0.7	1.7	1.3	3.3	0.4	0.8	0.9	1.7
Cardiovascular	1.4	1.6	7.4	8.4	12.2	12.1	33.5	30.0	45.7	48.6	25.3	25.2
Respiratory diseases	0.6	0.6	1.6	1.8	2.8	3.8	9.9	11.9	9.1	8.1	5.7	5.3
Neurological	0.6	0.6	2.1	1.2	3.1	1.3	1.5	1.3	2.6	2.6	1.9	1.6
Diabetes	0.1	0.1	0.6	0.4	0.7	0.6	2.2	2.5	2.5	2.5	1.5	1.4
Injuries	4.1	2.3	27.0	21.7	18.3	14.2	9.0	8.4	3.9	4.0	7.7	6.9
Cancer	0.6	0.6	3.7	3.6	4.9	7.7	8.4	14.2	11.4	10.6	6.7	7.0
Digestive diseases	1.0	2.4	3.7	5.8	3.9	4.8	5.8	5.9	3.3	2.9	3.1	3.4
Others	50.5	52.2	39.4	44.4	36.0	39.2	15.0	13.0	7.2	11.2	25.8	27.2

Source: Annual report of survey of causes of death (rural India), 1998.

Age Group 30 years and Above

From the age of 30 years, the paradox, as observed in developed nations, of lower level of mortality in females despite their higher morbidity compared to males has been observed in India too. Like the developed nations, the explanation for the emerging paradox in India also follows the same line—greater prevalence of life-threatening diseases among males seems to be the main cause of higher mortality rate in males. In general, it has been observed that prevalence rate of females was higher than males for both communicable as well as non-communicable diseases. Only exception is injury, where prevalence rate for males was higher compared to that of females. Nevertheless, when leading diseases in terms of causes of mortality is considered, males are more exposed to those diseases. For the age group 30-44 years, the top four leading causes of deaths (covering around 40 per cent of all deaths) were injury, tuberculosis, cardiovascular diseases and cancer. For these diseases, males experienced greater prevalence rate than females. The only exception was cancer where prevalence rate as well as percentage share of mortality from cancer was higher for females compared to that of males. However, the percentage share of cancer to the total number of deaths was much lower compared to that of cardiovascular diseases, tuberculosis and injury. Therefore, it can be presumed that higher prevalence of cancer among females was not enough to balance the mortality rate between male and female against the other life-threatening diseases where males were at a disadvantage.

For the age group 45-59 years, the leading causes of death were cardiovascular diseases, respiratory infection, respiratory diseases, tuberculosis, diabetes, cancer and injury—covering around 80 per cent of all deaths. These killer diseases were found to be more prevalent among males. On the other hand, diseases from which females experienced higher prevalence rate compared to males were fever, eye ailment, disorder of bones and cancer. Except cancer, other diseases were less life-threatening. Therefore, similar to the earlier age group, it can be concluded for even this age group that males suffered from diseases that were life threatening in majority and that in combination with males' higher severity of illness in general resulted in higher mortality than females.

Similarly, it can be seen that old males had higher mortality rate than that of females due to the higher prevalence of life-threatening diseases and higher severity in illness than females. The life threatening diseases from which older men reported higher prevalence rate than older women were cardiovascular diseases, diabetes, asthma (respiratory diseases), kidney disorders and tuberculosis. On the other hand, diseases like fever, eye ailments and disorders of bones were less life threatening and females suffered from these more than males. The only life-threatening one was cancer from which old-aged females suffered more compared to old-aged males.

Factors Influencing Gender Differential in Life Threatening Diseases

Apart from biological differences between a male and a female, there are some other underlying factors to influence gender differential in mortality as has been noted earlier. The factor that can lead to life-threatening diseases in males as well as greater tendency of death is gender differential in acquired risk through different lifestyle behaviour, perception about sickness and healthseeking behaviour. This section deals with two aspects: gender differential in healthseeking behaviour and gender differential in lifestyle through risk behaviour. Other factors relating to the psychological aspects were not taken into account in this study due to the non-availability of data.

First, gender differential in healthcare utilisation was observed through both inpatients as well as outpatient care. Then, gender differential in risk behaviour was examined through alcoholism, smoking and chewing tobacco. After examining gender differential in risk behaviour, attempts were made to understand how gender differential in risk behaviour affected that in health in terms of asthma and tuberculosis. These two diseases were included in the analysis mainly because of availability of data and they account for a significant proportion of total death count in India too.

Gender Differential in Healthcare Utilisation

The gender differential in healthcare utilisation was examined with data on both inpatients and outpatients healthcare found in the 60th round of the NSS. In this survey, respondents were asked about their sickness followed by healthcare in the last 15 days prior to the date of the survey. Further, all respondents were asked whether they were admitted to any hospital in the last one year prior to the date of survey.

Table 10.4 presents the percentage of people reported as seeking healthcare when they fell sick. Around 85 per cent of people sought healthcare when they fell sick and there were no noticeable gender gap. The pattern of gender differential in healthcare seeking behaviour also remained same across the different stages of life.

Table 10.4

Gender Differential in Outpatient Healthcare by Age Groups

Age group	*Male*	*Female*	*Female/male*
0-14	85.6	85.1	0.99
15-29	83.3	84.5	1.01
30-44	86.9	87.9	1.01
45-59	87.6	88.7	1.01
60+	83.7	82.2	0.98
Total	85.2	85.2	1.00
N	18790	19963	

Source: NSS 60th round data, 2004;

This picture of gender equality has appeared contrary to the existing literature. India was known for gender discrimination against females in terms of food, healthcare, etc., and that discrimination resulted in excess female mortality particularly during the childhood and early adulthood periods. With this recent appearance of gender equality in outpatient care, it can be said that females are not restricted from seeking at least outpatient care and that easing of gender discrimination might have reduced female mortality.

Another measure of healthcare, i.e., hospitalisation rate for the last one year prior to the survey date, has been presented in

Table 10.5 by age groups and sex. It is seen that except for the age group of 15-29 years, males were admitted to hospital in a greater numbers than females. The age group of 15-29 years is the prime reproductive age group and it can be assumed that reproductive health problems may cause some extra burden for females and accelerate their hospitalisation. Therefore, in general, females used less healthcare in terms of hospitalisation as has been observed from the NSS survey. Nevertheless, a higher hospitalisation rate can be interpreted in a different way—it may be one indicator of severity of disease because hospitalisation takes place after onset of serious illness only. Therefore, higher hospitalisation rate of males for most of the age groups may indicate that they suffered more severe illnesses and higher mortality compared to females.

Gender Differential in Food Consumption and Nutritional Status

Balanced diets with adequate amounts of protein, fat, carbohydrates, vitamins and minerals are required to ensure better health of both males and females. Balanced diets can also help a person avoid life-threatening diseases. Therefore, with the appearance of gender differential in life-threatening diseases across the different stages of life, it is worthwhile to check the gender differential in food consumption as well as nutritional status.

Table 10.5

Gender Differential in Inpatient Healthcare by Age Groups

Age group	*Male*	*Female*	*Female/male*
0-14	5.3	3.4	0.64**
15-29	5.3	6.6	1.25**
30-44	7.9	9.7	1.23**
45-59	14.2	11.5	0.81**
60+	16.2	12.3	0.76**
Total	7.8	7.3	0.94*
N	18790	19963	

Note: ** denotes $p<0.01$, * denotes $p<0.05$

Source: NSS 60th round data (2004).

In NFHS-3, both women and men were asked how often they consumed various types of food (daily, weekly, occasionally or never). It was found that the pattern of food consumption was more or less similar for males and females for pulses, vegetables and fruits. The variation appeared for only in regular consumption of milk or curd, egg, fish and chicken. Men were forced to consume more of these foods compared to women. Nevertheless, it is required to mention here that NFHS-3 gives information about consumption for various types of foods by different time intervals, and it was difficult to draw firm conclusions about the gender differential in food consumption pattern. To get a single indicator of food consumption, an index was constructed with eight food items and frequency of food consumption. Information on eight food items was collected under four categories. For example, for the consumption of milk, the four categories were daily, weekly, occasionally and never with scores of 3, 2, 1 and 0 respectively. The total score of all food items was taken to represent the amount of food consumed.

Table 10.6 presents the average food consumption index for males and females by age groups. It can be seen that females were likely to consume less food compared to males: the constructed index based on frequency of eight food items showed that food consumption was 6-7 per cent lower for females compared to males. Therefore, it can be interpreted that females were discriminated as far as intra-household food allocation is concerned. However, this differential could be due to mere differential in food habits of males and females. The perception that there was no as such gender discrimination in food allocation gets stronger when we look at gender differential in nutritional status. NFHS-3 has shown that except for the age group 20-39 years, there was no gender differential in the percentage of thin population (BMI<18.5). In the age group 15-19 years, males were thinner than females and in the age group 40-49 years, no differential was found. Therefore, better nutritional status of females in the age group 15-19 years indicates that gender discrimination in food against females did not exist and the poorer nutritional status of females in the age group 20-39 years could have been caused by child-bearing activity. Similarly, the childhood period also reveals no remarkable gender discrimination, as far food allocation is concerned.

NFHS-3 gives information about vitamin A and iron supplements in the children aged 6-59 months. The reports shows that gender differential in vitamin A and iron supplements is very marginal. While 18.4 per cent male children received Vitamin A supplements, 17.4 per cent female children received the same. On the other hand, the percentage of males and females that received iron supplements was 4.9 per cent and 4.4 per cent respectively.

Table 10.6

Average Score of Food Consumption by Sex and Age Groups

Age Groups	*Male*	*Females*	*Males/Females*
15-19	12.13	11.28	0.93**
20-29	12.50	11.59	0.93**
30-39	12.34	11.44	0.93**
40-49	12.07	11.31	0.94**
Total	12.28	11.44	0.93**

Note: **denotes $p<0.01$

Source: NFHS-2, 2005-06.

Looking at the nutritional status through anthropometric indicators of health (NFHS-3 Report, 2005-06), it was found that females did not differ from males in terms of all three indicators: height-for-age, weight-for-height and weight-for-age. Therefore, it can be said that gender discrimination in food allocation or nutritional status has changed. The earlier picture that females are discriminated in intra-household resource allocation has not appeared recently, and it might have been one of the reasons for the lowering of female mortality during the childhood period.

Summary and Conclusions

The results presented above explain the recently apparent paradox in India regarding gender differential in health. Why has female mortality reduced despite higher level of morbidity particularly from the age of 30 years? First it was observed that gender differential in disease pattern played an important role in explaining this paradox. Except for the childhood period, females experienced greater morbidity than males in total. Except for injury, females also suffered more from both communicable as well as non-communicable diseases. However, when it comes to the diseases those cause greater toll with respect to occurring deaths, males are in upper front. From childhood to old age, diseases causing majority of deaths in any particular age group is more rampant among males compared to females. For example, prevalence rate of diarrhoea and respiratory illness in childhood and the prevalence rate of cardiovascular diseases, tuberculosis, respiratory diseases (asthma), and diabetes during the adult and old age periods were higher among males; these diseases were the leading cause of death in the respective age groups. Another important fact that causes excess mortality among males is injury or accident. Across all the age groups, it was found that males faced injury or accident to much greater extent than females.

However, it is seen that, unlike in the developed nations, biological advantages in mortality of females do not appear in India for the childhood and early adulthood periods, despite greater prevalence of life-threatening diseases and injury among males. In this context, it can be assumed that discrimination against females in the early ages of life persists in India and denies them the biological advantage in reducing mortality. However, in terms of food and healthcare (outpatient care), significant discrimination has not been observed.

Another important factor, i.e., severity of illness measured through duration of illness episode, restricted days and bedridden days due to illness also seems to be important for excess male mortality. In all stages of life, males reported greater restricted days as well as bedridden days and that in turn seems to lead to excess male mortality and vulnerability to life-threatening diseases.

This study also tried to find out pathways through which high prevalence rate of life-threatening diseases in males appeared by analysing gender differential in healthcare utilisation and gender differential in risk behaviour. Studies in developed nations have shown that females use more healthcare or visit doctors more frequently compared to males, which made females more aware of illness, thereby resulting in more reporting of sickness compared to males. Again, greater healthcare utilisation is assumed to help females avoid life-threatening diseases. Nevertheless,

India is known for gender discrimination in terms of healthcare utilisation, food, etc. Studies conducted during the 19th century have envisaged that females were restricted from seeking healthcare and that caused poorer health (Das Gupta, 1995; Basu, 1989; Sen, 1988; Miller, 1981). Therefore, it was expected that behaviour of Indian women would not be similar to that of women belonging to the developed nations. Rather, it was expected that health-seeking behaviour of females would be less compared to males. However, recent data paints a different picture. It was found that females were no more discriminated in seeking at least outpatient healthcare. Across all the stages of life, the percentage of females seeking outpatient healthcare was equal with that of males. Given this picture of gender equality in outpatient care, it can be said that the current gender discrimination in terms of healthcare utilisation might have been helpful in establishing the biological advantage in mortality of females in the adult age group. Another measure of healthcare utilisation, i.e., hospitalisation rate in last one year, has also been considered. In terms of hospitalisation, it is found that males' rate of hospitalisation was higher than females' for all the age groups. This greater percentage of hospitalisation among males can be attributed to greater severity of diseases among men since hospitalisation occurs after severe illness in most cases.

Along with healthcare utilisation, relaxation of gender discrimination has also been observed in food consumption or allocation. For the childhood period and age group 15-49 years, it was observed that females were no more discriminated over their male counterparts in consuming food. A similar picture was noticed in some nutritional standards: percentage of thin population and anthropometric indicators. With this picture, it can be said that relaxation of gender discrimination in food consumption as well as healthcare utilisation might have been helpful in avoiding excessive female mortality.

The most convincing pathway for experiencing life-threatening diseases across the different stages of life course is the gender differential in risk behaviour. Pronounced gender differential in risk behaviour in terms of smoking, alcoholism and chewing tobacco is well known across the globe. The percentage of females indulging in risk behaviour is much lower than that of males. This study supports the existing fact that males use more narcotic substances, drink alcohol and chew tobacco compared to females. For the two chronic and life-threatening diseases—asthma and tuberculosis—prevalence rates were significantly higher among risk-takers. Chewing pan-masala and smoking have strong association with the prevalence of tuberculosis and asthma respectively. Given the lower risk-taking behaviour among females, the prevalence rate of asthma and tuberculosis among them was lower than that among males.

Nevertheless, this study could not take into account all type of life-threatening diseases in relation to risk-taking behaviour because of non-availability of data, but association with the asthma and tuberculosis provides some indication regarding the effect of life-threatening diseases on males. Again, it could be possible that fatality of any particular disease may happen to be greater in males than females, because of the higher incidence of risk-taking behaviour among males.

Appendix Table A-10.1

Prevalence Rate (Per 1000) of Asthma and Tuberculosis by Gender and Age Groups

Age Groups	*Asthma*			*Tuberculosis*		
	Male	*Female*	*F/M*	*Male*	*Female*	*F/M*
0-14	12	10	0.83**	2	2	1.00
15-29	10	11	1.10*	4	4	1.00
30-44	21	22	1.05	10	8	0.80**
45-59	51	51	1.00	13	9	0.69**
60+	114	87	0.76**	18	10	0.56**
Total	25	23	0.92**	7	5	0.71**

Note: ** denotes p<0.01, * denotes p<0.05

Source: NFHS-2 data, 1998-99.

References

Amin, S. (1990). "The Effect of Women's Status on Sex Differentials in Infant and Child Mortality in South Asia", *Genus* 46(3-4): 55-69.

Basu, A.M. (1989). "Is Discrimination in Food Really Necessary for Explaining Sex Differentials in Childhood Mortality", *Population Studies* 43: 193-210.

Das Gupta, M. (1987). "Selective Discrimination Against Female Children in Rural Punjab, India", *Population and Development Review* 13(1): 77-100.

———. (1995). "Life Course Perspectives on Women's Autonomy and Health Outcomes", *American Anthropologist* 97(3): 481-91.

Davis, M.A. (1981). "Sex Differences in Reporting Osteoarthritic Symptoms: A Socio Medical Approach", *Journal of Health and Social Behaviour* 19: 77-84.

Gajalakshmi, V., R. Peto, S. Kayak and S. Balasubramanian (2002). "Verbal Autopsy of 48000 Adult Deaths Attributable to Medical Causes in Chennai (formally Madras), India", *BMC Public Health* 2: 7.

Gajalakshmi, V. and R. Peto (2004). "Verbal Autopsy of 80,000 Adult Deaths in Tamil Nadu. South India". *BMC Public Health* 4: 47.

Goldman, N., S.S. Kovenman and R. Weinstein (1995). "Marital Status and Health Among the Elderly", *Social Science and Medicine* 12: 1717-30.

Gove, W.R. and M. Hughes (1979). "Possible Causes of the Apparent Sex Differences in Physical Health: An Empirical Investigation", *American Sociological Review* 44: 126-46.

Gove, W.R. (1985). "Gender Differences in Mental and Physical Illness: The effects of Fixed Roles and Nurturant roles", *Social Science and Medicine* 19: 77-84.

International Institute for Population Sciences (2007). *National Family Health Survey (NFHS-3), 2005-06.* Mumbai.

Joshi, R., M. Cardon, S. Iyengar, A. Sukumar, C.R. Raju, K.R. Raju, K. Raju, K.S. Reddy, A. Lopez, and B. Neal (2006). "Chronic Diseases Now a Leading Causes of Death in Rural India-Mortality Data from the Andhra Pradesh Rural Health Initiative", *International Journal of Epidemiology* 35: 1522-29.

Macintyre, S. (1993). "Gender Differences in the Perceptions of Common Cold Symptoms", *Social Science and Medicine* 36(1): 15-20.

Macintyre, S., G. Ford and K. Hunt (1999). "Do Women Over Report Morbidity? Men's and Women's Responses to Structured Prompting on a Standard Question on Long Standing Illness", *Social Science and Medicine* 48(1): 89-98.

McDonough, P., G.J. Duncan, D. Williams and J. House (1997). "Income Dynamics and Adult Mortality in the U.S, 1972-1987", *American Journal of Public Health* 87: 1476-83.

Miller, B.D. (1981). *The Endangered Sex: Neglect of Female Children in Rural North India*. Ithaca: Cornell University Press.

Naeye, R.L., L.S. Burt, D.L. Wright, W.A. Blanc, D. Tatter (1971). "Neonatal Mortality, The Male Disadvantage", *Pediatrics* 48: 902-6.

Nathanson, C.A. (1978). "Sex Roles as Variables in the Interpretation of Morbidity Data: A Methodological Critique", *International Journal of Epidemiology* 7: 253-62.

———. (1984). "Sex Differences in Mortality", *Annual Review of Sociology* 10: 191-213.

National Sample Survey Organisation (NSSO) (1998). "Survey Results on Consumption of Tobacco in India: NSS 50th Round (1993-94)", *Sarvekshana* 74: 259-387.

———. (2006). "Morbidity, Healthcare and the Condition of the Aged", Report 507, *NSS 60th Round*. January-June 2004. New Delhi: Ministry of Statistics and Programme Implementation, Government of India.

Omran, A.R. (1971). "The Epidemiologic Transition: A Theory of the Epidemiology of Population Change", *Milbank Memorial Fund & Quarterly* 49: 509-38.

Preston, S.H. (1976). *Mortality Pattern in National Population with Special Reference to Recorded Causes of Death*. New York: Academic Press.

Registrar General of India (2007). *Sample Registration System Statistical Report 2006*. New Delhi, India

———. (1998). Survey of Causes of Death (Rural) in India. Ministry of Home Affairs, Vital Statistics Division, New Delhi.

Sen, A. (1988). "Family and Food: Sex Bias in Poverty". Pp. 453-80 in T.N. Srinivasan and P.K. Bardhan (eds.) *Rural Poverty in South Asia*. Delhi: Oxford University Press.

Sen, Gupta, S.K. and P.N. Kapoor (1970). Principal Causes of Death in India. DGHS, Ministry of Health and Family Planning, New Delhi.

Verbrugge, L.M. (1982). "Sex Differentials in Health", *Public Health Reports* 97: 417-37.

———. (1985). "Gender and Health: An Update on Hypotheses and Evidence", *Journal of Health and Social Behaviour* 26: 156-182.

Waldron, I. (1976). "Why Do Women Live Longer than Man?", *Social Science and Medicine* 10: 349-362.

———. (1983). "Sex Differences in Illness Incidence, Prognosis and Mortality: Issues and Evidence", *Social Science and Medicine* 17: 1107-1123.

Williams, D.R. and C. Collins (1995). "U.S. Socio Economic and Racial Differences in Health: Patterns and Explanation". *Annual Review of Sociology*, 21: 349-86.

World Bank. (2006). *Global Burden of Disease and Risk Factors.* New York: Oxford University Press.

WHO (1997). *Tobacco or Health: A Global Status Report*. Geneva.

———. (1992). *International Statistical Classification of Diseases and Related Health Problems.* Geneva.

11

BULA BHADRA

Unequal Exchange

A Tale of Surrogacy and Indian Women's Health

> The Baby M case could be the forerunner of the use of poor third-world women's wombs to produce children for economically advantaged European-American couples.
>
> (Harding, 1991: 203)

> On January 29, 2014, 26 year old Yuma Sherpa, died in the aftermath of a surgical procedure to harvest eggs from her body, as part of the egg donation programme of a private clinic based in Lajpat Nagar, New Delhi.
>
> (Peoples Democracy, 2015)

Prelude

Gene Corea (1985: 276) in her *The Mother Machine* predicted a world where wombs of "nonvaluable" women are used as "breeders" for the embryos of "valuable" women. These predictions are difficult to discount when one looks at the fact that India's rent a womb enterprise has become a two-billion-dollar industry (Bhatia, 2012). This huge industry of transnational surrogacy has been realisable by real life national boundaries of a globalised world along with a partner in ICTs (information and communication technologies). The intended infertile couple, mediated through agencies and fertility clinics, engaged in transnational reproductive commerce, meet its service provider the Indian surrogate women. This has successfully generated with the shifting reality of a globalised often online marketplace where babies have been added to the shopping cart. Consequentially, it reinforces neo-colonial power hierarchies where the globalised North, the developed world maintains its hegemony over South, the so-called developing world. Some analysts think that the intended mothers' expressions, sentiments and language use make them a 'nation' that apparently exhibits many of the features of 19th century European colonisers. In a sense , this "cybernetic nation" naturalises the relationships between IM (intended mothers) residing in Europe, the United States (US), Australia, etc., and the foetus residing in the wombs of surrogates in India (Dasgupta and Dasgupta, 2013: 70). That is to say, the unequal exchange is reborn and this time, categorically in reproduction!

On the other side of the coin, this super capitalism centring on reproductive arena makes reproduction, reproductive capability and reproductive health as the Aunt Sally of much of these technological novelties and experimentation. India has long been a place for experimentation and implementation of old and new reproductive technologies, which are at best problematic and at worst hazardous. In 1980s, poor Indian women were targeted for promotion of Norplant, the infamous hormonal contraceptive. If health is defined 'as a state of complete physical, mental and social well-being and not merely the absence of disease or infirmity' except for a rhetorical concern for reproductive health, then women's health and well-being in India has certainly been a backbencher and a neglected issue. If India is an international destination for infertile couples seeking low-priced IVF (in vitro fertilisation), and surrogacy services, then it also has one of the highest maternal mortality and pregnancy-related morbidity rates in the world. The Center for Reproductive Right's report on maternal mortality in India estimates that around 117,000 maternal deaths occur here every year (CRR, 2008: 9). From a global perspective, India accounts for 19 per cent of all live births and 27 per cent of all maternal deaths (Saha and Saha, 2010: 2). The high incidence of maternal death in India continues to threaten the well-being of families, decimate economic productivity, and perpetuate health disparities. The dismal picture of majority women's health makes it abundantly clear that those majority women themselves along with larger section of society, do neither have any perception nor any initiative to cater to almost half of their citizens' health and welfare. Although life expectancy is same during the time of birth of both men and women, deeply entrenched patriarchal norms and values of India manifests itself in both the public and private spheres of women's lives in the country, determining the 'life chances' of women resulting in their qualitatively inferior status in every sphere and indubitably in health. This inferior health status starting from the conception where girls are regularly killed in the womb continuing with malnutrition, discriminatory family biases of preferential distribution of food and other circumstances culminating in marriages and pregnancies with high mortality rates, particularly during childhood and in their reproductive years. Since health is socially determined and to a considerable extent access to healthcare, is almost fully so. This being so, the 'lived experiences' of women in India are replete with potential risk factors that have implications for their lives and well-being. On top, this new international division of labour inculcates the redistribution of reproductive work that has divided potential gendered allies by conscripting migrant and subaltern classes of women in the service of metropolitan, citizen, and bourgeois women.

This paper, thus, interrogates the globalisation of reproductive inequalities and women's right to self-determination over their own bodies by using these technologies, focusing on their other distinct social identities by applying intersectionality especially focusing on women of urban India. Here an attempt is made to demonstrate that what appears to be freedom of 'choice' for white and rich women seems to translate into further commodification of the body of economically disadvantaged women. The paper addresses the question of what it means to practice intersectionality sociologically as a theoretical and methodological approach to 'unequal exchange in reproduction' with special reference to the thriving 'supermarket of reproductive alternatives' especially in the zenith of globalisation. The possibilities of selling body parts like eggs, or renting organs like wombs, define new types of social relations, created by the technologies of assisted reproduction. Artificial insemination, IVF and ovum transfer, although in actuality only marginally successful, along with surrogacy are widely practiced. Thus, the female body's generative capacity has now been discovered as a new 'arena of investment' and profit-making for scientists, medical engineers and entrepreneurs in the convivial ambiance of globalisation and ICTs. This study brings to the fore certain issues: do these technologies discriminate between women in terms of race, social class and developed/developing nations? Does there now exist another variety of 'division of labour and concomitant inequality' also in reproduction—between poor women who 'sell eggs or rent their uteruses' and affluent women who pay for them through the conduit of gigantic biomedical engineering and pharmaceutical companies, genetic and drug industries and research institutes and hospitals? In particular, is women's use of technologies for assisted conception, and the local and global transactions a classic testimony of erosion of the boundaries between reproductive body parts in the era of globalisation? Does this assisted reproductive arena create further new telling burdens on marginalised women's health? Have these repositioned women in a new system of inequality more subversive and invisible than even before?

Intersectional Perspective and New and Assisted Reproductive Technologies (NRTs and ARTs)

Global fertility industry or transnational surrogacy, whatever the taxonomy may be, is a prime example where intersectional paradigm is the most pertinent one. So, to begin with what does an intersectional approach entail? It is posited on the study of a matrix of power relations. It involves the simultaneous analyses of multiple, intersecting sources of subordination/oppression and is based on the premise that the impact of a particular source of subordination may vary, depending on its combination with other potential sources of subordination (or of relative privilege) (Denis, 2008: 677) It can be used in both quantitative and qualitative work (McCall, 2005), which examines the micro level of lived experiences (Smith, 1987; Shields, 1987), the meso level of organisations (Acker, 2006) or social structures (Risman, 2004), and the macro level (McCall, 2005) including internationally. What kinds of intersectionalities help to understand women's lives e.g., in terms of reproductive rights of women including the complexities of context notably economic location, place and time? While gender, class and race have become a widely accepted (though sometimes critiqued) triad of socially relevant locations for study (whose meaning is influenced by their very interconnection), they are not the only ones. Also of interests are ethnicity, religion/religious practice, nationality/citizenship, marital status, country of residence generation, class (whether class of origin or current class) languages, age, heterosexuality and able-bodiedness. Intersectionality addresses the most central theoretical and normative concern within feminist scholarship, namely, the acknowledgement of differences among women. The very fact of differences among women has become the leading subject of feminist theories in recent years. For Maria Mies (1986: 114-16), an increasing convergence of the sexual and international division of labour, a division where the women of the former colonies are mostly producers and women of the developed world mainly consumers is clearly manifest especially in transnational surrogacy and in case of migrant paid domestic workers (Hochschild, 2000). By addressing the issue of differences among women, intersectionality makes perceptible the multiple positioning that constitutes everyday life and the power relations that are central to it. Thus, intersectionality not only promises to address the 'fundamental and pervasive concern' of difference and diversity, but it does so in such a way that it is able to problematise the theoretical hegemony of gender and also provides a platform for feminist theory as a shared enterprise. In the context of this paper, to approach a policy problem (related to reproductive rights, for example) with an intersectional design (in order to ask questions about differences in constructions and experiences of reproductive freedoms according to class, race, national boundaries, sexual orientation and diverse ability) is to declare that reproductive freedom and rights ought to be examined for their differential, contradictory and contested entitlements and burdens.

In 2004, the European Commission—which allowed 'egg donation'—had to face a scandal around cases of economic abuse of eastern European women as egg producers. A clinic in Bucharest, Romania, named Global Arts and some laboratories in the United Kingdom (UK) were proven to be involved in traffic of eggs. Poor and uneducated women were paid $250 for every 'donation' (a worker's salary in Romania was in 2004 around $100 per month) and were not informed about health risk. They were asked to sign an illegal contract in order to protect the clinic from consequences. The whole issue was known because of journalists' inquiries about women who had severe health problems after 'donating' to Global Arts. A resolution was taken by the European Parliament against the traffic of human ova. Eggs were re-defined as body parts, and the ban on commercialisation of organs was approved, voted by 307 deputees; 199 contrary; and 25 abstained. Yet, heterologue forms of fertilisation are still possible by using forms of compensation masked as expense reimbursements. An extra-legal market seems to be operating alongside the legal one, and women who produce eggs or rent, their uteruses may become victims of criminal networks that work at the transnational level. Moreover, the legislative divide between countries in the world gave birth to forms of 'reproductive tourism' from the less permissive countries to the more accommodating ones. In some countries, sex selection, as well as the selection of other characteristics, are not permitted—but affluent couples fly overseas where they can shop for these services. Some have argued that NRTs have brought 'new freedoms' in the form of opportunities for some women—for instance, to prevent unwanted pregnancy and births through contraception and abortion; to some extent, the prevention of birth of undesired children through prenatal diagnosis technologies; and the possibility of motherhood for infertile women/couples and single and lesbian women through artificial insemination or IVF. Concomitantly, they have also brought 'new dependencies', on technologies and at a heavy price, not only financially, but also in terms of adverse effects on women's physical and mental health. While for some women, use of these technologies has meant a shift from being 'objects' and 'victims' to 'knowing subjects' and 'agents' of control over their own bodies, for others they have brought more outside control and expropriation. Considering the divisions between women who profit from NRTs and those exploited by them, medicalisation of women's bodies and the adverse effects of these technologies are unquestionably attested. Since not all women have the same interests regarding NRTs, coming from different socio-economic and cultural circumstances, the increasingly global hegemony of enterprise culture, the rise of fundamentalism, increasing disparities characterising various forms of domestic and international inequalities, and a woman's right to choose can be seen to be in crisis. This crisis is perhaps nowhere sharper than in relation to the transactions in reproductive body parts and reproductive services made possible through the globalisation of NRTs on the one hand, and ICTs (including the Internet) on the other. Previous feminist analyses have shown that under patriarchy, women has always been an object, but in the new reproductive technologies she is no longer one whole object but a series of objects which can be isolated, examined, recombined, sold, hired or simply thrown away, like ova that are not used for experimentation or fertilisation. Combined with the scientific method of analysis and synthesis, the woman has become less than a human person, bringing about her vivisection into a mass of reproductive matter. At bottom, as Mies (1988: 11) reminds us so aptly that "What is left is an assembly of parts. The bourgeois individual has eliminated itself." Thus ARTs and surrogacy are the latest additions to the long list of services that are offered in medical tourism and fertility industry, which portrays it as a win-win situation for the intended parents as well as the surrogate, with the clinics and the providers being the nucleus of the arrangement.

Personal is Global in the Supermarket of Reproductive Alternatives

Briefly, globalisation is marked in particular by transnational capital and trade liberalisation. Neoliberal economic policies facilitate the globalisation of technologies (through the import of high-tech equipment) and ideas (through the global electronic media, including satellite television), also made possible by faster modes of transport of goods, persons (through aviation) and knowledge (through the Internet). The global development of capitalism is nothing new, but what characterises its most recent phase is the 'cultural convergence' of cultures and lifestyles around the world in the societies it impacts. Although the market is the primary motor of globalisation, its implications are not limited to the commercial arena alone. In the field of biological reproduction, globalisation—understood as the rapid growth of global capitalism—has brought in its wake an extension of consumer culture creating 'new regimes of consumption'. Not only have women's whole bodies been thrown onto the world market for trafficking, the human body and its parts (organs, tissues, and cells) have been turned into commodities that are exchanged and traded. Initially confined to solid organs such as kidneys, livers and hearts, with the development and expanded use of IVF technology, the last decade of the 20th century saw this extended to reproductive body parts, such as sperm, ova and embryos, which have become discrete entities—commodities that can be donated or traded. These can be done by individuals themselves as well as infertility specialists, IVF brokers, etc., for profit. There is an unregulated trade in body parts and fertility tourism within and across countries; in particular, increasing access to the Internet has contributed immensely to the trade's further proliferation. Several centers all over the world, mainly in the US and Europe, but also in India, are profiting from the 'fertility business', including the commercial transactions in reproductive body parts. Globalisation involves an interaction between economic and cultural factors whereby changes in production and consumption factors can be seen as producing new shared identities. High-tech reproductive technologies are available in many developing countries, too. Since globalisation and new technologies make possible a beyond border, an experience of stateless citizenship the very personal matter of giving birth to babies or pregnancy, and the sanctification of biological motherhood has been trampled by transnational surrogacy to an enormous extent. The birth of babies, through surrogacy arrangements has graduated to "a public issue from a personal trouble" with all fanfare. The difference with this outsourcing is that it is emotionally mediated as childbirth, which is a highly emotional aspect of human lives and thus in the era of this super-capitalism the personal is not only public, it is a global issue. The difference is elsewhere. Here a customised baby is ordered by the affluent intended parents like commodities in the global supermarket of reproductive alternatives but in case of natural birth there hardly exists even a remote possibility of this variety.

The purpose here is not be condemnatory about the intended parents or intended mothers, but "purpose is to explain how such a consumer-driven commodity chain comes to exist, being shaped, while simultaneously shaping individual's experiences of infertility, feeling of loss and potential for recovery" (Rudrappa, 2013: 129). Karla Momberger (2000: 1-2, 32) a graduate student at Columbia law school, relates her story:

> I began my feminist/activist career trying to escape the confines of my body, and that now I take refuge in the solid reality of me-ness that my body brings... I donated ova to pay for law school. That's what I did. I am the mythical $50,000 woman. My finishing law school and becoming a lawyer depended, quite literally, on my body and how much it is worth.

Also, specialised agencies mediate between infertile women and potential egg donors (primarily college girls recruited through ads on college notice boards and the Internet) to choose from, with photos and complete profiles regarding IQ (intelligence quotient) and other characteristics. However, attempts to set up commercial transnational surrogacy bureaus have been largely unsuccessful in most Western European countries and UK, due to restrictive legislation, where also the sale of human gametes is banned by law. Since July 2003, Baby Donors, an Amsterdam-based company, claiming to be the first in Europe, has been advertising its services on its website, operationalised in September 2003. It offers to act as an intermediary for the sale of tailor-made, personalised sperm insemination and egg donor packages through the internet. It seeks entrepreneurs from around the world for franchising or joint venture partners at a license fee of €5,000. The global manifestations of ARTs are varied. Consumers of ARTs as reproductive aid range from infertile couples to couples who want children with special characteristics to same sex couples and women beyond their reproductive ages. Although the playing ground of ARTs remains uneven, it is the developed capitalist countries who remain the consummate consumer, and the global South continues to be the source of raw materials and suppliers of service. Interestingly enough, India, where most of the medical facilities for majority ordinary Indians wallow in utter miserable conditions, the presence of skilled intermediaries and cutting-edge technologies, cheaply accessible ample wombs for assisted reproduction has made India world's capital of transnational gestational and/or traditional surrogacy.

Transnational Surrogacy and Indian Surrogates: Unequal Exchange?

> All kinds of US jobs are being outsourced to India, from telemarketing to computer programming. Now you can add one more service to that list: child-bearing. Yes you heard right. Some childless couples in Europe and US are hiring Indian women as surrogate mothers (World Vision Report, 2009).

> Women of the South...are increasingly reduced to numbers, targets, wombs, tubes and other reproductive parts by the population controllers (Mies and Shiva, 1993).

The larger context in which surrogacy is practiced today is fundamentally propelled by commerce within the globalised economy. It has also become an essential component of the flourishing larger fertility industry. This is hardly a revelation that commercial surrogacy has assumed transnational industrial proportion and India has emerged as the global destination for not only ART practices like IVF, but also for traditional and gestational surrogacy arrangements. In fact, India is well-positioned to lead the world in making especially commercial gestational surrogacy a viable industry: labour is cheap, doctors are well-qualified, no problem of English being spoken as all the intermediaries know or are well-versed in it, adoptions are closed, and the government has worked hard to establish an infrastructure for medical tourism. Under Indian Council of Medical Research (ICMR) 2005 guidelines, there was no legal bar for the use of ART (assisted reproductive technology) by a single or an unmarried woman, and the child born would have legal rights on the woman or man concerned. Thereafter, partly due to pressure from campaigns because of absence of law on surrogacy, the draft ART Bills of 2008, 2010 and 2013, stated to be revised based on recommendations of the Ministry of Law and Justice, which have consistently proposed that ART in India would be available to all persons including single persons and foreign couples. The Ministry of Home Affairs (MHA), according to the guidelines of 9 July 2012, restricted surrogacy to foreign nationals; i.e., a man and a woman married for at least two years would be required to take a medical visa for surrogacy in India. As of now, even though surrogacy is an administrative concern, it has been decided that until the enactment of a law on the ART Bill, 2013, the guidelines issued by the MHA will prevail.[1] Further women in India cannot act as surrogates for more than three successful births, including that of their own children, is one of the landmark provision part of the proposed draft ART Bill, which the government plans to bring to the Cabinet before introducing in the Parliament for passage (PTI news reported in *The Hindu*, 5 August 2013). This in a sense is 180-degree turnaround for the anti-natal Indian state to turn pro-natal in case of ARTs and NRTs. But in all these, there is one clear convergence that it was the Indian woman who has been the target of both anti-natal population control campaigns and pro-natal pro-technology programmes. Further interesting is: how the use of ARTs like surrogacy is congruent with the anti-natal dialogue and hard-line population control programmes in India? Some have termed it "revised eugenic scripts". The negative eugenics has aimed the lower income groups and minorities with voluntary or coerced sterilisation, whereas the rhetoric of so-called "individual choices" tactically highlight ARTs as options for upper class and of course, white couples desperate to reproduction of a baby under their privatised surveillance. Not unexpectedly, these current forms of eugenics are matching to and probably product of neoliberal ideologies and policies (Pande, 2014: 27-32). Hartmann (2006) accurately explains the association between concepts of 'waste' and 'burden' with negative eugenics and the concept of 'consumer choice' as central to positive eugenics and the endorsement of ARTs and NRTs. This revised eugenics scripts is writ large in the policies of Government of India (GoI). It is ironic that the Government expenditure is decreasing on public health facilities and state-run hospitals where poor women access are mostly in dismal conditions barring a few and also rather

1. *http://www.thehindu.com/opinion/op-ed/ending-discrimination-in-surrogacy-laws/article5970609.ece*, Visited on 4 July 2014.

confounding that the country which has the highest absolute number of maternal deaths and 51 doctors for every 100,000 people, there many Indian scientists and doctors are investing in NRTs and ARTs. That is to say, the history of reproductive politics in India is not only a saga of state's surveillance and control of women's fertile bodies, but also carries a tale of contradictions (Pande, 2014: 35).

India's surrogacy explosion began when in 2004, when Radha Patel gestated and delivered twins for her UK-based daughter at Dr Nayna Patel's Akanksha Ferility Clinic in Anand, Gujarat (Ruparelia, 2007). This small town established its reputation as the surrogacy outsourcing center of the world. Due to the non-existence of any national registry, no authentic and reliable information can be given on the number of such clinics in India but information from ICMR and National Commission for Women (NCW) provide an approximate number of 3000 clinics that are in operation (Smerdon, 2008; Sama, 2009a). Surrogates are recruited through different procedures. For example, Dr Rama Devi's hospital in Mumbai sends infertile couples pictures of their surrogate and accept special request for 'Muslim eggs' and 'Hindu surrogates' and recruits surrogacy workers from among her employees' families and acquaintances (Schultz, 2008). Multinational corporate hospital like Planet hospital and corporate five-star hospitals like Rotunda Medical Center in Mumbai recruit surrogates through newspaper advertisement and are less personal compared to Dr Patel's Akanksha Ferility Clinic. The Rotunda offers a DHL-Cryo-Ship programme for couples to send frozen gametes and embryos to India for implantation. They were supposed to start a Skype Surrogate Connect video-conference programme so that the parents are able to have a clear notion of how well the pregnancy is going and whether or not the surrogate is looked after (Medical Tourism Corporation, 2009). Furthermore, there is no fixed fee for surrogacy in India, but the costs are significantly less. The entire surrogacy process in the US costs between $40,000 and $150,000. Surrogate workers receive between $20,000 and $30,000 of this sum. In India, the complete medical procedure, surrogate's fee, airline tickets, and hotel stay for two trips to India costs around $25,000, but prices can go as low as $12,000. Of that total cost, Indian women are paid between $2000 and $10,000 for their services (Gentleman, 2008). The demand for surrogacy is high, but applicant pools are deep. Some critics of globalisation fear that surrogacy services will follow the 'race to the bottom' pattern paved by previously outsourced industries. Shweta Khanna worked as a surrogate once before and was looking for another opportunity. Initially, she asked for about $2000, but when another woman offered $1500, Shweta had to settle half her original amount (Niazi, 2009: 1). In other cities, the demand has driven up the price! In 2004, surrogate workers received about $3000 for a successful delivery, but the going rate in Delhi was $10,600 (Wade, 2009). Every major city in India, such as Mumbai, Delhi, Chennai, Bengaluru and Kolkata, now are partners in surrogacy trade and proffer gestational surrogacy to those who can afford to pay the price (Wade, 2009).

The international press usually reinforces connections between poverty and surrogacy work creating the impression that it is the opportunity of a lifetime. The median family income in Anand, for example, is about ₹2,500 per month (about $52.00) putting most surrogacy worker's income at the poverty line (Pande, 2008; 2009). Many women earn enough to pull their families temporarily out of poverty or debt. Suman Dodia will buy a house with the $4500 that she earns from carrying a British couple's child. It would have taken her fifteen years to earn that sum as a maid (Schultz, 2008). Najima Vohra moved to Anand to work as a surrogate. She has no job, but helps her husband with his scrap metal business. They earn about $1.20-$1.45 a day. She worked in the wheat fields growing up, was married when she was 16, and has little education. The amount of $5500 that she earned as surrogate will buy the family a brick house, pay for her children's education, and help grow her husband's business. Sofia Vohra became a surrogate because she earns $25 a month as a glass-crusher, her husband is a drunk, and she must pay her daughter's dowries. "I'll be glad when this is over," she says, and quickly adds, "This is not exploitation. Crushing glass for 15 hours a day is exploitation. The baby's parents have given me a chance to make good marriages for my daughters. That's a big weight off my mind" (Haworth, 2007). This is Prayanka Sharma's second contract pregnancy. She thinks that this is just a means of survival in an unequal world; she argues, "there is nothing wrong with this. We give them a baby and they give us much-needed money. It's good for them and it's good for us" (Scott, 2007). Surrogacy is also a growing opportunity for single mothers. Rekha left an abusive marriage and her husband took the children because she could not support them. She became a surrogate to get her children back. A good number of salaried middle-class women have become surrogates to pay for family medical expenses. Anita, a bank worker, became a surrogate for a Korean-American couple, because her son has a heart condition and needed an expensive operation (Subramanian, 2007). The recent global recession also has had an impact on the fertility industry. Dr Patel has noticed an increase in middle-class women turning to surrogacy work as their husbands lose jobs (Chandran, 2009). This is how the global press presents surrogate workers' stories. The rhetorical focus here is on opportunity, choice and fair exchange, not unequal exchange, commodification of women's body, body parts or impact on health and risks. Rudy Rupak, President of Planet Hospital, says the client demand for ova from fair-skinned women is so high that he's flying donors from the former Soviet Republic of Georgia to clinics in India. A Planet Hospital surrogacy package that includes an Indian egg donor costs $32,500. One that includes eggs from Georgian donors costs $37,500 (Cohen, 2009). Colour and caste also play a central role in a surrogacy worker's negotiating power. As one clinician admits: "Brahmans get paid more than so-called 'untouchables' or lower castes. A fair-skinned, educated middle-class Brahman who speaks English will fetch that much more" (Subramanian, 2007: 9). According to another source many childless couples are interested in the women from northern India because "they are healthy and whitish in colour. Foreign couples are eager to have a white child" (Roy, 2008). One surrogate agent explains how he could not find work for a south Indian woman because she was too dark (Sama, 2006: 75). Dr Rama's Institute has a "Criteria for Selection of Surrogate" handout that she gives to customers, so that they know that "planned children are in good wombs."

> ...The surrogate mother should be no smaller than 1.60 meters (5'3") and should weigh between 50 and 60 kilograms (110 and

132 pounds). She should be married, have her own children and a regular period, be free of sexually transmitted and hereditary diseases, be tested for ovarian problems and chromosomal analyses, be emotionally stable ....The skin color should not be too dark, and the appearance should be "pleasant" (Schultz, 2008: 3).

In Sama's (2006: 74) analysis of 33 surrogacy-related advertisements, about 40 per cent specified that intended parents were looking for surrogates that were "fair, good-looking, and beautiful." But it must be kept in mind that these criteria are for gestational and not traditional surrogates. The surrogate is not genetically related to the fetus. So, worries about skin color are more likely worries about moral character. It appears that the racial markers that have historically marked light-skinned women as good mothers and dark-skinned women bad mothers have been extended to mark 'good' and 'bad' wombs. This is distinctly a characteristic mark of neo-racial and neo-colonial attitudes where patriarchy and super capitalism, i.e., globalisation intersect.

In the website of Medical Tourism Corporation of India, it is clearly stated: "What are the screening criteria for surrogate¿ How is a surrogate chosen in India¿"

Medical Tourism's network of hospitals in India has very meticulous and stringent criteria for choosing a surrogate. The surrogates are between 21-35 years of age. They are married with previous normal deliveries and healthy babies. Detailed medical history, surgical history, personal history, and family history is looked into. History of blood transfusion and addiction is also taken. It is made sure that the surrogate has an uneventful obstetric history (no repeated miscarriages, no antenatal, intra-natal and postnatal complications during previous pregnancies). The surrogate and her partner are screened for infectious diseases like sexually transmitted diseases, Hepatitis B, Hepatitis C, HIV, and VDRL. Thalassemia screening is also done. Detailed pelvic sonography and other tests for uterine receptivity are performed to ensure maximum chances of success. A detailed financial and legal agreement is then drawn up between the surrogate and the commissioning couple.[2]

Choice is a real complicated and probably most contentious word in case of commercial surrogacy. Pande (2014: 134) tells us that "Ironically, while supporters of surrogacy emphasise the element of choice (i.e., that is the woman has the right to choose what to do with her body) most of the surrogates' narratives indirectly downplay choice as part of their decision, as if to say, 'it was not only in my hands, so I cannot be held responsible, and should not be stigmatised'." One of Pande's surrogate said that she knows that surrogacy is unethical but it is absolutely necessary for survival or to fill the empty stomach. It is obvious that as surrogates become conduits to give birth to children, their autonomy, choice, and freedom are all redefined and reconstructed within the framework of negotiation, discipline, control and surveillance; thus ultimately transforming their bodies into 'docile bodies'. In other words, a surrogate is not at all free to interpret her pregnancy or her life during this period. In actual reality, "the surrogacy contracts, ideally created to protect the rights of all parties, are undoubtedly skewed toward protecting the interests and rights of the intended parents, rather than the surrogate" (Nayak, 2013: 16). It is well-nigh impossible for the surrogates to defy the decisions of the intended parents reiterating their subordinate status and lack of power to take decisions freely. With or without the written contract, the surrogate is almost totally subservient to the clinic and the intended parents. This is indisputably clear when staying arrangements of the surrogates are taken into consideration.

Portrayals about surrogate workers staying arrangement during their pregnancy are also not encouraging and glorious. I will present some research findings here. Questions have been raised about surrogate workers' autonomy under these contracts. One of the fears is that under so-called "third world conditions" surrogates would be coerced into accepting living conditions, where their pregnancies could be more strictly monitored. Most surrogacy programmes have hostels where nurses and nutritionists attend to

2. *http://www.medicaltourismco.com/low-cost-surrogacy-in*. Visited on 23 December 2014.

their daily needs. Some clinics allow children to live with surrogates and permit family visits, and others regulate interactions. Surrogates in residence at Patel's clinic routinely get visits from family and friends, and "are happy never to leave the premises: meals are catered, kids are in the care of husbands or parents, and jobs are on hold. They will get better care for these pregnancies than they had for their own...and for many it's the first time they have not had to work" (Subramanian, 2007) Another Mumbai hospital offers a voluntary hostel programme, which according to Dr Gautam Allahbadia, does not confine surrogates forcefully. "Right in the beginning, some surrogates move in to the hostel sometimes with their children and some surrogates who have family compulsions stay at home" (Medical Tourism Corporation, 2009). Under the contract Nagadurga signed at Dr Rama's clinic, she has agreed to put her children into a home and to avoid sexual intercourse with her husband during the pregnancy (Schultz, 2008). Surveillance and regulation are sometimes used as selling points. Julie has tried five times to conceive. She is hiring an Indian surrogate because most surrogates stay either in the clinic or in supervised homes, and "that kind of control would just not be possible in the United States." In the US, "you have no idea if your surrogate mother is smoking, drinking alcohol, doing drugs. You have no idea what she's doing. You have a third party agency [in India] as a mediator between the two of you" (Scott, 2007). Madge's (2013: 16) work on a private medical clinic in Gujarat tells us that:

> The surrogates were placed in a surrogate hostel during the nine months of pregnancy. The hostel at the clinic was a two-story bungalow, which, originally, was the house of Dr Nita. There were eight rooms with iron beds and the belongings of the women were scattered around. The only source of entertainment for the women was television, one on each floor. Initially these surrogates found the idea of being away from family fascinating and a break from their daily routine. They chatted and laughed with each other. But slowly their 'controlled' life in the hostel due to their 'delicate pregnancies' ('soft', 'delicate', and 'fragile' were terms often used by the clinic staff and some surrogates also) rankled and took a toll on them. The women were not allowed to step out of the

house and their only trips for nine months were to the clinic and back. Though family members could visit on Sundays, the women missed their homes and children. I witnessed some of the women weeping uncontrollably for their families.

Surrogacy hostels, therefore, are contested spaces and the power hierarchy of the medical establishment, and intended parents pose restriction for surrogates' real autonomy. For example, a surrogate had received a mobile phone from an intended parents and had to deal with the inquiries about her health thus turning the advantage of having a mobile phone into a means of surveillance. The surrogate said:

> Madam calls me every day, and asks about my health telling me what to eat and not. Like yesterday, she told me to eat lots of green vegetables, as it would be good for my health. Anyways, I follow what the doctor asks me to do (Sama interview, surrogate Rita).

At a surrogacy hostel at Garv, Tina, a surrogate, describes the daily routine in the following way:

> Everything works like clockwork. We wake up at 8 am, have tea take our medicines and injections and go back to sleep. Then wake up at noon, bathe and eat lunch. We basically rest. That's what is required for us. We are allowed visitors but not for the night. In evening we pray. Then the English tutor comes and teaches us how to speak in English. We will be learning how to use a computer next (Quoted in Pande, 2014: 64).

The obedience to the clinic and to the intended parents is a clear case of power inequity in the surrogacy arrangement and life in surrogacy hostel can be added to the catalogue of "total Institutions", which Erving Goffman did not have the fortune to experience. In a real sense, the surrogate mothers have very few rights in India and are often stigmatised. Unlike pregnancy of a married woman which is often a matter of celebration, a surrogate pregnancy is veiled in secrecy and hence strict surveillance and exploitation are structurally embedded in Indian surrogacy arrangement. Also pregnancy in surrogacy is treated like an ailment as the pregnant women needed to be separated from the rest of the world. This certainly reminds of child birth practices up to early

20th century in several countries in terms of inclusion-exclusion dichotomy.

Indian Surrogates and their Health: Who Cares?

What is striking about surrogacy and other ARTs and NRTs is that how smoothly the global capitalist patriarchy accepts gendered globalised labour along with different body parts of women as commodities, whereas women had to struggle acrimoniously to get even an iota of their rightful dues, e.g., right to education, entry in different professional fields, like medicine, right to ancestral property, right to abortion, equal pay for equal work, right to divorce, etc.—both legally and socially. As mentioned earlier, India has a dismal track record as far maternal mortality and general health of women are concerned. In the 2014 Human Development Report (HDR) released on 24 July in Tokyo, India is ranked at 135 out of 187 countries (*Times of India*). In India, where women are portrayed as Matrishakti (mother power) paradoxically face huge social, economic and cultural barriers to good healthcare lifelong, of course subject to their class location. Indian women's lived experiences as gendered beings result in multiple and, significantly, interrelated health needs. The multiple burdens of 'production and reproduction' borne from a position of disadvantage has telling consequences on women's well-being. Every five minutes an Indian woman dies of pregnancy-related causes, and for every women that dies, 30 more develop chronic and debilitating conditions that affect her quality of life (CRR, 2008: 11). Maternal deaths are causally linked to poverty, education, and social status. In India 70 per cent of women are poor and women continue to earn half of what men earn (CRR, 2008: 17). The CRR attributes this to a range of gendered medical, socio-economic, caste, age-related and health-system-based factors including inadequate nutrition, early marriage, lack of access to medical care and family reluctance to seek out medical care for women and girls (CRR, 2008: 14-20). The Indian government has come under severe criticism in an UN-sponsored study for losing its focus on broader sexual and reproductive health of women while attempting to achieve the Millennium Development Goals (MDGs). The Eleventh Five Year Plan (2007-2012) in its 27 national targets has an aim to reduce incidence of anaemia amongst women and girls, which has a direct bearing on maternal health and maternal mortality. The reality shows that 55 per cent of the women in India are anaemic and that the number of anaemic women is increasing. The risks of anaemia (a condition associated with poor nutrition) are greater in India than anywhere else in the world. Anaemic women are more susceptible to communicable diseases such as tuberculosis and malaria. They also face additional risks of falling into a cycle of multiple pregnancies in their efforts to have children that survive. Unfortunately the persistence of gender-based discrimination in food, nutrition, and healthcare has increased anaemia rates over the past 10 years. The National Human Rights Commission (NHRC) reports that merely 30 per cent of the population receives services through the public health system, less than 50 per cent of women give birth with the assistance of a skilled attendant, and only 40 per cent of births happen in a hospital setting. Although the Indian government has promised to ensure that women get four antenatal examinations through the National Rural Health Mission (NRHM), less than three quarters receive any antenatal care at all. The National Family Health Survey (NFHS) reveals that only about 36.4 per cent of women across the country receive any postnatal care within two days of giving birth. For every maternal death in India, an estimated 30 more women suffer injury, infection, and pregnancy-related disabilities (NFHS-3).

The country where majority women's of the general health and welfare are so severely neglected, the surrogate women's health is not even considered in the discourses on women's health in public domain. The website of Medical Tourism Corporation, India, does not mention anything about the health of surrogates after delivery of the baby or if the pregnancy is unsuccessful. What happens to those who get ill during the pregnancy? Or, what happens if there are complications due to side effects of drugs or surgical procedure? A lull exists on all these. All the pamphlets and propaganda are about how 'normal, safe the procedure is, and how the 'surrogates are taken good care during their pregnancy' in spite of the fact that most surrogates come from lower socio-economic background with minimal educational qualification and also along with almost no understanding or consciousness about health. Commercial surrogacy, though has become a gargantuan industry, is inundated with possible harms and risks to surrogate women. The foremost risk stems from the financial burdens surrogates are under, and the pressure from the families for quick money. "Among the most common reasons for engaging in surrogacy that women cite are children's education, purchase of a house, marriage in the family and husband's inability to work" (Nayak, 2013: 7). Additionally, if family members are ill, which involve heavy financial responsibility, women enter into surrogacy. In fact, the website of Texas-based Medical Tourism Corporation has an entire page dedicated to 'low cost surrogacy' in India.

> Overall, one glance over the page promising 'low cost' surrogacy procedures for people from US, UK, Australia and other European countries gives a sense that the surrogacy in India is a procedure clearly designed to benefit those who will rent a womb in India, not the Indian women renting their wombs out.[3]

The healthcare needs of a surrogate are measured only in terms of giving birth to a child. Once she has delivered the coveted child, she is on her own. The narratives of different surrogates make it amply clear that they feel a bounden duty to support their families' financial interest or share the economic burden. One surrogate said, "My husband said your life should not be in danger. I said, it's okay, it doesn't matter. We have problems at home. Anyway, whatever is God's will, shall happen. Earlier people used to give births to 5-6 children." (Surrogate Anita, Sama interview). Another surrogate Rita said, "There has also been a change in the attitude of my husband from earlier (before surrogacy). Before, he was not considerate about my diet or health" (Sama interview). Thus, the one and only focal point of the surrogacy arrangement is to have a baby successfully, for which, the surrogate is nothing but a medium. Many surrogates have expressed feelings about neglect of the surrogates' health by the clinics, by the doctors and even by the

3. *http://www.firstpost.com/living/health-minister-harsh-vardhan-bats-adoption-surrogacy-1785103.html*. Visited on 5 December 2014.

intended parents after the birth. This disregard is of course the hall mark of the business that decides the transactions in this industry.

> The general attitude of the couples and the doctors is of carelessness with respect to their health. I am not saying this only for myself, but happens with other surrogates also. Everywhere the attitude is similar. The couples treat the surrogates only as a means of having a child. The health of the surrogate is the least of their concerns. (Surrogate Savita Sama interview).

Sunita had been a surrogate and an egg donor by the age of 26 and now a surrogate agent for recruiting possible potential surrogates. She was supposed to get ₹250,000 (approximately USD 5,000) for the surrogacy arrangement, but received only ₹30,000 (approximately USD 600) as she had miscarried after two and a half months (Sama interview). Sunita was unaware of the number of eggs that have been retrieved from her when she was the egg donor. Likewise, many of the surrogates were ignorant of the number of embryos that had been implanted in their wombs. Thus, there was no question of "informed consent' in this matter. Such situations clearly attest to the fact that in regard to bodily harm, the surrogates were minimally informed or completely uninformed about adverse effects of the process of surrogacy. The possibility of miscarriage in surrogacy arrangements are hardly considered risks by the clinics involved. To attain pregnancy, the body of the surrogate is artificially prepared by altering her natural menstrual cycle by inducing hormones. Some well-established side effects are hot flashes, mood swings, headaches, bloating, spotting, uterine cramping, fullness of breasts, light-headedness, and vaginal irritation. In addition to these, there is a very high possibility that the surrogate will undergo CS (caesarean section) as the doctors and the intended couples want a safe and controlled delivery of the baby. In most cases of commercial surrogacy, the majority of which are transnational, the intended couples prefer to be present at the time of delivery, requiring CS to be conducted. The potential risks of CS, however, are barely considered, *viz.*, infection of the incision or the uterus, heavy blood loss, injury and damage to the adjoining tissues of the uterus, injury to the fetus and problems from anaesthesia are only a few. In many instances, women are not given adequate time for recovery from CS or vaginal births, thus adding to the health risk of the surrogate.

It is not only the physical risks that a surrogate woman faces but also societal stigmatisation which has deep emotional impacts on her. In surrogacy, birth is not a matter of celebration like marriage as the former is done in utter secrecy. Mostly the husband knows as he signs the contract for the surrogate and then the women move to surrogacy hostels or homes which are again within locked doors and barbed wires. Rita said only she and her husband knew about it and they did not tell anyone. But there is a tension also about hiding it from everyone. I don't enter hospital from the front gate. It is a small place, you never know if somebody from our village is here, and also sees us! (Sama Interview).

This insider-outsider, emic-etic scenario is a telling one on the surrogates' mental health. They develop a guilt feeling and legitimise this by self-consoling that they are doing it for their families. But the whole situation is an unhealthy one from the point of view of an expecting woman.

This proves that the medical process and the establishment engaged in this business are hardly transparent. Majority of the surrogates being unaware of the drug effects and of the painful injections are just mere signatories without having sometimes faintest idea about the biomedical technologies and professional medicine used in childbirth related to different types of ARTs. Sama, the Delhi-based women's health group, has pointed out that the proposed surrogacy Bill has lots of health related loopholes and biased in favour of clinics and clients. The Bill tries to ensure that the surrogate goes through IVF even if her eggs are viable to keep a separation between the egg donor and the traditional surrogate so the that the latter cannot get attached to the baby. The Bill gives even right to ask for abortion and fetal reduction to the intended parents and the surrogate is bound to carry out this mandate (Pande, 2014: 177-78). Interestingly, but not surprisingly, health implications of surrogacy are rarely reported in the media. A rare media report on a 30 year old surrogate, who was attempting surrogacy for the third time ended up with innumerable health complications and a hysterectomy, received only ₹15,000 (approximately USD 300) for surrogacy, but not any compensation for her treatment (Srivastava, 2011). Ergo, surrogacy, thus, is exercised through coerced consent where the choice is limited or nil for the surrogate women as their healthcare needs are measured only in terms of giving birth to a child. So, who cares after the birth of the child what happens to the surrogates?

In Lieu of a Conclusion

At this point, it must be asserted that in response to the rising demand for surrogates in the fertility industry, two issues can be highlighted. First, when a child is born to a surrogate mother using sperm and eggs from anonymous donors because the infertile couple was unable to create their own embryo using the IVF techniques, the child then has five people who could lay claim to parenthood—a genetic mother, a commissioning mother, a surrogate mother, a genetic father and a commissioning father. If the intended parents are divorced (baby Manji case), then who is the legal mother of the baby? Does the child born to a surrogate mother automatically get the citizenship of the surrogate mother or the legal parents? In surrogacy nothing guarantees one's status as the parent: not egg, sperm, womb or breast milk and a whole new arena of kinship status is being redefined and reconstituted. Second, gestational surrogacy in India has supplied us with a lens to explain the ways specific technologies and materialisations continue to utilise the poor woman's body and body parts and her reproductive labour for the transnational market. In this supermarket of alternatives, surrogates giving birth to babies are no longer considered as mothers but simply contractual labourers/workers whose products can be sold to those who can afford it. These surrogate workers, like all other workers are mostly controlled by the owners, and obliviously cannot prevail upon the latter. Accordingly, surrogacy has led to the pushing of the boundaries of reproductive labour from the realm of the private to the public within a larger globalised paradigm. Commercial surrogacy lies at the intersection of patriarchy and capitalism and of a low-tech workforce with high-tech sophisticated reproductive technologies whose control is in the hands of massive biomedical engineering and pharmaceutical companies, genetic and drug industries and research institutes, hospitals and a new group of negotiators with highly skilled and ambitious hegemonic medical regime. What prayers do these surrogates alias contractual labours have since they need this new job of renting their wombs for their sustenance? Surrogates belong to industry's most unorganised sector who do not seem to have a chance even to organise themselves until and unless the state comes to the rescue, which has not happened yet and it seems there is not a slim chance even in the distant future!

The two central issues thus haunts: should commercial surrogacy in any form be promoted in a country like India with such an abysmally poor record on women's health? And, why is surrogacy preferred to adoption? Why are adoptions suddenly a dirty process and the adopted child the unholy baby? One response is preference for genetic ties as authentic, primordial ties in one way or the other for a strong, unmediated pure family. Are we going back or this eugenic propensity is late modern? (Becker, 2000).

Note: Names of all surrogates have been changed.

References

Acker, Joan (2006). *Class Questions: Feminist Answers*. Lanham, MD: Rowman & Littleffield Publishers.

Becker, G. (2000). *The Elusive Embryo: How Women and Men Approach New Reproductive Technologies*. Berkeley: University of California Place.

Bhatia, Shekhar (2012). "Revealed: More and More Britons are Paying Indian Women to Become Surrogate Mothers". 26 May. *http://www.telegraph.co.uk/health/healthnews/9292343/Revealed-how-more-and-more-Britons-are-paying-Indian-women-to-become-surrogate-mothers.html*. Visited on 12 August 2014.

Center for Reproductive Rights (CRR) (2008). *Maternal Mortality in India: Using International and Constitutional Law to Promote Accountability and Change*. New York: Center for Reproductive Rights. *http://reproductiverights.org/en/document/maternal-mortality-inindia-using-international-and-constitutional-law-to-promote-accountab*. (accessed: 11 November 2012).

Chandran, Rina (2009). "As Crisis Bites: Indian Women Turn to Surrogacy", *Reuters*. *http://www.reuters.com/article/idUSTRE53705T20090408* (accessed: 17 April 2010).

Cohen, Margot (2009). "A Search for a Surrogate Leads to India", *Wall Street Journal*, (October 9).

Corea, Genea (1985). *The Mother Machine: Reproductive Technologies from Artificial Insemination to Artificial Wombs*, New York: Harper and Row.

Dasgupta, Sayantani and Shamita Dasgupta (2013). "Shifting Sands", in S. Dasgupta and S. Dasgupta (eds.), *Globalisation and Transnational Surrogacy in India*. UK: Lexington. pp.67-84.

Denis, Ann (2008). "Intersectional Analysis. A Contribution of Feminism to Sociology", *International Sociology* 23.5: 677-94.

Gentleman, Amelia (2008). "India Nurtures Business of Surrogate Motherhood", *New York Times*, 10 March. p.A9

Harding, Sandra (1991). *Whose Science? Whose Knowledge? Thinking from Women's Lives*. Ithaca, NY: Cornell University Press.

Hartmann, Betsy (2006). "Eugenics of the Everyday: Some Preliminary Reflections", Background paper for the *Consultation on New Reproductive and Genetic Technologies and Women's Lives*. New Delhi. June.

Haworth, Abagail (2007). "Surrogate Mothers: Wombs for Rent", in *Marie Claire*. *http://www.marieclaire.com/world-reports/news/international/surrogate-mothers-india* (accessed: 16 January 2010).

Hoschschild, A.R. (2000). "Global Care Chains and Emotional Surplus Value", in W. Hutton and A. Giddens (eds.), *On the Edge: Living with Global Capitalism*. London: Jonathon Cape.

Madge, V. (2013). "Surrogacy in India: A Case Study of Clinic in Anand, Gujarat", Unpublished PhD. Dissertation.

McCall, Lesli (2005). "The Complexity of Intersectionality." *Signs: Journal of Women in Culture and Society* 3(30): 1771-800.

Medical Tourism Corporation (2009). "Interview with Dr Gautam Allahbadia—Surrogacy Expert India". *http://www.medicaltourismco.com/assisted-reproduction-fertility/dr-Gautam-Allahbadia-India-Surrogacy-Expert.php* (accessed: May 27, 2012).

Mies, Maria (1986). *Patriarchy and Accumulation on a World Scale: Women in the International Division of Labour.* London: Zed Books.

———. (1988). "From the Individual to the Individual: in the Supermarket of Reproductive Alternatives", *Reproductive and Genetic Engineering: Journal of International Feminist Analysis* 1(3): 1-13.

Mies, Maria and Vandana Shiva (1993). *Ecofeminism*. Melbourne: Spinifex.

Momberger, Karla (2000). "Breeder at Law", *Columbia Journal of Gender and Law* 11(2): 1-51.

Nayak, Preeti (2013). "The Three Ms of Commercial Surrogacy in India", in S. Dasgupta and S. Dasgupta (eds.), *Globalisation and Transnational Surrogacy in India*. UK: Lexington, pp.2-22.

Niazi, Shuriah (2009). "Surrogacy Boom", *Boloji.com*. 14 October. *http://www.boloji.com/wfs6/wfs1027.htm* (accessed: 23 March 2010).

Pande, Amrita (2009). "Not an 'Angel', Not a 'Whore'", *Indian Journal of Gender Studies* 16(2): 141-73.

———. (2008). "Commercial Gestational Surrogacy in India: Nine Months of Labor?, in Kenji Kosaka and Masahiro Ogino (eds.), *A Quest for Alternative Sociology*. Nishinomiya, Japan: Trans Pacific Press. pp.71-88.

Pande, Amrita (2014). *Wombs in Labour*. New York: Columbia University Press.

Peoples Democracy (2015). *Peoples Democracy*. 11 January . Accessed on 15 December 2014.

Risman, Barbara J. (2004). "Gender as a Social Structure: Theory Wrestling with Activism",*Gender & Society* 18(4), 429-50.

Roy, S. (2008). "Surrogate Motherhood: Should it be Allowed?", Merinews. com, 30 June.

Rudrappa, Sharmila (2013). "Mother India", in S. Dasgupta and S. Dasgupta (eds.), *Globalisation and Transnational Surrogacy in India*. UK: Lexington. pp.125-44.

Ruparelia, Rakhi (2007). Giving Away the "Gift of Life": Surrogacy and the Canadian assisted human reproduction act. In *Canadian Journal of Family Law* 23(1): 11-54.

Saha, U.C. and K.B. Saha (2010). A Trend in Women's Health in India—What Has Been Achieved and What Can Be Done", *Rural and Remote Health* 10: 1260..

Sama (2006). *ARTs and Women: Assistance in Reproduction or Subjugation?* New Delhi: Sama Resource Group for Women's Health.

——. (2009a). "Assisted Reproductive Technologies: For Whose Benefit?", in *Economic and Political Weekly* 46(18): 25-31.

——. (2009b). "Unravelling the Fertility Industry: Challenges and Strategies for Movement Building". *http://samawomenshealth.wordpress.com/2009/11/27/unraveling-the-fertility-industrychallenges-and-strategies-for-movement-building/* (accessed: 17 April 2010).

Schultz, Sandra (2008). "In India, Surrogacy Has Become a Global Business", *Der Spiegel Online (*trans. Christopher Sultan). *http://www.spiegel.de/international/world/0,1518,580209,00.html* (accessed: 23 March 2011).

Scott, Amy (2007). "Wombs for Rent" Grows in India"", *Marketplace NPR*. 27 December [MP3 file]

NFHS-3. Available: *http://www.nfhsindia.org/factsheet.html*. Data is listed by state. Visited on August 17, 2014.

Shields, Stephanie (1987). "Gender: An Intersectionality Perspective", *Sex Roles* (2008) 59: 301-11.

Smerdon, U.R. (2008). "Crossing Bodies, Crossing Borders: International Surrogacy Between the United States and India", *Cumberland Law Review* 39: 15-85.

Smith, Dorothy (1987). *The Everyday World as Problematic: A Feminist Sociology*. Boston: North-eastern University Press.

Srivastava, K. (2011). "Women-Loses-Uterus-After-Becoming-Surrogate-Mother-Thrice", *Daily News & Analysis*, 27 December. *http://www.dnaindia.com/mumbai/report_ women-loses-uterus-after-becoming -surrogate-mother-thrice,* visited on 19 February 2012.

Subramanian, Sarmishta (2007). "Wombs for Rent: Is Paying the Poor to Have Children Wrong When Both Sides Reap Such Benefits?", in *Maclean's* 2 July.

Wade, Matt (2009). "Take Away Baby Boom", in *Brisbane Times*. *http://www.brisbanetimes.com.au/news/world/the-takeaway-babyboom/2009/01/30/1232818725697.html* (accessed: 10 April 2011).

World Vision Report (2009). *Indian Surrogates, 2009. http://broadcast-silas.worldvision.org/worldvision/radio.nsf/469f9e233bacf93887256dbf00650330/ed1e72059d09300888257179005d0fbf.* Accessed on 9 October 2014.

Part IV

The Status of the Indian States

12

U.V. SOMAYAJULU

Infrastructure and Human Resources in Empowered Action Group (EAG) States

Progress Under NRHM and Issues

Introduction

The Hon'ble Prime Minister launched the National Rural Health Mission (NRHM) on 12 April 2005 throughout the country with special focus on 18 states, including eight EAG states, the northeastern states, Jammu & Kashmir (J&K) and Himachal Pradesh (HP).

The NRHM seeks to provide accessible, affordable and quality healthcare to the rural population, especially the vulnerable sections. It also seeks to reduce the MMR (maternal mortality ratio) in the country from 407 to 100 per 100,000 live births; IMR (infant mortality ratio) from 60 to 30 per 1,000 live births and the TFR (total fertility rate) from 3.0 to 2.1 within the seven-year period of the Mission.

The key features in order to achieve the goals of the Mission include making the public health delivery system fully functional and accountable to the community, human resources management, community involvement, decentralisation, rigorous monitoring and evaluation against standards, convergence of health and related programmes village level upwards, innovations and flexible financing and also interventions for improving the health indictors.

NRHM aims at improving the health status of the people in general and women and children in particular. The success of NRHM depends to a large extent on the infrastructure and human resources available at various levels.

Objectives and Data Sources

An attempt is made in this paper to understand the progress made in improving infrastructure as well as human resources at the health facilities in the EAG states *viz.,* Uttar Pradesh (UP), Madhya Pradesh (MP), Bihar, Chhattisgarh, Jharkhand, Rajasthan, Odisha and Uttarakhand. The union government identified these states as EAG states as they need special attention in terms of development inputs as they are weak in terms of public health indicators and public health infrastructure.

The paper uses the available secondary data and reports such as Common Review Mission Reports, Rural Health Statistics and other secondary sources.

Discussion of Results

Financial Allocations

The Government of India's (GoI) allocation for Ministry of Health and Family Welfare (MoHFW) increased from ₹14,974 crores in 2007-08 to ₹37,330 crores in 2013-14. In 2013-14, allocation for NRHM was ₹19,120 crores accounting for 51 per cent of the total MoHFW's budget. GoI's allocations for NRHM increased by 73 per cent during 2007-08 to 2013-14. There also have been improvements in utilisation of the allocated funds. When NRHM was launched, in 2005-06, only 72 per cent of the total released funds (GoI and state) were spent, while in 2011-12, 86 per cent of the released funds were spent. In 2012-13, per capita (rural) NRHM expenditure was ₹213 and ₹131, if the total population (urban and rural) is taken into account.

Financial allocations for enhancing human resources in public health facilities have increased considerably in the recent past. For instance, the allocation increased from ₹769 crores in 2010-11 to ₹2,179 crores in 2012-13.

Number of Facilities and Human Resources at National Level

Table 12.1 gives the progress in health infrastructure at the national level. There is considerable improvement in physical infrastructure at various levels. Although number of Health Sub-centres (HSCs) increased by 1.6 per cent during the reference period, the HSCs in government buildings increased from 50 per cent to 64 per cent. The number of Auxiliary Nurse Midwifes (ANMs) at HSCs increased by 34 per cent.

Table 12.1

Health Infrastructure: All India

Infrastructure	*2005*	*2012*	*% change*
HSCs	146,026	148,366	1.6
HSC in government building (%)	50	64	28
ANMs at HSCs	139,798	187,902	34
PHCs	23,236	24,049	3.5
PHCs in government building(%)	78	90	15
24×7 PHCs		8236-34%	
Allopathic Doctors at PHCs	20,308	28,984+ 6,323 Ayush	74
CHCs	3,346	4833	97
24×7 CHCs		4321-89%	
Specialists at CHCs	3,550	5062	42
CHCs in government building (%)	92	97	5.4
Nurse midwife at PHC/CHC	28,930	46,903	62
Lab Technician at PHC/CHC	12,284	12,941	5.3
Pharmacist at PHC/CHC	17,708	21,003	19
Radiographer at PHC/CHC	1,337	1,886	41

Source: Government of India, 2012.

The number of Primary Health Centres (PHCs) increased by 3.5 per cent, while PHCs in government building increased from 78 per cent to 90 per cent. Thus, most of the PHCs have own building. Another significant improvement is in terms of the number of 24×7 PHCs, where one-third of the PHCs in 2012 becoming operational 24×7. The number of doctors at PHCs increased from 20,308 to 35,307 (74% increase from 2005).

The number of Community Health Centres (CHCs) increased by 97 per cent and 89 per cent of these are operational 24×7 and 97 per cent have own government building. The number of specialists at CHCs increased by 42 per cent, which is a good sign as specialist services are needed at this level.

Increase in the number of ANMs and radiographer at PHC/CHC level is high with 62 per cent and 41 per cent respectively, while that of lab technicians was about 5 per cent, and this perhaps needs attention as it affects the diagnostic services provided at PHC/CHC. Availability of pharmacists at PHC/CHC increased by 19 per cent.

Number of First Referral Units (FRUs)

FRUs play vital role in the health service delivery as the cases that need specialist care or services are referred to these facilities by the providers at PHC level. Increase in the number of FRUs *viz.,* district hospitals, sub-divisional hospitals, and CHCs at the national level can be understood from the analysis presented in Table 12.2. The total number of FRUs increased by 2.8 times in the reference period of 2005-06 to 2012-13. The biggest increase was recorded in case of CHCs, followed by that of district hospitals, with the lowest increase of 1.9 fold in case of sub-divisional hospitals. Overall, the FRUs increased by 2.8 fold in the reference period.

Table 12.2

Number of FRUs: All India

Number of FRUs	*2005-06*	*2012-13*	*Increase*
District Hospital (DH)	213	620	2.9 fold
Sub-divisional Hospital (SDH)	364	708	1.9 fold
CHC	343	1313	3.8 fold
Total	940	2641	2.8 fold

Source: Government of India, 2012.

Population Coverage by Health Facilities

Table 12.3 gives the population coverage by various health facilities at all-India level. In spite of improvements in financial allocations and the total number of facilities, the population covered by the facilities is higher than the prescribed norm in case of HSCs, PHC and CHCs. The sub-centres cover an average population of 5,615 and 4 villages, while the PHCs cover 27 villages and population of 34,641. The CHCs cover, on an average, 133 villages and population of 1.73 lakh. State-wise analysis (not presented in Table 12.3) reveals that the average population covered by PHCs is high in some of the states—68,442 in West Bengal and 75,870 in Jharkhand—much higher than the national average. This needs attention as this would have implications in terms of quality of care.

Table 12.3

Population Coverage by Health Facilities: All India

Facility	*Population Norm*	*Population Coverage*	*Average Number Villages*
SC	3,000-5,000	5,615	4
PHC	20,000-30,000	34,641	27
CHC	80,000-120,000	1.73 lakh	133

Source: Government of India, 2012.

Having understood the national scenario, we will now focus on the situation in the EAG states.

Progress in Facilities during 2005-2010

As Table 12.4 indicates, there was considerable increase in the number of 24×7 PHCs during 2005-2010 across the states. The improvement in terms of number of 24×7 PHCs was considerable in Bihar and Jharkhand in particular. Same holds good for the number of FRUs as well. The improvement in number of FRUs was also considerable in most of the EAG states such as MP, Bihar and Rajasthan as the situation improved from nil. While UP has the highest number of 24×7 PHCs, Odisha has the lowest number.

Table 12.4

Progress in Number of 24×7 PHCs and First Referral Units 2005-2010

State	*Number of 24×7 PHCs*		*Number of FRUs*	
	2005	*2010*	*2005*	*2010*
Bihar	0	533	0	76
Chhattisgarh	125	418	48	56
Jharkhand	0	194	0	19
Madhya Pradesh	180	212	0	87
Odisha	-	64	0	48
Rajasthan	-	500	0	100
Uttar Pradesh	225	648	42	136
Uttarakhand	8	94	29	72

Source: Government of India, 2012.

Even MP has less number of 24×7 PHCs. seems to be having less number of 24×7 PHCs. UP has the highest number of FRUs, while Jharkhand has the lowest number, with Odisha having less number of FRUs.

Number of Health Facilities Functioning

One can understand the changes in health infrastructure in terms of number of functioning Sub-Centres (SCs), PHCs and CHCs across the EAG states during 2005-2012 from the Table 12.5. The number of SCs increased in Uttarakhand, Rajasthan, Odisha and Chhattisgarh, while it reduced in Bihar, Jharkhand and MP. In UP, the number of SCs remained same during 2005-2012. Increase in number of PHCs was recorded in Bihar, Chhattisgarh, Uttarakhand and UP, while decline was recorded in Jharkhand, MP, Odisha, and Rajasthan. In case of CHCs, Chhattisgarh, Jharkhand, MP, Odisha, Rajasthan, Uttarakhand and UP recorded increase, while Bihar recorded decline. UP had the highest number of SCs, PHCs and CHCs, while Uttarakhand had the lowest number of these facilities. Bihar has less number of CHCs.

Table 12.5

Number of Functioning SCs, PHCs and CHCs: 2005-2012

	State	2005			2012		
		No. of SCs	*No. of PHCs*	*No. of CHCs*	*No. of SCs*	*No. of PHCs*	*No. of CHCs*
1	Bihar	10337	1648	101	9696	1863	70
2	Chhattisgarh	3818	517	116	5111	755	149
3	Jharkhand	4462	561	47	3958	330	188
4	Madhya Pradesh	8874	1192	229	8869	1156	333
5	Odisha	5927	1282	231	6688	1226	377
6	Rajasthan	10512	1713	326	11487	1528	382
7	Uttarakhand	1576	225	44	1848	257	59
8	Uttar Pradesh	20521	3660	386	20521	3692	515

Source: Government of India, 2012.

Building for SCs, PHCs and CHCs

Table 12.6 gives the status of building availability for the SCs in the states. In Bihar, Chhattisgarh, Odisha and Jharkhand, half of the SCs was functioning in government buildings in 2012. In Rajasthan,

Table 12.6

Building Status of Sub-Centres 2005-2012

State	2005				2012				
	Total No. of Functioning SCs	No. of SCs Functioning in			Total No. of Functioning SCs	No of SCs Functioning in			Buildings Under Construction
		Government Building	Rented Building	Rent Free Panchayat/ Voluntary Society Building		Government Building	Rented Building	Rent Free Panchayat/ Voluntary Society Building	
Bihar	10,337	NA	NA	NA	9,696	4,848 (50%)	4,848	0	2616
Chhattisgarh	3,818	1,458 (38%)	0	2,360	5,111	2,740 (54%)	906	1,465	1320
Jharkhand	4,462	NA	NA	NA	3,958	1,969 (50%)	1,066	923	612
Madhya Pradesh	8,874	3,996 (45%)	4,878	0	8,869	7,254 (82%)	1,035	580	956
Odisha	5,927	2,542 (43%)	3,385	0	6,688	3,570 (53%)	2,708	410	1344
Rajasthan	1,0512	8,211 (78%)	0	2,301	11,487	,10391 (90%)	509	587	249
Uttarakhand	1,576	562 (36%)	1,014	0	1,848	NA			
Uttar Pradesh	2,0521	6,494 (32%)	14,027	0	20,521	1,6187 (79%)	4,334	0	3,538

Note: NA= Not Available

Source: Government of India, 2012.

MP and UP, situation in terms of availability of government building for the SCs was better in 2012. During 2005-2012, UP recorded higher increase in the availability of government SC building. While Bihar and Jharkhand recorded the lowest proportion of SCs located in government building, Rajasthan recorded the highest proportion. In most of the states, construction of the SC building was in progress as on 2012 and situation should improve with completion of the construction activities.

Table 12.7 gives the status of building availability for the PHCs in the EAG states. The building status of PHCs in Chhattisgarh has not improved during 2005-2012, while in MP, Rajasthan and UP, situation in terms of PHCs functioning from government building has improved. About one-fourth of the PHCs in Jharkhand and Uttarakhand were functioning in non-government buildings and this needs attention. Although Chhattisgarh did not record much improvement in terms of government building, the completion of construction would be helpful.

Table 12.8 gives the status of building availability for the CHCs in the EAG states. The building status of CHCs is better in Bihar, Jharkhand, Odisha, Rajasthan, and UP as all the CHCs were functioning in government building. Rajasthan recorded significant improvement during 2005-2012 in terms of provision of government building. MP is one state where the situation needs to be improved.

Table 12.9 gives the status of building construction for various facilities. Across the states, the number of health facilities with complete construction and that with construction work in progress varied. In UP, upgradation of the building was in progress. In Bihar and Jharkhand, construction work was in progress in case of SC, APHC/(Additional Primary Health Centres) PHC and CHC. Perhaps the time taken to complete the construction of buildings needs attention, so that all the health facilities function from own building.

Human Resources

Availability of Female Health Worker/ANM

Table 12.10 gives the data an improvement of availability of female health workers/ANMs in PHCs and SCs during 2005-2012.

Table 12.7

Building Status of PHCs, 2005-2012

State	2005				2012				
	Total No. of PHCs Functioning	No. of SCs Functioning in			Total No. of PHCs Functioning SCs	No. of SCs Functioning in			No. of Buildings Under Construction
		Government Building	Rented Building	Rent Free Panchayat/ Voluntary Society Building		Government Building	Rented Building	Rent Free Panchayat/ Voluntary Society Building	
Bihar	1648	NA	NA	NA	1863	NA	NA	NA	NA
Chhattisgarh	517	326 (63%)	0	191	755	477 (63%)	35	243	210
Jharkhand	561	NA	NA	NA	330	252 (76%)	30	48	62
Madhya Pradesh	1192	746 (63%)	446	0	1156	1047 (90%)	109	0	51
Odisha	1282	1282 (100%)	0	0	1226	1161 (95%)	32	33	33
Rajasthan	1713	1446 (84%)	0	267	1528	1518 (99%)	3	7	4
Uttarakhand	225	182 (81%)	43	0	257	195 (76%)	62	0	0
Uttar Pradesh	3660	1835 (50%)	1825	0	3692	3303 (90%)	389	0	0

Note: NA= Not Available

Source: Government of India, 2012.

Table 12.8

Building Status of CHCs, 2005-2012

State	2005				2012				
	Total No. of CHCs Functioning	CHCs Functioning in			Total Number of CHCs Functioning	CHCs Functioning in			Buildings Under Construction
		Government Building	Rented Building	Rent Free Panchayat/ Voluntary Society Building		Government Building	Rented Building	Rent Free Panchayat/ Voluntary Society Building	
Bihar	101	NA	NA	NA	70	70 (100%)	0	0	0
Chhattisgarh	116	116 (100%)	0	0	149	135 (91%)	0	14	11
Jharkhand	47	NA	NA	NA	188	188 (100%)	0	0	0
Madhya Pradesh	229	229 (100%)	0	0	333	221 (66%)	111	1	58
Odisha	231	231 (100%)	0	0	377	377 (100%)	0	0	0
Rajasthan	326	256 (79%)	0	70	382	382 (100%)	0	0	0
Uttarakhand	44	44(100%)	0	0	59	55 (93%)	NA		
Uttar Pradesh	386	386(100%)	0	0	515	515(100%)	0	0	50

Note: NA= Not Available

Source : Government of India, 2012

Although Chhattisgarh and UP recorded vacancy of ANM posts, there was substantial improvement during 2005-2012. UP had the severest shortfall. In Bihar, Jharkhand, Odisha and Rajasthan, more number of health workers are in position than the number of sanctioned posts.

Availability of Doctors at PHCs

Table 12.11 indicates, UP, Chhattisgarh, MP, Odisha and Uttarakhand recorded vacancy of doctor's posts in PHCs. In most of the states, the number of vacant posts increased during 2005-2012 and this needs attention. UP recorded the highest shortfall and vacancies, followed by Chhattisgarh. In case of Chhattisgarh, the number of vacant posts increased from 406 to 1,075 during 2005-2012, while in case of Odisha, it increased from 0 to 248. Perhaps the medical graduates are not evincing interest in working in the rural areas.

Table 12.9

Construction Status of Buildings

Facility	*Bihar*		*Chhattisgarh*		*Jharkhand*	
	No. of New Buildings Completed	*Work in Progress (No.)*	*No. of New Buildings Completed*	*Work in Progress (No.)*	*No. of New Buildings Completed*	*Work in Progress (No.)*
SC	767	1583	1173	1430	166	244
APHC	1	216	-	-	-	-
PHC	94	41	117	188	28	73
CHC	0	201	94	11	15	134
DH	10	2	7	1	21	15

Facility	*Odisha*		*Uttar Pradesh-Upgradation*	
	No. of New Buildings Completed	*Work in Progress (No.)*	*Planned*	*Completed*
SC	22	0	2908	2824
APHC	-	-		
PHC	55	55	942	908
CHC	156	75	50	50
DH	32	-	129	12

Source: Common Review Mission Reports.

Availability of Specialists at CHCSs

Table 12.12 gives the availability of specialists such as surgeon, OB and GY (obstetrician and gynaecologist), physicians and pediatricians at the CHCs. All the states recorded increase in the sanctioned posts of specialists at CHCs and vacancies and short falls during 2005-2012. MP, Rajasthan and Odisha recorded higher volume of shortfall and these need urgent attention. The number of vacant posts increased in Chhattisgarh (446 to 525), MP (204 to 568), and Uttarakhand (92 to 159). Rajasthan is the only state that recorded decline in the number of vacant posts (from 230 to 150). Given the importance of specialists in providing healthcare services to patients requiring the special care at this FRU, there is an urgent need to fill the vacancies.

Availability of Laboratory Technicians at PHCs and CHCs

Availability of laboratory technicians at PHCs and CHCs is essential so as to facilitate diagnosis at the facility. As Table 12.13 indicates, the shortfall in case of laboratory technicians increased during 2005-2012 in Chhattisgarh and Odisha, and declined in MP and Uttarakhand. The concern is that UP, Bihar, Odisha and MP recorded huge shortfall in 2012. Increase in the number of vacant laboratory technician posts was recorded in Chhattisgarh (285 to 460), MP (68 to 207), and Odisha (33 to 105). The diagnostic services would get affected with the vacancy of laboratory technicians and hence this needs attention.

Availability of Pharmacists at PHCs and CHCs

As Table 12.14 indicates, Bihar, Rajasthan and MP recorded huge shortfall in the number of pharmacists available at PHCs and CHCs. Increase in the number of vacant pharmacist posts was recorded in Chhattisgarh (282 to 442), Odisha (56 to 304) and Uttarakhand (12 to 39). In case of MP, the number of vacant pharmacist posts declined during 2005-2012. The vacancies in pharmacist posts across the states need attention.

Concluding Remarks

The analysis indicates considerable increase in bed strength in government health institutions (upto CHC level) in Bihar and UP during 2005-2009. Regarding the infrastructure development, the progress in completion of the works taken up seems to be slow in most of the states. DLHS 3 data, though not so recent, indicates gaps in ANM staying in quarters where the facility is available.

The recent common review mission reports also indicate significant improvement in number of PHCs and HSCs (health sub centres) in Bihar and also a huge need for CHCs, additional PHCs and HSCs in the state. In view of the huge shortfall in the human resources, innovative strategies should be adopted to ensure physical infrastructure at the health facilities at various levels.

In spite of considerable improvements, gaps exist in HR in terms of doctors, specialists, paramedics, staff nurses, pharmacists, *et al.* In most of the states, 24×7 health facilities are not functional due to shortage of staff and vacancies.

Construction and renovation of the health facilities also need attention to ensure speedy action and this applies to SCs and staff quarters as well.

Outsourcing has been tried successfully in some of the states for recruitments and there is a need to document the outcome/benefits for adopting the same in other states. There is also an urgent need to address human resource related gaps in view of increasing OP/IP (outpatient/inpatient) case load.

Non-availability of basic amenities such as running water, electricity, toilets, etc., needs attention.

There is also need for data on progress and outcomes of the various initiatives.

References

Government of India (2012). *Rural Health Statistics in India 2012.* New Delhi: Statistics Division, Ministry of Health and Family Welfare. *www. mohfw.nic. in/WriteReadData/l892s/492794502RHS%202012.pdf*

Others:

"Accountability Initiatives: Tracking India's Social Sector Budgets", *http://www.accountability.india* (accessed on 28 November 2013).

Fifth Common Review Mission Report, Bihar 2011.

Fifth Common Review Mission Report, Chhattisgarh 2011.

Fifth Common Review Mission Report, Jharkhand 2011.

Fifth Common Review Mission Report, Odisha 2011.

Fifth Common Review Mission Report, Rajasthan 2011.

Fifth Common Review Mission Report, Uttar Pradesh 2011.

Fifth Common Review Mission Report, Uttarakhand 2011.

National Rural Health Mission, Mission Document 2005-2012.

NRHM Framework for Implementation, *www.nrhm.gov.in* accessed on 28 November 2013

Table 12.10

Female Health Worker/ANM Availability, 2005-2012

State	2005					2012				
	Health Worker (Female)/ANM					Health Worker (Female)/ANM				
	Required	Sanctioned	In Position	Vacant	Shortfall	Required	Sanctioned	In Position	Vacant	Shortfall
Bihar	11985	NA	NA	NA	NA	11559	NA	16943	NA	*
Chhattisgarh	4335	4335	3667	668	668	5866	6408	5468	940	398
Jharkhand	5023	NA	NA	NA	NA	4288	4288	6574	*	*
Madhya Pradesh	10066	10027	9345	682	721	10025	8376	10204	*	*
Odisha	7209	7121	6768	353	441	7914	7442	8211	*	*
Rajasthan	12225	11425	11425	0	800	13015	14348	17638	*	*
Uttarakhand	1801	1660	1486	174	315	2105	2077	2016	*	*
Uttar Pradesh	24181	18577	18146	431	6035	24213	25190	22464	2726	1749

Note: NA= Not Available

Source: Government of India, 2012.

Table 12.11

Doctor's Availability at PHCs , 2005-2012

State	*2005*					*2012*				
	Doctors at PHCs					*Doctors at PHCs*				
	Required	*Sanctioned*	*In Position*	*Vacant*	*Shortfall*	*Required*	*Sanctioned*	*In Position*	*Vacant*	*Shortfall*
Bihar	1648	NA	NA	NA	NA	1863	2078	3532	*	*
Chhattisgarh	517	1034	628	406	*	755	1510	435	1075	320
Jharkhand	561	NA	NA	NA	NA	330	330	407	*	*
Madhya Pradesh	1192	1278	839	439	353	1156	1238	814	424	342
Odisha	1282	1353	1353	0	*	1226	1317	1069	248	157
Rajasthan	1713	1517	1506	11	207	1528	1824	1755	69	*
Uttarakhand	225	272	182	90	43	257	299	205	94	52
Uttar Pradesh	3660	NA	NA	NA	NA	3692	4509	2861	1648	831

Note: NA= Not Available

Source: Government of India, 2012.

Table 12.12

Specialists Availability at CHCs, 2005-2012

State	2005					2012				
	Surgeons, OB & GY, Physicians, Pediatricians					Surgeons, OB & GY, Physicians, Pediatricians				
	Required	Sanctioned	In Position	Vacant	Shortfall	Required	Sanctioned	In Position	Vacant	Shortfall
Bihar	404	NA	NA	NA	NA	280	280	151	129	129
Chhattisgarh	464	464	18	446	446	596	596	71	525	525
Jharkhand	188	NA	NA	NA	NA	752	124	86	38	666
Madhya Pradesh	916	253	49	204	867	1332	835	267	568	1065
Odisha	924	496	NA	NA	NA	1508	908	317	591	1191
Rajasthan	1304	811	581	230	723	1528	298	148	150	1380
Uttarakhand	176	163	71	92	105	236	210	51	159	185
Uttar Pradesh	1544	NA	NA	NA	NA	2060	2060	1740	320	320

Note: NA= Not Available

Source: Government of India, 2012.

Table 12.13

Availability of Laboratory Technicians at PHCs and CHCs

State/UT	2005					2012				
	Laboratory Technicians					Laboratory Technicians				
	Required	*Sanctioned*	*In Position*	*Vacant*	*Shortfall*	*Required*	*Sanctioned*	*In Position*	*Vacant*	*Shortfall*
Bihar	1749	NA	NA	NA	NA	1933	683	498	185	1435
Chhattisgarh	633	633	348	285	285	904	904	444	460	460
Jharkhand	608	NA	NA	NA	NA	518	518	371	147	147
Madhya Pradesh	1421	454	386	68	1035	1489	816	609	207	880
Odisha	1513	344	311	33	1202	1603	476	371	105	1232
Rajasthan	2039	2153	2065	88	*	1910	1818	2639	*	*
Uttarakhand	269	90	32	58	237	316	89	81	8	235
Uttar Pradesh	4046	NA	NA	NA	NA	4207	1116	1836	*	2371

Note: NA= Not Available

Source: Government of India, 2012.

Table 12.14

Availability of Pharmacists at PHCs and CHCs

State/UT	2005					2012				
	Pharmacists					Pharmacists				
	Required	*Sanctioned*	*In Position*	*Vacant*	*Shortfall*	*Required*	*Sanctioned*	*In Position*	*Vacant*	*Shortfall*
Bihar	1749	NA	NA	NA	NA	1933	989	439	550	1494
Chhattisgarh	633	749	467	282	166	904	1053	611	442	293
Jharkhand	608	NA	NA	NA	NA	518	518	298	220	220
Madhya Pradesh	1421	1419	216	1203	1205	1489	1443	678	765	811
Odisha	1513	2040	1984	56	*	1603	1819	1515	304	88
Rajasthan	2039	2375	2355	20	*	1910	362	551	*	1359
Uttarakhand	269	293	281	12	*	316	331	292	39	24
Uttar Pradesh	4046	NA	NA	NA	NA	4207	6472	5582	890	*

Note: NA= Not Available

Source: Government of India, 2012.

13

P. SATYA SEKHAR

Implementing the RMNCH+A Interventions in the States of Telangana and Andhra Pradesh

Introduction

The MMR (maternal mortality ratio) and IMR (infant mortality rate) are two key health indicators of maternal and child health, where India falls far behind the international estimates. Figure 13.1 illustrates MMR across the emerging BRICS countries (Brazil, Russian Federation, India, China, and South Africa), and also plots MMR for Andhra Pradesh (AP), India. It is clear that while India has the highest MMR across the BRICS group, AP has recorded a lower MMR. AP is the fourth state in the country after Kerala, Tamil Nadu (TN), and Maharashtra which will reach Millennium Development Goals (MDG) 5.

Figure 13.1

Maternal Mortality Ratio, 2013

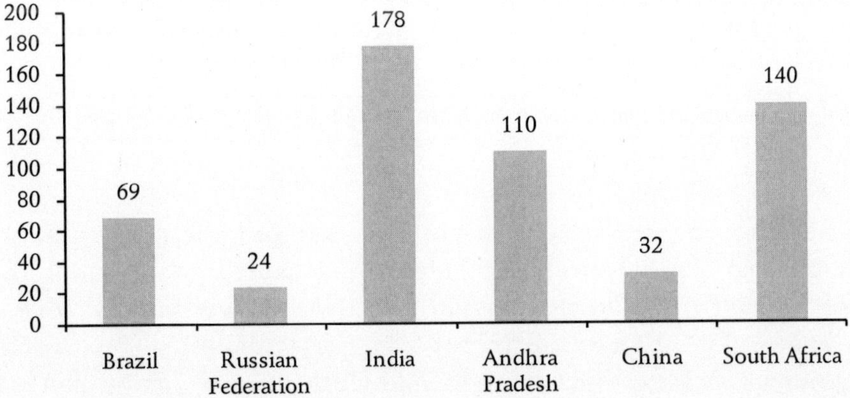

Source: BRICS (2014) and SRS (2014).

Similarly in the case of CMR (child mortality ratio) across the BRICS economies, one can see that India has the highest rates, and AP continues to contribute to this high national burden. Among the southern states of India, AP recorded highest IMR as compared to Kerala (12), Tamil Nadu (21) and Karnataka (32). However, recent evidence indicate that 85-95 per cent of the deliveries are conducted in health facilities under skilled attendant supervision and roughly 58-62 per cent neonate children die within one month of their birth in many states (SRS, 2014). Studies reported wide variations in infant and child mortality among mothers with rural residence; mothers with no education as compared to mothers who have completed 10 years of schooling, adolescent mothers in the age group pf 15-19 years and mothers from low SLI (standard living index) (NFHS-3, 2005-06).

Figure 13.2

Child Mortality Ratio, 2013

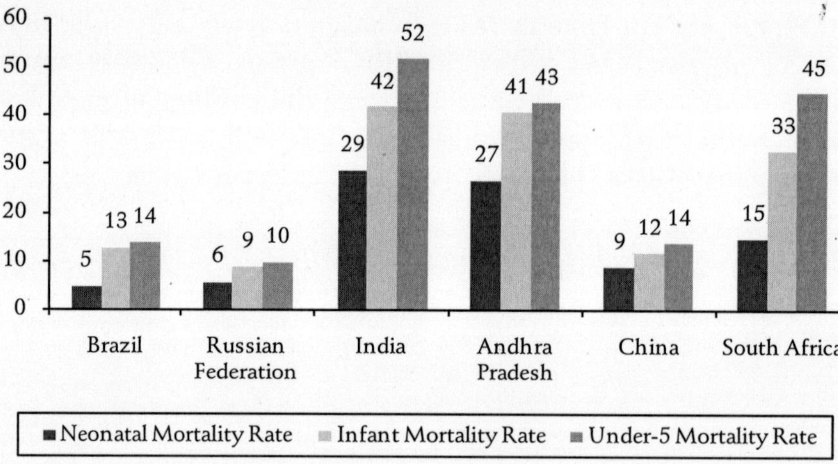

Source: BRICS (2014) and SRS (2014).

Improving maternal and child health and their survival are central to the achievement of national health goals under the National Rural Health Mission (NRHM) as well as the MDGs 4 and 5. The substantial increase in the availability of financial resources for Reproductive and Child Health (RCH), and expansion of healthcare infrastructure and workforce since 2005 under NRHM led to significant improvements and was reflected in IMR, MMR and other outcome indicators across high-focus as well as non-high focus states in India.

The Ministry of Health and Family Welfare (MoHFW), Government of India (GoI, 2013), initiated a strategic approach to RMNCH+A (Reproductive, Maternal, Newborn, Child Health plus Adolescent Health) in the country to attain the goal of healthy mother and children with a coordinated approach to maternal and child health in the 12th Five Year Plan Period (2012-2017) bringing equity in quality health services addressing vulnerable and remote rural groups and urban slum dwellers.

This RMNCH+A strategy embodies a vision for comprehensive and integrated health services by ensuring a "Continuum-of-Care" throughout the "lifecycle" (using a life-stage approach) for all adolescents, mothers and children in India. The 12th Five Year Plan has defined the targets of health outcomes for undivided AP with the following goals:

- Reduction of IMR from 39 (SRS, 2013) to 25 per 1,000 live births by end of 2017.
- Reduction in MMR to 61 from 110 per lakh live births (2010-2012) by end of 2017.
- Reduction of anaemia from 62.93 per cent (NFHS, 2005-06) to 30 per cent by end of 2017.

The population projections (2001-2026) of undivided AP reported 62-66 per cent working group population in the age group of 15-59 (RGI, 2006). Further, projected female population (in age group 15-49) indicated marginal decline and is expected to remain around 53-55 per cent until the end of the projected year of 2026. Thus, for both the states, it is required to extend the same extent of MCH services in the coming decade also.

In this paper, an attempt has been made to analyse the situation analysis of RMNCH+A life stages for newly formed states of Telangana and AP. We have utilised available secondary data from national and state level data sets, such as National Family Health Survey (NFHS), District Level Household Survey (DLHS), Sample Registration System (SRS) reports and unpublished demographic and health reports conducted by Indian Institute of Health and Family Welfare (IIHFW).

Priority Behaviours Across RMNCH+A Life Stages

Reproductive Health

Overall awareness of contraceptive methods has increased among married women from 1998-99 to 2005-06, evident from universal awareness levels for female sterilisation (100%), followed closely by male sterilisation (89%), contraceptive pills (63%), condoms (48%) and intrauterine contraceptive device (IUCD) (46%) for the undivided state of AP (NFHS 3, 2005-06).

In terms of current utilisation, overall use stood at 61 per cent in Telangana and 69.7 per cent in AP. In both the states, most commonly used method was the female sterilisation (DLHS 4).

Unmet need for family planning is defined as the percentage of currently married women who either want to space their next birth or stop childbearing entirely, but are not using any contraception. The unmet need for contraception increased from 8.5 per cent (DLHS 3) to 23 per cent (DLHS 4, 2012-13) in Telangana. Less than one-fifth (17%) in AP reported unmet need (12% for spacing and 5% for limiting).

A gap of less than 3 years between two consecutive births increases the risk of maternal and child mortality. However as per the data reported in NFHS 3 (2005-06), a median interval between two consecutive births was 31 months in undivided AP, and 12 per cent of births took place within 18 months. The DLHS 4 (2012-13) reported prevalence of STI (sexually transmitted infections)/RTI (reproductive tract infections) among 16-17 per cent married women in both Telangana and AP; however 26 per cent in Telangana and 21 per cent in AP reported having knowledge of STI/RTI. The HIV/AIDS related knowledge levels were comparatively higher among all married women (77-79%) and 61-65 per cent married women know the place for testing HIV/AIDS (DLHS 4) in the two states.

Increasing women's uptake of need based modern contraceptive methods other than female sterilisation, increasing their awareness and knowledge levels about STI/RTI and HIV/AIDS and encouraging related treatment seeking behaviour remains priority areas.

Maternal Health

The proportion of women that received at least one ANC (antenatal care) check-up has varied across the years, from 95 per cent in 2005-06 to 96 per cent in 2009 (CES, 2010) in the undivided AP. However, pregnant women who had registered for ANC within the recommended first trimester marginally varied from 82 per cent in Telangana and 85 per cent in AP (DLHS 4). In both the states, more than three-fourth of pregnant women received ANC measurements, like blood pressure check-up, and blood examination for hemoglobin. Half of the pregnant women consumed 100 IFA tablets in both states with marginal inter-district variations. Research studies reported that pregnant women belonging to low wealth quintile, SC (scheduled caste) and ST (scheduled tribe) communities and women with no education as compared to their counterparts reported low coverage of first trimester registration and IFA consumption. DLHS 4 reported that 95-96 per cent of pregnant women made more than three visits and a higher proportion received 2 TT injections.

Less than two-fifth (38% in Telangana and 36% in AP) of pregnant women were informed about pregnancy complications by the health personnel. Studies conducted in undivided AP showed that women with higher education were more likely to have received advice on two ANC components, including expected date of delivery and breastfeeding (Murthy and Sekhar, 2012).

The proportion of institutional deliveries rose to 94-96 per cent in 2012-13 as compared to 74-76 per cent during 2007-08 in Telangana and AP. In 9 out of 10 institutional deliveries, private sector institutional deliveries accounted for 62 per cent of the deliveries, whereas 32 per cent were conducted in public institutions in Telangana. Private sector deliveries dominated in Hyderabad (80%) followed by Karimnagar (74%) district. In Telangana, higher domiciliary deliveries reported in Adilabad (13%) followed by Ranga Reddy (5.5%) and Mahabubnagar (5.4%).

In AP, higher private sector deliveries were reported from Kadapa (71%), followed by Guntur (63%), Nellore (66%) and Prakasam (67%) districts. However, 49-52 per cent of public institution deliveries was reported in Vizianagaram, Visakhapatnam and Chittoor districts. Higher proportion for domiciliary deliveries were reported in Kurnool (24%), followed by Vishakhapatnam (19%) and Anantapur (15%).

The mode of transport availed by pregnant women to reach health facility for delivery was auto rickshaw (63%), followed by government-run 108 ambulances (16%) (Murthy and Sekhar, 2012).

More than half (54%) of the deliveries in Telangana resulted in Caesarean sections (C-sections) and 46 per cent ended as normal deliveries. The C-sections are four times higher in private institutions compared to public institutions in Telangana. However, C-section interventions remained at 26 per cent in private institutions as compared to 9 per cent in public institutions in AP state.

A positive finding is that post-partum check-up within 48 hoursfor mothers have remained at 74 per cent in Telangana and 80 per cent in AP; however this service needs universal coverage.

Priority area in this life stage include encouraging ANC registration within first trimester, increasing consumption of IFA tablets, universal ANC advice on post-partum check-up, nutritious food and feeding practices.

Universal institutional deliveries is required in both the states, along with emphasis on public institution deliveries and increase in the number of Janani Suraksha Yojana (JSY) beneficiaries from below 25 per cent in both states. There is a need to check the high rates of C-section interventions in private sector. Also, there is a need to include sensitisation program for autorickshaw drivers with a check list of do's and don'ts on safe transport of pregnant women to health facility.

Newborn Care

A new/sterilised blade was used to cut the cord of the new born in 89 per cent of home deliveries. More than half (54%) mothers reported that newborn cord; was kept clean by the attendant, free of any application like powder and oil. Fifty-eight per cent women received advice about Kangaroo Mother Care (KMC). Correct newborn care practices must be encouraged for better child health outcomes in both the states (Murthy and Sekhar, 2012).

> With almost half (60%) of infant deaths in the undivided Andhra Pradesh occurring between 24 hours and 1 week (SRS report, 2012), encouraging correct newborn care practices such as cord, thermal and skin to skin care, early breastfeeding and mothers knowledge about danger signs in infants, are a priority issue.

Child Health

Less than half (48%) of the children in Telangana received full immunisation (including BCG, OPV3, DPT3 and Measles vaccines). The full immunisation figure decreased from 72 per cent in 2007-08 (DLHS 3) to 48 per cent in 2012-13 (DLHS 4). In terms of individual vaccine uptake, DLHS 4 (2012-13) showed that the BCG vaccine was almost commonly administered at 95 per cent, while DPT-3 and Oral Polio Vaccine (OPV3) had the lowest uptake at 63 per cent and 71 per cent respectively. The dropout rate from BCG to DPT3 and BCG to OPV3 remained at 32 per cent and 23 per cent respectively.

In AP, 61 per cent of children in the age group of 12-23 months were fully immunised and the coverage rates for individual vaccine uptake was DPT-3 (75%), followed by OPV-3 (82%) and Measles (87%). The dropout rate from BCG to DPT3 and BCG to OPV3 remained at 21 per cent and 14 per cent respectively.

Most commonly reported reasons for no or incomplete vaccinations are lack of perceived need (45%), inconvenient time (13%), inconvenient place (13%) and long waiting time (13%), in undivided AP (CES, 2009; N= 274).

Although breastfeeding is universal, DLHS 4 survey reported that 75 per cent in AP state and 63 per cent in Telangana state, children were exclusively breastfed for the first six months of life, while close to 54-56 per cent infants were breastfed within one hour of birth. Studies reported no major variation in early initiation of breastfeeding among mothers of different education groups; majority of infants from scheduled tribes and households with low SLI were breastfed within one hour of birth (Murthy and Sekhar, 2012).

In terms of illness among children, the prevalence of diarrhoea decreased from 6 per cent in 2007-08 to 5 per cent in 2012-13 and 61 per cent of cases in the reference 2 weeks were given ORS in Telangana. AP also reported a decline in prevalence of diarrhoea from 8 per cent in 2007-08 to 4.3 per cent in 2012-13 and about 53 per cent cases received ORS. The prevalence of Acute Respiratory Infection (ARI) was reported at 3.4 per cent in Telangana and 6.4 per cent in AP, and treatment wads were sought for 82 per cent in Telangana and 74 per cent in AP (DLHS 4).

> Priority areas in this life stage include universal coverage for full immunisation and identifying reasons for dropouts, encouraging exclusive breastfeeding, increasing mother's knowledge about illness management (including knowledge of ORS, food and fluid intake practices during illness) and encouraging appropriate care-seeking practices.

Adolescent Health

Women's age at marriage occupies a prominent place in demography as it is one of the proximate determinants of fertility. Between DLHS 3 and DLHS 4 survey period of five years, the proportion of currently married women aged 20-24 married below 18 years was 28 per cent in Telangana. Across districts, above 30 per cent of marriages before 18 years were reported in Mahbubnagar, Khammam and Nalgonda districts. Around 11 per cent of the marriage among girls is below the legal age of 18 years in Telangna as compared to 16 per cent in Andhra Pradesh.

Between the two waves of DLHS surveys (2007-08 and 2012-13), women who were married below the age of 18 years declined twofold from 28 per cent (2007-08) to 16 per cent (2012-13) in AP. Districts which required special behavioural change communication interventions stood at Guntur (22%), followed by Kurnool (20%) and Anantapur (19%). A significant decline was reported in adolescent childbearing declined from 15 per cent (DLHS 3) to 6 per cent (DLHS 4) in AP. However, special emphasis is required for Guntur (10%), East Godavari (8%), Kurnool (8%) and Nellore (7%).

Among adolescent age (15-19 years) anaemia was prevalent in 51 per cent in Telangana and 59 per cent in AP.

Priority areas in this life stage include delaying age at marriage and childbirth, increasing knowledge of family planning, STI/RTI and HIV/AIDS and encouraging anaemia prevention and reduction practices among adolescent girls.

References

BRICS (2014). *Joint Statistical Publication 2014.* Instituto Brasiliro De Geografiae Estatistica–IBEG.

Coverage Evaluation Survey (CES) (2009). *Andhra Pradesh Fact Sheet.* Ministry of Health & Family Welfare, Government of India, UNICEF.

Government of India (2013). *A Strategic Approach to Reproductive, Maternal, Newborn, Child and Adolescent Health (RMNCH+A) in India.* Ministry of Health and Family Welfare.

International Institute for Population Sciences (IIPS) and Macro International (2008). *National Family Health Survey (NFHS-3), India, 2005-06: Andhra Pradesh.* Mumbai: IIPS.

Murthy, S.R and P. Satya Sekhar (2012) *Evidence to Guide the Development of Social and Behavior Change Communication Strategy for Maternal and Child Health and Nutrition in Andhra Pradesh.* Hyderabad: National Rural Health Mission, Government of Andhra Pradesh, UNICEF.

Registrar General of India (RGI) (2006). *Population Projections for India and States 1996-2026.* Report of Technical Group on Population Projections, Government of India.

Sample Registration System (SRS) (2014). *Statistical Report 2013.* Registrar General & Census Commissioner Government of India.

Satya Sekhar, P., V. Uma Devi, N.V. Rajeswari and C.H.V.S.S. Rao (2007). *Baseline Survey on Reproductive and Child Health (RCH-II) in Andhra Pradesh.* Hyderabad: Indian Institute of Health and Family Welfare.

UNICEF and World Health Organization (2014). *Filling the Health Agenda for Women and Children.* The 2014 Report (Conference Draft), Countdown to 2015.

Others:

A Strategic Approach to Reproductive, Maternal, Newborn, Child and Adolescent Health (RMNCH+A) in India. Ministry of Health and Family Welfare, Government of India, New Delhi.

District Level Household and Fertility Survey (DLHS-4), Andhra Pradesh and Telangana Fact Sheets (2012-13). Ministry of Health and Family Welfare, Government of India, New Delhi and International Institute of Population Sciences. Mumbai: IIPS.

National Family Health Survey (NFHS-2), India, 1998-99: Andhra Pradesh 1992. Mumbai: IIPS and ORC Macro.

National Family Health Survey (MCH and Family Planning): Andhra Pradesh, 1992. Bombay: PRC, Visakhapatnam and IIPS.

Rapid Household Survey: Reproductive and Child Health Project, 1998-99. Ministry of Health and Family Welfare, Government of India, New Delhi and Population Research Centre, Visakhapatnam.

14

M. BENSON THOMAS and K.S. JAMES

Regional Disparities in Mortality and its Causes in Kerala

An Epidemiological Exploration

Introduction

Achievement in health indices even with low per capita income and less nutrient intake is a noted feature of Kerala's development experience. This is widely considered as unique since it goes against the essential pre-requirement of improvement in economic and nutrition condition for better health status of many development theories. The mortality rates of infants, children and mothers were low and the life expectancy was considerably higher in Kerala than the rest of India and those are even comparable with that of many developed countries in 1970s. However, recent evidence from developed countries indicate that further improvement in life expectancy leading to an advance stage of epidemiological transition could be achieved mainly through reducing adult mortality. It was achieved by adopting effective strategies against controlling mortality from chronic/degenerative diseases among the adult ages. But unlike the experience in developed countries, an unexpected slowdown in mortality decline mainly in the adult ages and consequent delay in life expectancy improvement is noted in Kerala, leading to delay in experiencing epidemiological transition to advance stages. Such slowdown was the result of escalating supremacy of chronic/degenerative diseases among the causes of deaths mainly circulatory diseases and neoplasm (cancer) (Thomas, 2012; Thomas and James, 2014). However, studies exploring such changes in detail at different levels are scarce.

Studies in many countries, found disparities among different subgroups in epidemiological transition. Although these countries have better performance in overall mortality decline, there were high disparities at the micro level where some subgroups are far below the national averages (Huynen *et al.*, 2005; Arriaga, 1984). In effect, the disparities affected the overall pace of mortality decline by neutralising the achievement of other groups. Such disparities in epidemiological transition are largely noted in the developing countries (Arriaga, 1984). Notably, most of the causes of disparities in the death rates and its causes are due to an unequal distribution of healthcare institutions as well as discrepancy of risk exposure among subgroups in these countries. A bunch of reports suggest possible disparities in the prevalence of mortality rates and causes of deaths across different regional and socio-economic groups in Kerala also (RGI-CDSR, RGI-MCCD, RGI-SRS, Various Years; Shyjan, 2010; Navaneetham *et al.*, 2009 and Navaneetham and Kabeer, 2005). But these reports are insufficient in measuring such disparities in death rates as well as causes of deaths by its rate of prevalence and proportional contributions. In other words, contribution of the sub-population to the overall mortality decline by deaths rates and its causes is still unexplored. Moreover, most of these reports are based on surveys where the representations of subgroups are narrowed down to little clusters. Apart from all, the lack of reliable information about the disparities across the subgroups becomes a lacuna, while examining the competence of existing health policies in the state.

Considering the importance of understanding the difference in the mortality and causes of death in subgroups and the role of each subgroup in the overall mortality level for healthcare intervention, the paper analyses the difference in mortality and causes of deaths in Kerala. It focuses on regional subgroup population by taking districts as subgroup category for a cross-sectional analysis.

Methodology and Data

Both the theoretical and the empirical studies of epidemiological transition point out the possibility of disparities in epidemiological transition across various subgroups even within a society. According to Omran (1971), the disparities in epidemiological transition can be visible for different factors such as socio-economic and health infrastructures, etc. This can be due to the disparities in the consumption pattern where the affluent people are more prone to lifestyle diseases than the poor. However, later studies highlighted that such disparities are subject to the possibility of risk exposure and also the availability of healthcare facilities. Notably, experience of many countries indicates that epidemiological transition shows polarisation or delay in transition due to the discrepancy in its cause factors (Mesle *et al.*, 2002; Vallin and Mesle, 2004). Such variations can be seen in their pattern of mortality and also in cause of death.

However, very few studies trace out the difference in mortality and cause of death across the sub-population in Kerala as mentioned above. This paper examines such differences by analysing the experience of mortality and causes of death among various subgroups in the state. In the first section, the paper measures the differences in mortality by using indicators such as CDR (Crude Death Rates), LE (Life Expectancy), and the TLE (Temporary Life Expectancy). The second section focuses on the variations in the prevalence of causes of deaths. It specifically investigates the proportion of major group of death causes as well as Age Cause Specific Death Rates (ACSDR) of major diseases across the districts in Kerala.

The analytical part of the study uses the data on registered death in the state which is collected from the Vital Registration System[1] (VRS) for the year of 2008. However, the major lacunae of VRS data are under-reporting, especially in infant ages and also the massive level of age misreporting towards the older ages. To minimise such errors, the study has used indirect estimation of under-5 mortality rate across the districts for the year 2012 provided by Ram *et al.* (2013), keeping in mind the high possibility of misreporting of deaths in those ages. Similarly, the study has grouped the maximum age as 85+ to reduce the bias of age misreporting at the oldest ages. The study has used estimated population in different age group

1. The data was collected from VRS office, Thiruvananthapuram. Authors are thankfully acknowledging the same.

levels in the year 2008 for analysis. The study extrapolated total population at 2008 from the population growth in the inter-censual period between 2001 and 2011. Later, the total population of 2008 was divided into different age intervals in accordance with the proportion of population in different age intervals at 2001.

Regional Difference in Mortality and Mortality Pattern

Crude Death Rates

The difference in mortality across districts can be identified from the CDR in Kerala. The CDR refers to the number of deaths to the total population living at all ages in the mid-year of the calendar year. Figure 14.1 reflects the CDR of Kerala and different districts. It can be seen that the average CDR is 6.3 per thousand population in the state. However, the rate varies across districts. Pathanamthitta district (8.2) recorded the highest CDR, followed by Thrissur (7.2), Kottayam (7.1), and Alappuzha (7.1) in the year 2008. Malappuram (4.6) has the lowest CDR followed by Wayanad (4.7), Kasaragod (4.9), Idukki (5.7) and Kozhikkode (5.9). Rest of the districts is more or less close to the state average.

Figure 14.1

Crude Death Rates in Kerala, 2008

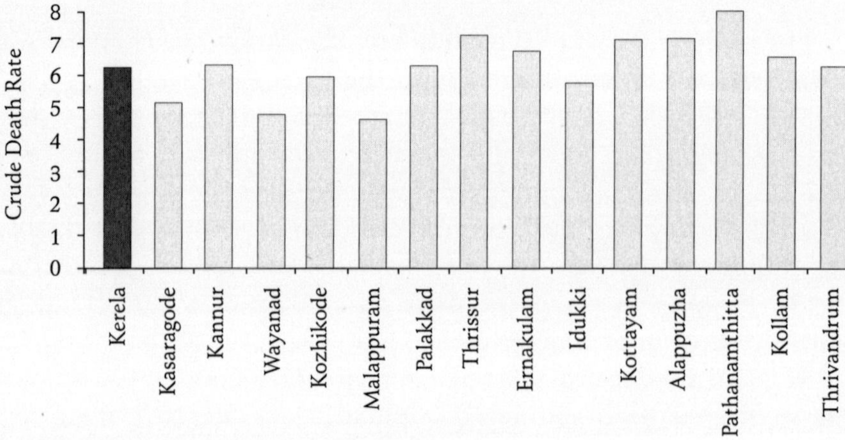

Source: Author's Calculation from VRS Data, 2008.

It should be noted that all the southern districts except Idukki have higher CDR which is more than the state average. But the northern districts are below the state level of CDR. However, the CDR is biased with the weightages of populations' age composition. And therefore, the south-north disparities in CDR may be due to the difference in age structures, where the northerners have relatively more young population. Nevertheless, the status of CDR across the districts indicates that relatively, more deaths are happening in the southern districts in Kerala.

Life Expectancy Among the Districts

The level of life expectancy at birth (e_o) is often used as a convenient measurement to understand the mortality level across different populations. It indicates the expected years of life of a person at birth and whether he/she is subjected to the current level of death rates in different age intervals during his/her life. Figure 14.2 shows life expectancy at birth (e_0) for males and females among the districts in Kerala in the year 2008. It shows that Kerala has achieved 70.7 years of life expectancy for males and 77.6 years for females. Notably, the level of life expectancy has improved in the state where it was only 25.5 for males and 27.4 for females in the first decade of the last century. However, this figure indicates that the life expectancy varies across the districts. For males, Alappuzha stands highest with life expectancy at 71.8 years and Thrissur with 69.6 years clocks lowest in life expectancy. Kottayam district has recorded 79.1 years of life expectancy for female, while Thiruvananthapuram and Kasargode districts have only 76.5 years. It should be kept in mind that the difference in life expectancy between the lowest and the highest is greater among females.

The prevalence of sex disparities in the life expectancy is a notable feature in Kerala. Similar to the state level averages of life expectancy of males and females, the difference is also shown across the districts. It indicates that the females are much more advanced in the mortality reduction, while it stands at lower level among the males in Kerala. This means that the females enjoy more favourable health status in all the districts than the males. It is also interesting that the districts with high female life expectancy are no different from those with low female life expectancy in terms of gender difference. In other words, there is no reason to believe that the gender difference will be reduced when the life expectancy moves to the highest levels.

Figure 14.2

Life Expectancy Across the Districts in Kerala, 2008

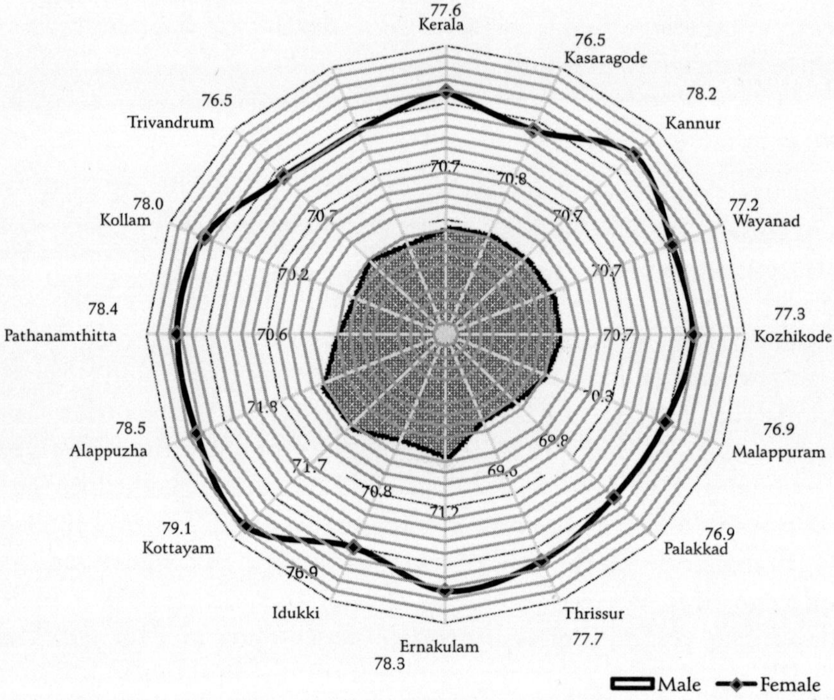

Source: Author's Calculation from VRS Data, 2008.

A major lacuna of life expectancy indicators is that it is restricted by the problems of relative magnitudes, i.e., a possible change in life expectancy indicators depends upon the level of already achieved life expectancy (Arriaga, 1984). Apart from that, the life expectancy estimation is also constrained by technical problems like unreliability of information that is older than 65 years. Moreover, there is a possibility of a counteracting effect that neutralises the contribution of different age groups, where a high mortality increase experienced by one group is offset by a reduction in the other group in the general life expectancy indicator (Arriaga,

1984; Dutton, 1979). To overcome these lacunas, the paper uses TLE indicators to examine the changes in mortality reduction among different age groups.

Temporary Life Expectancy

The TLE at selected exact age intervals by sex across the districts in Kerala is shown in Table 14.1 and Table 14.2. A temporary life expectancy from age x to (x + i) can be interpreted as the average number of years that a 'group of persons' alive at exact age x will live from age x to (x+ i) years (Arriaga, 1984).

$$\text{i.e.,} \quad {}_{i}e_{x} \quad \frac{T_{x} \quad T_{x\ i}}{l_{x}}$$

where, ${}_{i}e_{x}$ represents the TLE from age x and $x+n$. T_x and T_{x+i} are the number of person-years lived at age l_x and older, $x+i$ and older, respectively. l_x is the number of survivors at age x in a life table (as radix) of 100,000.

Table 14.1

Temporary Life Expectancy across the Districts in Kerala, 2008 (Male)

State/District	*0-80*	*0-15*	*15-40*	*40-60*	*60-80*
Kerala	68.5	14.8	24.7	18.8	14.7
Thiruvananthapuram	68.4	14.8	24.7	18.8	14.7
Kollam	67.9	14.8	24.7	18.6	14.5
Pathanamthitta	68.2	14.8	24.6	18.6	14.9
Alappuzha	68.8	14.7	24.7	18.8	15.1
Kottayam	68.8	14.8	24.7	18.8	15.2
Idukki	68.5	14.7	24.7	18.9	14.8
Ernakulam	68.9	14.8	24.7	18.8	14.8
Thrissur	67.9	14.8	24.7	18.6	14.5
Palakkad	68.0	14.8	24.7	18.7	14.4
Malappuram	68.7	14.8	24.8	18.8	14.3
Kozhikode	68.5	14.7	24.8	18.9	14.4
Wayanad	67.6	14.7	24.7	18.8	14.7
Kannur	68.7	14.8	24.7	18.8	14.4
Kasargod	68.7	14.7	24.8	18.9	14.8

Source: Author's Calculation from VRS Data, 2008.

The Tables 14.1 and 14.2 reflects that TLE between the ages of 0-80 has ample room to be filled mainly because of low attainment in the mortality reduction at the old adults and the older ages across the districts. It shows low attainment for males (68.5 years) and high for females (73.4 years) in terms of TLE in between the ages 0-80. All the districts have greater or lesser achievement of TLE in those ages. Among the males, Ernakulam, Kottayam and Alappuzha have achieved higher levels, while Thrissur, Kollam and Wayanad are at the bottom. For females, Kannur, Kottayam and Ernakulam are ranked as high achievers and at the same time Thiruvananthapuram, Idukki and Wayanad stand at lower than the state average.

Table 14.2

Temporary Life Expectancy Across the Districts in Kerala, 2008 (Female)

State/District	*0-80*	*0-15*	*15-40*	*40-60*	*60-80*
Kerala	73.4	14.8	24.8	19.5	17.1
Thiruvananthapuram	72.5	14.8	24.7	19.4	16.7
Kollam	73.6	14.8	24.9	19.5	17.0
Pathanamthitta	73.3	14.9	24.8	19.4	17.0
Alappuzha	73.8	14.7	25.0	19.5	17.3
Kottayam	74.2	14.8	25.0	19.5	17.6
Idukki	72.9	14.7	24.7	19.5	17.1
Ernakulam	74.0	14.9	24.9	19.5	17.1
Thrissur	73.6	14.8	24.9	19.5	16.9
Palakkad	73.2	14.8	24.8	19.5	16.9
Malappuram	73.3	14.9	25.0	19.4	16.5
Kozhikode	73.4	14.7	24.9	19.6	17.1
Wayanad	72.4	14.6	24.7	19.5	17.1
Kannur	74.5	14.9	24.9	19.6	17.2
Kasargod	73.3	14.7	25.0	19.4	17.0

Source: Author's Calculation from VRS Data, 2008.

The TLE between the ages (0-15) and (15-40) shows that they have achieved close to the maximum possible levels. Moreover, no district shows a significant variation from this pattern. This shows that the state has achieved almost maximum mortality reduction from the young (0-15) and the young adult age groups (15-40). In regards to the old adult ages (40-60), males have 18.8 years and the females have 19.5 years of TLE. But males have only 14.7 years, whereas the females have 17.1 years of expected life in between the old ages of 60-80 years. Notably, males are lagging in these age groups in attaining higher life expectancy compared to the females. It clearly indicates the gap in attaining TLE in the ages 0-80 years, which can be due to delay of that in the ages 40-60 years and 60-80 years in Kerala.

In short, the analysis of pattern and the levels of mortality indicate variations in the death pattern across the districts in Kerala. Both life expectancies at birth and the TLE in the ages 0-80 years reflect such difference. The TLE analysis shows that, even though there is difference among the districts, it is very small and is mainly the result of variations in the 60-80 age group. But the sex difference in mortality, which appears mainly among the age group 40-60 years and 60-80 years, is a matter of concern.

Structure of Causes of Deaths Across the Districts

A major feature of epidemiological transition is the changes in the causes of deaths mainly from infectious/parasites to chronic/degenerative diseases (Omran, 1971). Such change in diseases can result in drastic reduction in mortality rates among younger ages and consequent increase in mortality in the older ages. However, the advanced theory propounded by Olshansky and Ault (1986) argued for a further possibility of change in the pattern of death by shifting the deaths to the oldest ages, while keeping the chronic/degenerative diseases as main causes of death. It should be remembered that studies have already found that the causes of deaths have shifted to the dominance of chronic/degenerative diseases; however there is a delay to the shift in mortality decline among the adult ages in the state as a whole as mentioned in the introductory section. The following section of this paper analyses status of such transition in the causes of deaths across the districts in Kerala.

Two major analyses have been carried out to understand the changes in the causes of death. In the first part, the study analyses the proportion of major causes of death across the districts to identify the status of epidemiological transition at the macro level. Consequently in the second part, it looks at the Age Cause Specific Death Rates (ACSDR) of major diseases in the state to understand the intensity of individual diseases.

Proportion of Major Causes of Deaths Across the Districts

Table 14.3 shows the proportional share of three major groups in terms of cause of deaths across the districts in Kerala during the year 2008, which is available from the VRS. The group of cause of deaths has been classified according to the nature of causes from the 46 classified reasons of deaths available from the VRS.

Table 14.3

Proportion of Major Causes of Deaths Across the Districts in Kerala, 2008

District/State	*Male*				*Female*			
	Group 1	*Group 2*	*Group 3*	*Others*	*Group 1*	*Group 2*	*Group 3*	*Others*
Kasargode	5.1	71.3	6.3	17.4	6.6	70.8	2.5	20.1
Kannur	2.0	67.7	5.6	24.8	1.3	72.7	3.1	22.9
Wayanad	2.2	61.6	10.5	25.7	2.6	68.3	5.5	23.6
Kozhikode	1.5	57.6	6.6	34.3	1.3	62.6	3.3	32.7
Malappuram	2.0	68.1	5.2	24.7	2.5	70.9	2.9	23.6
Palakkad	3.8	69.3	7.3	19.5	3.7	70.7	3.8	21.7
Thrissur	2.5	70.0	6.9	20.6	2.4	74.8	3.5	19.4
Ernakulam	2.0	70.2	9.0	18.8	2.0	77.1	3.8	17.1
Idukki	2.9	66.8	9.9	20.4	3.5	72.3	5.6	18.6
Kottayam	2.8	61.0	6.6	29.6	2.7	66.2	2.9	28.2
Alappuzha	2.6	72.4	7.4	17.7	2.2	78.2	2.3	17.2
Pathanamthitta	4.6	74.9	6.0	14.5	4.5	79.9	2.2	13.4
Kollam	3.4	71.5	9.1	16.0	3.4	76.7	3.7	16.1
Thiruvananthapuram	4.3	72.1	6.1	17.5	3.5	78.8	2.5	15.1
Kerala	2.9	68.4	7.1	21.6	2.8	73.4	3.2	20.6

Source: Calculated by using VRS Data, 2008.

The first group includes infectious/parasites, maternal and perinatal deaths. It comprises of infectious/parasites such as cholera, typhoid, food poisoning, dysentery, tuberculosis, leprosy, diphtheria, whooping cough, tetanus, poliomyelitis, measles, rabies, malaria, meningitis, pneumonia, influenza, jaundice, syphilis genitourinary, and also AIDS; maternal and perinatal injuries are death due to abortion, pregnancy and child birth, birth injuries and also the premature deaths. Second group is chronic/degenerative diseases consisting deaths due to cancer, diabetes, anaemia, heart attack, asthma, liver disease, ulcer, appendicitis, paralysis, senility, old age, hysteria, blood pressure and also kidney trouble. the third group is accidents and injuries consisting of deaths due to venomous animal bites, burns (accidental), drowning, falls, poisoning, accident (traffic/vehicles), other accidents, suicides and also homicides. The group 'Others' represent other causes of deaths, which are not included in any of the above groups.

The information furnished in Table 14.3 indicates clear dominance of Group 2 causes of deaths. Such dominance can be visible for males (68.4%) and females (73.4%) at the state levels. Second dominant group was Group 3 causes, which accounts for 7.1 per cent of male deaths and 3.2 per cent female deaths. But Group 1 causes are at the third position where 2.9 per cent of males and 2.8 per cent of females are dying due to such causes in Kerala. This distribution of causes of deaths is almost similar across the districts except at Kasargod, Pathanamthitta and Thiruvananthapuram where Group 1 causes are at the second position among the females. On the other hand, the proportion of prevalence of all the group of causes is more or less similar across the districts. However, relatively more disparities are visible in Group 2 causes across the districts.

The Tables 14.4 and 14.5 record the prevalence of major causes of death in Kerala for the year 2008. It can be seen that heart attack is a major cause of death, followed by asthma and cancer in the state. Both of these diseases are prevailing at higher rates (ACSDR) among the males than females in the state. The death rates due to heart attack are 222 and 122 for males and females respectively. The death rates are only 84 and 65 for asthma for one lakh population in Kerala. However, the rate of deaths varies across the districts. It can be seen that ACSDR of heart attack is much higher in the districts of Pathanamthitta (380, 209), Kollam (285, 149), Alappuzha (272, 143) and Thrissur (243, 134) for males and females. At the same time, the death rates due to asthma are relatively higher in

Table 14.4

ACSDR of Males across the Districts in Kerala, 2008 (Per 100,000 Population)

Area	*Infects/ Parasite*	*Cancer*	*Heart Attack*	*Asthma*	*Paralysis*	*Blood Pressure*	*Accidents and Injuries*	*Diabetes*
Kasargode	29	51	170	58	34	20	37	12
Kannur	14	61	220	105	27	15	41	6
Wayanad	10	50	123	64	23	20	59	7
Kozhikode	10	66	175	51	34	14	46	11
Malappuram	10	48	171	66	24	11	28	4
Palakkad	27	53	213	100	22	12	53	12
Thrissur	20	64	243	81	19	12	59	12
Ernakulam	15	72	235	102	14	14	71	12
Idukki	18	43	169	97	14	25	69	19
Kottayam	24	57	232	107	9	12	56	23
Alappuzha	20	65	272	104	16	19	61	16
Pathanamthitta	46	70	380	69	23	37	61	64
Kollam	24	61	285	73	18	17	73	18
Thiruvananthapuram	26	55	221	91	14	13	44	23
Kerala	20	59	222	84	21	15	53	15

Source: Calculated by using VRS Data, 2008.

Table 14.5

ACSDR of Females across the Districts in Kerala, 2008 (Per 100,000 Population)

Area	Infects/ Parasite	Cancer	Heart Attack	Asthma	Paralysis	Blood Pressure	Accidents and Injuries	Diabetes
Kasargod	24	28	86	45	24	19	10	9
Kannur	6	34	117	81	36	17	15	5
Wayanad	7	29	57	45	15	22	19	14
Kozhikode	5	40	97	43	36	16	16	8
Malappuram	7	24	92	49	28	14	11	4
Palakkad	16	33	111	69	25	15	20	13
Thrissur	11	36	134	61	17	14	20	13
Ernakulam	9	44	133	87	16	20	20	13
Idukki	14	27	78	52	11	27	24	24
Kottayam	14	33	131	78	11	14	16	23
Alappuzha	12	41	143	97	20	27	13	17
Pathanamthitta	29	40	209	45	23	40	15	75
Kollam	14	40	149	54	16	20	19	18
Thiruvananthapuram	15	36	137	78	14	16	13	23
Kerala	12	35	122	65	22	18	16	16

Source: Calculated by using VRS Data, 2008.

Kottayam (107, 78), Alappuzha (104, 97) and Ernakulam (102, 85) for one lakh males and females. The ACSDR from cancer are also dominant in the state, making it the third major cause in state. However, the dominance of remaining major causes of deaths varies among males and females. Notably, fourth and fifth major causes of death are from accidents and injuries, and paralysis among males, while they are paralysis and blood pressure among females.

Summary

The major aim of the paper is to examine the status of epidemiological transition across districts in Kerala. In the first section, the paper analysed CDR, LE and the TLE to identify the mortality differences across the districts. The analysis of CDR has given an impression that its prevalence is very low in Kerala, with an average of 6.3 deaths per 1000 people in the state level. Almost all districts have more or less similar death rates. Nevertheless, the northern districts have slightly lower CDR than southerners which can be because of the age structure of their population. The life expectancy at birth in Kerala from the VRS data also shows males have 70.7 and females have 77.6 expected years at their birth. All the districts have almost similar years of life expectancy, which indicates that there is no significant disparity between the districts in terms of life expectancy. However, the gender disparity in life expectancy can be visible in all districts with more or less similar difference.

The study also calculated TLE for all the districts to understand the level of mortality difference in major age intervals. It was found that for the TLE between the age group 0 to 80, males have achieved 68.4 and females 73.6 years respectively. There are very small disparities between TLE across the districts with the state averages. However, the study found that the disparity was a result of 60-80 age groups where 0-15 years, 15-40 years and 40-60 years has almost achieved their maximum in those intervals (except the males at 40-60 years). Moreover, the study found a similar sex difference in TLE in all the districts because of delay in completion of male TLE among the ages 40-60 and 60-80 years.

In the second section, the study analysed causes of death to understand if any significant disparity is prevailing across the districts. Analysis was done by taking the proportion of major causes of deaths and ACSDR of major diseases. The analysis of proportion of causes of death in Kerala shows that the major proportional share of death have happened because of Group 2 causes which is followed by Group 3 and Group 1 diseases. Notably, the share of Group 1 causes, which were the major causes in the earlier decades, became very small indicating that the state has gone through a significant level of epidemiological transition over the decades. The dominance of Group 2 diseases followed by Group 3 causes can be visible throughout the state, indicating that all the districts in Kerala are advanced in epidemiological transition without much disparity. The analysis on ACSDR of major causes of death in Kerala indicates that heart attack is the prominent cause of death followed by asthma, paralysis, and accidents and injuries. But the death rates from infectious diseases have fallen considerably. Such pattern is visible in all the districts. In short, the epidemiological transition across the districts in Kerala has almost similar pattern in their mortality and causes of deaths across the districts.

The high prevalence of chronic/degenerative diseases as causes of death in all the districts particularly for the males in the adult and older age groups requires a significant concern. Apart from making delay in attaining the advance stages of epidemiological transition, these diseases are responsible for high socio-economic burden in the state. High death rate due to these diseases especially for males in the adult age group leads to financial crisis as they are the breadwinners of their families. It should be noted that several studies including various rounds of NSS reports (mainly 52nd and 60th Rounds) are in confirmation that the morbidity due to chronic/degenerative diseases are on rise in Kerala and also becomes a major cause for spiraling healthcare spending and even catastrophic healthcare burden. Considering the same, this is a high time for the state to bring adequate policies by various aspects of preventive/promotive and curative care for chronic/degenerative diseases. Such initiations in all the districts can help the state to achieve the advance stage of epidemiological transition, without disparities as in the developed countries.

References

Arriaga, E.E. (1984). "Measuring and Explaining the Change in Life Expectancies", *Demography* 21(2): 83-96.

Bhende, A. and T. Kanitkar (1977). *Principles of Population Studies*. New Delhi: Himalaya Publishing House.

Dutton, J. (1979). "Changes in Soviet Mortality Pattern 1959-1977", *Population Development Review* 5: 267-91.

GoK-VRS (2008). *Vital Statistics*. Thiruvananthapuram: Department of Economics and Statistics, Government of Kerala.

Huynen, M.M., L. Vollebregt, P. Martens and B.M. Benavides (2005). "The Epidemiologic Transition in Peru", *Rev panam salud Publica/Pan AMJ Public Health* 17(1): 51-59.

Mesle, F., J. Vallin, A. Zoe (2002). "Mortality in Europe: The Divergence between East and West", *Population* (English Edition), 57(1): 157-97.

Navaneetham, K., M. Kabeer (2005). *Health Status of Kerala: A Life Course Perspective*. Project by CDS, Trivandrum and IDPAD, New Delhi.

Navaneetham,K., M. Kabeer, V. Santhakumar (2009). "Emerging Morbidity Patterns in Kerala", in A. Ashokan (ed.), *Perspective of Health Economics*. New Delhi: Serial Publication.

Olshansky, A., A. Brian (1986). "The Fourth Stage of Epidemiological Transition; The Age of Delayed Degenerative Diseases", *The Milbank Quarterly* 64(3): 355-91.

Omran, A.R. (1971). "The Epidemiological Transition; A Theory of Epidemiology of Population Change", *Milbank Quarterly* 49: 509-38.

Ram, U., P. Jha, F. Ram, K. Kumar, S. Awasthi, A. Shet, J. Pader, S. Nansukusa, R. Kumar (2013). "Neonatal, 1–59 Month, and Under-5 Mortality in 597 Indian Districts, 2001 to 2012: Estimates from National Demographic and Mortality Surveys" Articles, *Lancet* 1: 219-26.

RGI-CDSR. (Various Years). *Report on Cause of Death Survey: Rural*. New Delhi: Office of the Registrar General and Census.

RGI-MCCD. (Various Years). *Report on Medical Certification of Cause of Death*. New Delhi: Office of the Registrar General and Census.

RGI-SRS. (Various Years). *Report of the Sample Registration System*. New Delhi: Office of the Registrar General and Census.

Shyjan, D. (2009). *Human Development Report of the Fisherfolks in Kerala*. Published jointly by UNDP, Planning Commission and Kerala State Planning Board, Thiruvananthapuram.

Thomas, M.B. (2012). "Changes in Mortality in Kerala, India: Some Emerging Concerns", *Universal Journal of Education and General Studies* 18: 234-41.

Thomas, M.B., K.S. James (2014). "Changes in Mortality and Human Longevity in Kerala: Are They Leading to the Advanced Stages", Special Issue: *Epidemiological Transition: Beyond Omran's Theory, Global Health Action* 7: 1-12.

Vallin, J., F. Mesle (2004). "Convergence and Divergence in Mortality: A New Approaches to Health Transition", *Demographic Research, MPDR On-line Journal*, Germany.